Third Edition

Appleton & Lange's Review of
MICROBIOLOGY
& IMMUNOLOGY

Third Edition

Appleton & Lange's Review of
MICROBIOLOGY
& IMMUNOLOGY

William W. Yotis, PhD
Professor Emeritus of Microbiology
Loyola University of Chicago
Stritch School of Medicine
Maywood, Illinois

Tadayo Hashimoto, MD, PhD
Professor of Microbiology
Loyola University of Chicago
Stritch School of Medicine
Maywood, Illinois

Harold J. Blumenthal, PhD
Professor Emeritus of Microbiology
Loyola University of Chicago
Stritch School of Medicine
Maywood, Illinois

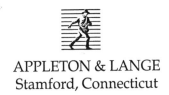

APPLETON & LANGE
Stamford, Connecticut

Copyright © 1997 by Appleton & Lange
A Simon & Schuster Company
Copyright © 1993 and 1989 by Appleton & Lange

97 98 99 00 01 / 10 9 8 7 6 5 4 3 2 1

Prentice Hall International (UK) Limited, *London*
Prentice Hall of Australia Pty. Limited, *Sydney*
Prentice Hall Canada, Inc., *Toronto*
Prentice Hall Hispanoamericana, S.A., *Mexico*
Prentice Hall of India Private Limited, *New Delhi*
Prentice Hall of Japan, Inc., *Tokyo*
Simon and Schuster Asia Pte. Ltd., *Singapore*
Editora Prentice Hall do Brasil Ltda., *Rio de Janeiro*
Prentice Hall, *Upper Saddle River, New Jersey*

Library of Congress Catalogue Card Number: 96-085346

Acquisitions Editor: Marinita Timban
Production Service: Rainbow Graphics, Inc.

ISBN   0-8385-0273-3

Contents

Preface

Like any other medical science, microbiology has been enriched with new information that appears in the United States Medical Licensing Examination Step 1 (USMLE Step 1), state board, or other microbiology examinations. The abundance of novel findings in the field of microbiology, although useful and exciting, nevertheless presents problems in determining what one has to know in order to pass a qualifying examination in medical microbiology. Faced with this situation, the individual who is scheduled to take such a test tries to locate past examinations, which may or may not be up to date and appropriate. During our 31 years as medical microbiologists, we have been frequently asked by medical and other microbiology students to provide them with samples of examination questions. Many of these students have found these examination samples valuable and have urged us to write a medical microbiology and immunology review book. To comply with the wishes of our students, we decided to write this book in 1989 and have updated it with every edition.

The third edition contains approximately 25% new material. Additional material has been added in immunology, molecular biology, diagnostic microbiology, and the application of basic concepts for the diagnosis, control, and prevention of microbial diseases. Some of these changes address pertinent suggestions made by reviewers of the first and second editions, to whom we express our appreciation. Furthermore, the third edition includes figures as part of several of the examination questions. This new edition attempts to include updated knowledge in all relevant areas of medical microbiology and immunology and will expose the reader to the types of examination questions that are now used in the USMLE Step 1. Ours will be the first book that will familiarize the reader with the examination format for the USMLE. The format of the examination questions include single best answer, negatively phrased single best answer, and matching sets to reflect the current USMLE. The references given as part of the answers to the questions have been updated.

Serious attempts have been made to compose more than 1000 examination questions, answers, and explanations of the highest caliber in the USMLE style, and we hope these will be of assistance in reviewing medical microbiology and immunology.

There are other competing microbiology review books on the market. The main differences between our book and the others are that ours attempts to include recent significant developments in the field, omits outdated or irrelevant test questions, tests the student in all the germane areas of medical microbiology and immunology, and familiarizes the student with the types of examination questions that are now encountered in the USMLE Step 1.

Introduction

This book is designed to help you review microbiology and immunology for your course and for the United States Medical Licensing Examination Step 1 (USMLE Step 1). Here in one package is a comprehensive review resource with over 1000 exam-type questions with referenced paragraph-length discussions of each answer. In addition the last 100 questions have been set aside as a practice test for self-assessment purposes. The entire book has been designed to help you assess your areas of relative strength and weakness.

ORGANIZATION OF THIS BOOK

This book is divided into nine chapters. Eight chapters provide a review of the major areas of microbiology and immunology. The last chapter is a practice test, which integrates all of these areas into one simulated examination.

This introduction provides information on question types, test-taking strategies, various ways you can use this book, and specific information on the USMLE Step 1.

Questions
The USMLE Step 1 contains three different types of questions (or "items," in testing parlance). In general, about 70% of these are "one best answer–single item" questions (A type), 20% are "one best answer–matching sets" questions (B type), and 10% are "extended matching set" questions (R type). In some cases a group of two or three questions may be related to a situational theme. In addition some questions have illustrative material that requires understanding and interpretation on your part. Moreover, questions may be of three levels of difficulty: (1) rote memory questions; (2) memory questions that require more understanding of the problem; and (3) questions that require understanding *and* judgment. In view of the fact that the USMLE is moving toward the judgment question and away from the rote memory question, judgment questions have been added throughout this text. Finally, some of the items are stated in the negative. In such instances, we have printed the negative word in capital letters (eg, "All of the following are correct EXCEPT," "Which of the following choices is NOT correct," and "Which of the following is LEAST correct").

Single best answer. This type of question presents a problem or asks a question and is followed by five choices, only one of which is entirely correct. The directions preceding this type of question will generally appear as follows:

DIRECTIONS: Each of the numbered items or incomplete statements in this section is followed by answers or by completions of the statement. Select the ONE lettered answer or completion that is BEST in each case.

An example for this item type follows:

1. An obese 21-year-old woman complains of increased growth of <u>coarse hair on her lip</u>, chin, chest, and abdomen. She also notes <u>menstrual irregularity with periods of amenorrhea</u>. The most likely cause is

    (A) polycystic ovary disease
    (B) an ovarian tumor
    (C) an adrenal tumor
    (D) Cushing's disease
    (E) familial hirsutism

In this type of question, choices other than the correct answer may be partially correct, but there can only be one *best* answer. In the preceding question, the key word is "most." Although ovarian tumors, adrenal tumors, and Cushing's disease are causes of hirsutism (described in the stem of the question), <u>polycystic ovary disease is a much more common cause</u>. Familial hirsutism is not associated with the menstrual irregularities mentioned. Thus, the *most* likely cause of the manifestations described can only be "(A) polycystic ovary disease."

**STRATEGIES FOR ANSWERING
SINGLE BEST ANSWER QUESTIONS***

1. Remember that only one choice can be the correct answer.
2. Read the question carefully to be sure that you understand what is being asked.
3. Quickly read each choice for familiarity. (This important step is often ignored by test takers.)
4. Go back and consider each choice individually.
5. If a choice is partially correct, tentatively consider it to be incorrect. (This step will help you lessen your choices and increase your odds of choosing the correct answer.)
6. Consider the remaining choices and select the one you think is the answer. At this point, you may want to scan the stem quickly to be sure you understand the question and your answer.
7. Fill in the appropriate circle on the answer sheet. (Even if you do not know the answer, you should at least guess. Your score is based on the number of correct answers, **so do not leave any blanks.**)

* Note that steps 2 through 7 should take an average of 50 seconds total. The actual examination is timed for an average of 50 seconds per question.

Negatively phrased single best answer. These questions always contain a capitalized focus of either LEAST, NOT, or EXCEPT. In order to answer these types of questions you must be able to identify a false or least likely answer choice. An example of this question format follows.

DIRECTIONS (Question 2): Each of the numbered items or incomplete statements in this section is negatively phrased, as indicated by a capitalized word such as NOT, LEAST, or EXCEPT. Select the ONE lettered answer or completion that is BEST in each case.

2. All of the following structures drain into the internal jugular vein EXCEPT the

    (A) lingual veins
    (B) facial veins
    (C) superior thyroid veins
    (D) interior petrosal sinus
    (E) azygos vein

The correct answer is E. This is an unusually vexing format because looking for a false or least likely answer choice runs counter to our normal thought processes which are more adept at finding "right" answers. With this type of format it is usually helpful to reread the negatively phrased question to be certain that you comprehend it. Next, read all the answer choices and mark **T** or **F** beside them if they are true or false, respectively. Consider any answer which you feel is only partially correct as a true. Choose your final answer only from those items identified as false. Remember, there is only one best answer which is the LEAST likely, FALSE, or NOT true. Always answer every question even if you have to guess.

Matching sets. These questions are essentially matching questions that are usually accompanied by the following general directions:

DIRECTIONS (Questions 2 through 4): Each group of items in this section consists of lettered headings followed by a set of words or phrases. For each numbered word or phrase, select the ONE lettered heading that is most closely associated with it. <u>Each lettered heading may be selected once, more than once, or not at all.</u>

Any number of questions (usually two to six) may follow the five headings:

Questions 2 through 4
For each adverse drug reaction in the following list, select the antibiotic with which it is most closely associated.

    (A) tetracycline
    (B) chloramphenicol
    (C) clindamycin
    (D) cefotaxime
    (E) gentamicin

  2. Bone marrow suppression *B*

  3. Pseudomembranous enterocolitis *C*

  4. Acute fatty necrosis of liver *A*

One best answer–extended matching sets. Questions 5 through 7

    (A) variable regions of light and heavy chains
    (B) constant regions of light and heavy chains
    (C) constant region of heavy chain
    (D) J chain
    (E) hinge region
    (F) HLA-A
    (G) HLA-B
    (H) HLA-C
    (I) C5a
    (J) Fc

  5. Macrophage and neutrophil attractant *I*

  6. Determines isotypes *C*

  7. Determines idiotypes *A*

Notice that, unlike the single-item questions, the choices in the matching sets questions *precede* the actual questions. As with the single-item questions, however, only **one** choice can be correct for a given question.

Answers, Explanations, and References
In each of the sections of this book, the question sections are followed by a section containing the answers, explanations, and references for the questions. This section (1) tells you the answer to each question; (2) gives you an explanation of why the answer is correct and why the other answers are incorrect, as well as background information on the subject matter; and/or (3) tells you where you can find more in-depth information on the subject

matter in other books and journals. We encourage you to use this section as a basis for further study.

If you choose the correct answer to a question, you can then read the explanation (1) for reinforcement and (2) to add to your knowledge about the subject matter (remember that the explanations tell not only why the answer is correct, but also often why the other choices are incorrect). **If you choose the wrong answer** to a question, you can read the explanation for an instructional review of the material in the question. Furthermore, you can look up the references at the end of the chapter and refer to the specific pages cited for a more in-depth discussion.

Practice Test

The practice test at the end of the book includes all the topics covered in Chapters 1 through 8. The questions are grouped according to question type (one best answer–single item, one best answer–matching sets, comparison matching sets, then multiple true–false items), with the subject areas integrated. Specific instructions for how to take the practice test are given on page 251.

The practice test is followed by a subspecialty list, which will enable you to analyze your areas of strength and weakness to help you focus your review. For example, in checking off your incorrect answers, you may find that a pattern develops, revealing that you answered most or all of the virology questions incorrectly. In this case you could note the references (in the Answers and Explanations section) for your incorrect answers and read those sources. You might also want to purchase a virology text or review book to do a much more thorough review. We think you will find this subspecialty list very helpful, and we urge you to use it.

HOW TO USE THIS BOOK

There are two logical ways to get the most value from this book. We will call them Plan A and Plan B.

In Plan A you go straight to the practice test and complete it according to the instructions given on page 251. Using the subspecialty list analyze your areas of strength and weakness. This analysis will be a good indicator of your initial knowledge

of the subject and will help to identify specific areas for preparation and review. You can now use the first eight chapters of the book to help you improve your relatively weak points.

In Plan B you go through Chapters 1 through 8 checking off your answers and then comparing your choices with the answers and discussions in the book. Once you have completed this process, you can take the practice test and see how well prepared you are. If you still have a major weakness, it should be apparent in time for you to take remedial action.

In Plan A, by taking the practice test first, you get quick feedback regarding your initial areas of strength and weakness. You may find that you have a good command of the material, indicating that perhaps only a cursory review of the first eight chapters is necessary. This, of course, would be good to know early in your exam preparation. On the other hand, you may find that you have many areas of weakness. In this case you could then focus on these areas in your review, not just with this book but also with textbooks.

It is, however, likely that you will do at least some studying prior to taking the USMLE Step 1 (especially since you have this book). Therefore, it may be more realistic to take the practice test after you have reviewed the first eight chapters (as in Plan B). This approach will probably give you a more realistic type of testing situation, since very few of us just sit down to a test without studying. In this case, you will have done some reviewing (from superficial to in-depth), and your practice test will reflect this studying time. If, after reviewing the first eight chapters and taking the practice test, you still have some weaknesses, you can then go back to the first chapters and supplement your review with your texts.

SPECIFIC INFORMATION ON THE STEP 1 EXAMINATION

The official source of all information with respect to USMLE Step 1 is the National Board of Medical Examiners (NBME), 3930 Chestnut Street, Philadelphia, PA 19104. Established in 1915, the NBME is a voluntary, nonprofit, independent organization whose sole function is the design, implementation, distribution, and processing of a vast bank of question items, certifying examinations, and evaluative services in the professional medical field.

In order to sit for the Step 1 examination, a person must be either an officially enrolled medical student or a graduate of an accredited U.S. or Canadian medical school. It is not necessary to complete any particular year of medical school in order to be a candidate for Step 1. Neither is it required to take Step 1 before Step 2.

In applying for Step 1, you must use forms supplied by the NBME. Remember that registration closes *ten weeks* before the scheduled examination date. Some U.S. and Canadian medical schools require their students to take Step 1 even if they are noncandidates. Such students can register as noncandidates at the request of their school. A person who takes Step 1 as a noncandidate can later change to candidate status, and after payment of a fee, receive certification credit.

USMLE EXAMINATION CONTENT

The test items in the USMLE examination focus on the following items:

Microbial structure and composition
- classification and its basis
- composition and fine structure of subcellular parts: cell wall, outer membrane, cytoplasmic membrane, capsule, flagella, spores, and cytoplasmic inclusions

Microbial cell metabolism, physiology, and regulation
- biochemistry and physiology of microbial growth (bacteria, chlamydiae, viruses, and fungi)
- chemotaxis and motility
- transport of nutrients
- mechanisms of resistance to environment
- regulatory mechanisms: transcriptional and translational regulation; end-product inhibition, global regulation

Bacterial pathogens
- structure, genetics, and chemistry of bacterial pathogens
- nature and mechanisms of the action of bacterial virulence factors
- physical and chemical properties of viruses

- replication schemes of classes of viruses
- genetics

Medical mycology, including structure and physiology of yeast and molds

Medical parasitology, including life cycles of major protozoan organisms and helminths

Scoring
Because there is no deduction for wrong answers, you should answer every question. Your test is scored in the following way:

1. The number of questions answered correctly is totaled. This total is called the raw score.
2. The raw score is converted statistically to a "standard" score on a scale of 200 to 800, with the mean set at 500. Each 100 points away from 500 is one standard deviation.
3. Your score is compared statistically with the criteria set by the scores of the second-year medical school candidates for certification in the June administration during the prior 4 years. This statistical comparison is what is meant by the term "criterion-referenced test."
4. A score of 500 places you around the 50th percentile. A score of 380 is the minimum passing score for Step 1; it probably represents about the 12th to 15th percentile. If you answer 50% or so of the questions correctly, you will almost certainly receive a passing score.

Remember: You do not have to pass all seven basic science components, although you will receive a standard score in each of them. A score of less than 400 (about the 15th percentile) on any particular area is a real cause for concern as it will certainly drag down your overall score. Likewise, a score of 600 or better (85th percentile) indicates an area of great relative strength. (You can use the practice test included in *Appleton & Lange's Review for USMLE Step 1*, Second Edition to help determine your areas of strength and weakness well in advance of the actual examination.)

Physical Conditions
The NBME is very concerned that all their exams be administered under uniform conditions in the numerous centers that are used. Except for several

No. 2 pencils and an eraser, you are not permitted to bring anything (eg, books, notes, calculators) into the test room. All examinees receive the same questions at the same session. The questions, however, are printed in different sequences in several different booklets, and the booklets are randomly distributed. In addition, examinees are moved to different seats at least once during the test. Of course, each test is monitored by at least one proctor. The object of these maneuvers is to discourage cheating or even the temptation to cheat.

The number of candidates who fail Step 1 is quite small; however, individual students as well as entire medical school programs benefit when scores on the examination are high. No one wants to squeak by with a 350 when a little effort might raise that score to 450. That is why you have made a wise decision to use the self-assessment and review materials available in the Third Edition of *Appleton & Lange's Review of Microbiology and Immunology.*

CHAPTER 1

General Microbiology
Questions

DIRECTIONS (Questions 1 through 48): Each of the numbered items or incomplete statements in this section is followed by answers or by completions of the statement. Select the ONE lettered answer or completion that is BEST in each case.

1. Prokaryotic cells

    (A) are all motile
    (B) contain 80 S ribosomes
    (C) lack nuclear membrane
    (D) contain ergosterol in the cytoplasmic membrane
    (E) generate adenosine triphosphate (ATP) in the mitochondria

2. The bacterial chromosome is best described as

    (A) a large circular strand of supercoiled double-stranded DNA
    (B) a large strand of single-stranded RNA
    (C) fragmented pieces of double-stranded DNA
    (D) strands that contain double-stranded DNA and histone
    (E) a large circular strand of double-stranded DNA surrounded by the membrane

3. Bacterial chromosome

    (A) is not attached to cell membrane
    (B) replicates bidirectionally
    (C) is attached to microtubules
    (D) cannot be visualized by electron microscopy
    (E) replicate unidirectionally

4. Bacterial H antigen is derived from

    (A) microtubule
    (B) hemolysin
    (C) haptenic oligosaccharide
    (D) endotoxin
    (E) flagellin

Questions 5 and 6 refer to the following figure, which shows the ultraviolet (UV) light death curve of *Escherichia coli* culture.

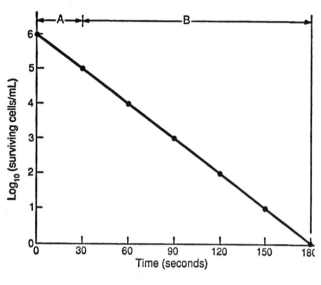

Figure 1–1

5. If during B, 10% of the cells survive any 30-second dose

   (A) the number of viable cells remaining after an additional 30-second dose is 1% of the original
   (B) the number of viable cells remaining at 1 minute is 0.1% of the original
   (C) 90% of the cells are killed with each additional 60-second dose of UV
   (D) the killing curve cannot be modified markedly by irradiating the cells with white light following UV irradiation
   (E) the killing curve can be modified markedly by irradiating the same number of cells in a larger volume of liquid

6. The observation that the death curve is straight from time zero indicates

   (A) mutants lacking nucleic acid
   (B) cells in the population having more than one enzyme are involved
   (C) mutants that do not require thymine
   (D) cells growing in pairs

(E) only a single target is inactivated in *Escherichia coli*

7. Two hundred fifty colonies were counted on a plate on which 0.1 mL of 10^{-3} dilution of a urine sample was inoculated. The number of bacteria per 1 mL of the urine is

   (A) 2.5×10^5
   (B) 25×10^5
   (C) 25×10^6
   (D) 2.5×10^6
   (E) 2.5×10^7

8. All of the following compounds are found in the cell walls of certain bacteria EXCEPT

   (A) teichoic acid
   (B) diaminopimelic acid
   (C) dideoxyhexose
   (D) chitin
   (E) peptidoglycan

9. The endotoxin of gram-negative bacteria is associated with

   (A) mesosome
   (B) cytoplasmic membrane
   (C) capsule
   (D) cell wall
   (E) pilus

10. Bacterial spores are characterized by

    (A) high-water content
    (B) the absence of calcium dipicolinate
    (C) resistance to heat, desiccation, and UV irradiation
    (D) the absence of the nucleoid
    (E) the absence of ribosomes

11. The most common stain used in the clinical microbiology laboratory for detecting the presence of bacteria and assessing the quality of specimens is the

    (A) auramine–rhodamine stain
    (B) Ziehl–Neelsen stain
    (C) Levaditi silver stain

(D) Giemsa stain

(E) Gram stain

Questions 12 through 14 refer to the following figure, which shows the growth curve of a gram-negative bacillus.

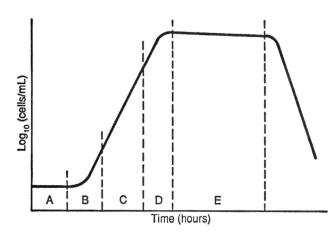

Figure 1–2

12. In general

  (A) cell numbers increase fourfold during each generation in phase C

  (B) cells are killed by penicillin most rapidly during phase C

  (C) no metabolic activity can be measured during phase E

  (D) cellular DNA is synthesized exponentially during phase B

  (E) cells die exponentially during phase E

13. In general

  (A) no metabolic activity can be measured during phase A

  (B) synchronized growth occurs during phase C

  (C) no metabolic activity can be measured during phase E

  (D) cell protein and RNA are synthesized exponentially during phase C

  (E) cells are very susceptible to antimicrobial agents during phase E

14. Phase A may be caused by

  (A) the need for the synthesis of an inducible enzyme

  (B) germination of the gram-negative bacillus

  (C) a large initial inoculum

  (D) an excess of necessary metabolic intermediates

  (E) an inoculum taken from the exponential phase of growth

15. The use of DNA probes for the direct detection of a pathogen from the patient's specimen sometimes lacks sensitivity. A technique to increase the sensitivity by amplifying the target could be to

  (A) use duplicate specimens

  (B) use a nonradioactive probe

  (C) perform more frequent assays

  (D) increase the incubation times

  (E) use a DNA probe directed at ribosomal RNA

16. Biologically, bacterial spore formation is an excellent model for studying

  (A) energy generation

  (B) differentiation

  (C) bacterial classification

  (D) immune mechanisms

  (E) bacterial pathogenicity

17. The phosphoenol–phosphotransferase system (PTS)

  (A) is used to transport fatty acids

  (B) is basically an example of a facilitated diffusion

  (C) phosphorylates the transported substances

  (D) does not require the heat-stable protein

  (E) requires adenosine triphosphate

18. Diffusion of the drug through the outer membranes is important in antimicrobial therapy directed against

    (A) gram-positive bacteria
    (B) gram-negative bacteria
    (C) all bacteria
    (D) bacteria in stationary phase
    (E) none of the above

19. Measurement of bacterial cell mass can most conveniently be accomplished by the use of

    (A) plate counts
    (B) turbidimetric measurements
    (C) estimation of oxygen consumption
    (D) a Coulter counter
    (E) a Petroff–Hauser counting chamber

20. *Pseudomonas aeruginosa* is growing exponentially in a culture medium with a generation time of 15 minutes. At 9:00 a.m. the medium contains 1×10^5 cell per milliliter. The number of cells per milliliter 90 minutes later is

    (A) 1.6×10^6
    (B) 1.6×10^5
    (C) 3.2×10^5
    (D) 6.4×10^6
    (E) 8.0×10^6

21. Bacteria commonly reproduce by

    (A) spore formation
    (B) bud formation
    (C) binary fission
    (D) host cell synthesis of bacterial components
    (E) elaborate mitotic divisions

22. Many bacteria use the two component–signal transduction system in order to respond to environmental change. This system involves

    (A) phosphorylation of protein kinase
    (B) disintegration of ribosome
    (C) new DNA synthesis
    (D) protein methylation
    (E) glycosylation

23. The uptake of iron is facilitated in bacteria by their production of

    (A) enzyme I
    (B) siderophores
    (C) carboxydismutase
    (D) nitrogenase
    (E) HPr

24. Bacteria respond to an upward shift in temperature or an imposition of certain chemical stresses by the production of

    (A) ribosomal proteins
    (B) flagellar proteins
    (C) heat-shock proteins
    (D) porin proteins
    (E) capsular polypeptides

25. The tolerance of facultative anaerobic bacteria to superoxide is caused by the

    (A) lack of cytochrome C oxidase
    (B) presence of cytochrome C oxidase
    (C) lack of peroxidase
    (D) presence of superoxide dismutase and catalase
    (E) inability to form the superoxide radical

26. Invasin proteins in the outer membrane of certain pathogenic gram-negative bacteria contribute to the

    (A) formation of endotoxin
    (B) adherence to the surface of host cells
    (C) immunity to bacteriophage infection
    (D) penetration into the host cell cytoplasm
    (E) rapid spread to other tissues and organs

27. All of the following are methods that some microbes may use for the regeneration of nicotinamide–adenine dinucleotide from its reduced form during glucose formation EXCEPT

    (A) ethanol production
    (B) butyric acid production
    (C) carbon dioxide reduction
    (D) lactate production
    (E) propionate production

28. Bacteria grown aerobically with acetate as the sole carbon and energy source will

    (A) use the glyoxylate cycle
    (B) not be able to use the tricarboxylic acid cycle biosynthetically
    (C) not contain cytochromes
    (D) not contain nicotinamide–adenine dinucleotide phosphate-linked dehydrogenases
    (E) not form alpha-ketoglutarate

29. All of the following are true statements about metabolism EXCEPT that the

    (A) reduced form of nicotinamide–adenine dinucleotide phosphate is the usual biosynthetic reducing coenzyme
    (B) hexose monophosphate (pentose phosphate) pathway is a cyclic pathway with independent oxidative and nonoxidative segments
    (C) Entner–Doudoroff glycolytic pathway is found both in animal and bacterial cells
    (D) Embden–Meyerhof (EM) pathway, with replacement of two EM enzymes, can be used to form glucose-6-phosphate biosynthetically from pyruvate
    (E) most cells are able to use the EM and hexose monophosphate (pentose phosphate) glycolytic pathways concurrently

30. All of the following are true statements about metabolism EXCEPT that

    (A) fructose diphosphate aldolase is an enzyme specific for the Embden–Meyerhof glycolytic pathway
    (B) thiamine pyrophosphate is the coenzyme for transketolase
    (C) under anaerobic conditions, there are many more different methods used by bacteria than by animal cells to reoxidize the reduced form of nicotinamide–adenine dinucleotide to nicotinamide–adenine dinucleotide
    (D) whenever there is an oxidase reaction, there is always generation of hydrogen peroxide (H_2O_2) and superoxide

    (E) the myeloperoxidase–hydrogen peroxide–halide ion system for killing bacteria is found in polymorphonuclear leukocytes

31. All of the following are true statements about microbial metabolism EXCEPT

    (A) heterotrophic carbon dioxide fixation, which is present in all cells, provides C4 acids such as oxaloacetate, so that the tricarboxylic acid cycle can continue to function during growth
    (B) the glyoxylate cycle is found in animal cells, as well as in bacteria
    (C) obligate anaerobes are killed when growing in the presence of oxygen because of the production of hydrogen peroxide (H_2O_2) and superoxide in the absence of catalase and superoxide dismutase
    (D) in Pasteur's effect, more glucose is utilized anaerobically than is used aerobically
    (E) if an amino acid, such as glutamate, is supplied to an *E. coli* growth medium containing glucose, *E. coli* will not make glutamate because of metabolic control mechanisms

32. All of the following are true statements about bacterial chemotaxis EXCEPT

    (A) in the presence of a substance that attracts bacteria (positive chemotaxis), bacteria tumble less frequently
    (B) bacteria have a temporal response, or "memory," about past and present concentrations of an attractant or repellent
    (C) methyl-accepting chemotaxis proteins play important roles in the bacterial sensory system
    (D) methyl groups on methyl-accepting chemotaxis proteins can be removed by a methylesterase
    (E) methyl-accepting chemotaxis proteins can be methylated by a specific methyl transferase using glutamate as the methyl donor

33. Lipopolysaccharides are correctly described as

    (A) found in gram-negative bacteria of all species
    (B) able to produce a febrile response
    (C) possessing somatic (O) antigen specificity
    (D) containing lipid A as an integral part of their structure
    (E) all of the above

34. Structures and substances that may enhance the virulence or invasiveness of a bacterium include

    (A) the capsule
    (B) hyaluronidase
    (C) M protein
    (D) lecithinase
    (E) all of the above

35. Bacterial cytoplasmic membranes (plasma membranes) are correctly described as

    (A) semipermeable membranes located inside the cell walls
    (B) containing receptors for chemotactic movement
    (C) associated with the basal body of bacterial flagella
    (D) containing respiratory enzymes
    (E) all of the above

36. The Gram stain distinguishes between

    (A) spheroplasts of *E. coli* and protoplasts of *Bacillus megaterium*
    (B) *Mycobacterium tuberculosis* and *Mycobacterium kansasii*
    (C) mycoplasmas and L forms
    (D) bacteria having essential differences in the structure of the cell wall
    (E) bacteria and fungi

37. Bacterial chromosome replication is believed to

    (A) be a bidirectional process
    (B) begin at the replicator site of the chromosome

    (C) require protein synthesis for initiation
    (D) begin when a fixed amount of the initiator protein has accumulated
    (E) all of the above

38. Properties that increase during the phagocytic respiratory burst include

    (A) oxygen uptake
    (B) hydrogen peroxide production
    (C) O_2^- (superoxide) production
    (D) hexose monophosphate pathway activity
    (E) all of the above

39. Counterclockwise rotation of bacterial flagella causes bacteria to

    (A) tumble
    (B) rest
    (C) swim forward
    (D) aggregate
    (E) sporulate

40. Bacterial proteins that are involved in murein assembly, expansion, shaping, and septum formation are

    (A) heat-shock protein
    (B) penicillin-binding proteins
    (C) Braun's lipoprotein
    (D) c-AMP binding protein
    (E) porin protein

41. Obligate anaerobes

    (A) require high oxidation and reduction potential for growth
    (B) can survive but cannot grow in the presence of oxygen
    (C) do not contain superoxide dismutase
    (D) cannot produce infections in humans unless aerobes are present simultaneously
    (E) never form spores

42. In bacteria, the frequency of initiation of chromosome replication varies with

    (A) the size of the bacteria
    (B) the size of the chromosome
    (C) cell growth rate
    (D) the shape of the bacteria
    (E) all of the above

43. Periplasmic space of gram-negative bacteria

    (A) refers to a space between the outer membrane and peptidoglycan layer
    (B) represents a part of the cytoplasm between the cytoplasmic membrane and the nucleoid
    (C) is a space between the peptidoglycan layer and the cytoplasmic membrane
    (D) is a space between the outer membrane and the cytoplasmic membrane
    (E) contains no enzymes or proteins

44. Complete killing of all living organisms from a particular location or material is accomplished by

    (A) pasteurization
    (B) disinfection
    (C) sterilization
    (D) boiling
    (E) all of the above

45. The alcohols are protein denaturants that rapidly kill vegetative bacteria when applied as aqueous solution in the range of

    (A) 10 to 20%
    (B) 30 to 40%
    (C) 40 to 60%
    (D) 70 to 95%
    (E) 100%

46. Protonmotive force

    (A) drives transport solutes by shock-insensitive system of active transport
    (B) powers the flagellar motors that rotate the filaments resulting in cell motility
    (C) generates ATP by coupling the phosphorylation of adenosine diphosphate

(ADP) to passage of protons inward through special channels in the cell membrane
    (D) does all of the above
    (E) does none of the above

47. Microorganisms that can grow best at low O_2 concentrations and can also grow without O_2 is called

    (A) aerobe
    (B) strict anaerobe
    (C) aerotolerant anaerobe
    (D) microaerophilic
    (E) facultative anaerobe

48. Lysozyme degrades

    (A) RNA polymerase
    (B) peptidoglycan
    (C) capsular polysaccharide
    (D) lipid A
    (E) flagellin

DIRECTIONS (Questions 49 through 60): Each group of items in this section consists of lettered headings followed by a set of numbered words or phrases. For each numbered word or phrase, select the ONE lettered heading that is most closely associated with it. Each lettered heading may be selected once, more than once, or not at all.

Questions 49 through 51

    (A) cell wall
    (B) cytoplasmic membrane (plasma membrane)
    (C) pilus
    (D) flagellum
    (E) plasmid

49. Confers a characteristic shape on a bacterium

50. H antigen of a bacterium

51. Surrounds the cytoplasm of a protoplast

Questions 52 and 53

   (A) N-acetylmuramic acid

   (B) teichoic acid

   (C) lipopolysaccharide

   (D) lipid-P–P-muramic acid pentapeptide

   (E) calcium-dipicolinic acid

52. Lipid A

53. Endospore (bacterial)

Questions 54 and 55

   (A) riboflavin

   (B) thiamine pyrophosphate

   (C) folic acid

   (D) pyridoxal phosphate

   (E) pantothenic acid

54. Required by some bacteria, which cannot synthesize it, for decarboxylation of keto acids

55. Plays a role in the transamination and racemization of amino acids

Questions 56 and 57

   (A) tricarboxylic acid cycle

   (B) hexose monophosphate (pentose phosphate) pathway

   (C) glyoxylate cycle

   (D) Embden–Meyerhof pathway

   (E) Entner–Doudoroff pathway

56. Isocitrate lyase

57. Transketolase

Question 58

   (A) glucose-6-phosphate dehydrogenase

   (B) glutathione reductase

   (C) myeloperoxidase

   (D) the reduced form of nicotinamide–adenine dinucleotide phosphate oxidase

   (E) nicotinamide–adenine dinucleotide phosphate-linked lactate dehydrogenase

58. Enzyme deficiency in leukocytes responsible for chronic granulomatous disease of childhood

Questions 59 through 60

The following diagram shows the moieties of a typical bacterial endotoxin that contains the items A through J. Repeating Outer Core Inner Core Unit O-Specific Chain Core Lipid A

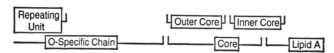

Figure 1–3

(A) 2-keto-3-deoxyoctonate (KDO)

(B) l-glycero-D-manno-heptose

(C) ethanolamine

(D) D-glucosamine

(E) phosphate

(F) lipid A

(G) outer core

(H) inner core

(I) O-specific chain

(J) 3-hydroxy-tetradecanoic acid

59. Component responsible for the production of pyrexia, hypotension, production of tumor necrosis, and interleukin-1

60. Component to be used as antigen for the diagnosis of a gram-negative bacterium that causes disseminated intravascular coagulation

General Microbiology
Answers and Explanations

1. **(C)** Some prokaryotic cells move by rotation of the flagella or by gliding. Some bacteria do not move at all. All prokaryotic cells contain 70 S ribosomes, not 80 S ribosomes. By far, the most important characteristic of prokaryotic cells is the lack of the nuclear membrane that surrounds the nuclear body (nuclei), which some people call "nucleoid." Bacteria does not contain ergosterol in their cytoplasmic membrane. The fungal cytoplasmic membrane invariably contains ergosterol, which makes fungi sensitive to polyene antibiotics. Bacteria generate ATP on the cytoplasmic membrane. Mitochondria are absent in bacteria. *(Ryan et al, pp 11–29)*

2. **(A)** The bacterial genome resides on a single chromosome and typically consists of about 4,000 genes encoded in one large circular molecule of double-stranded DNA containing about 5 million nucleotide base pairs. This moleculer is more than 1 mm long. Unlike eukaryotic chromosome, bacterial chromosome is not associated with histone and is not surrounded by the nuclear membrane. *(Ryan et al, p 33)*

3. **(C)** Bacterial spores have a highly dehydrated core (cytoplasm) which contains numerous ribosomes and one nucleus. The core is surrounded by the cortex and coats. Located in the core of bacterial spore is calcium dipicolinate which accounts for 10 to 20% of spore dry weight. Probably because of this unique structure and the compounds it contains, bacterial spores are highly resistant to heat, desiccation, and UV irradiation. *(Ryan et al, p 24)*

4. **(E)** Flagella, which are the locomotive organs of motile bacteria, are composed of proteins known as flagellin. The flagellar antigens are called H antigens. The H antigens are of two kinds: those shared by a number of species or types and those peculiar to a particular species or type. Many of the species or types are diphasic; that is, at one stage of a culture, the specific flagellar antigens may occur (specific phase), whereas at another, the group antigens may be present (group phase). H antigens are used in the serologic identification of various species of the genus *Salmonella* and *Escherichia*. Microtubules, hemolysin, haptenic oligosaccharide, and endotoxin do not contain H antigens. *(Jawetz et al, pp 214–215; Ryan et al, pp 322–344)*

5. **(A)** An examination of the death curve shown in the figure given indicates that there is a 90% reduction in the surviving cells for each 30-second exposure to UV light. That is, there is one log reduction of the cell population for every 30 seconds. That is, in 30 seconds the surviving cells were reduced from 1,000,000 cells (10^6) to 100,000 cells (10^5). Then, the number of viable cells remaining after an additional 30 seconds (1-minute total exposure) were reduced to 10,000 cells (10^4). Ten thousand cells represent 1% of the original cell population. UV light irradiation of bacterial cells causes them to form pyrimidine dimers that distort the shape of the

DNA and leads to inhibition of DNA synthesis. If, following UV light irradiation, the bacterial cells are exposed to visible light, the lethal effect of the UV light is significantly reduced. This phenomenon is called photoreactivation and is due to the activation of an enzyme that removes the pyrimidine dimers from the bacterial DNA. *(Jawetz et al, pp 43–44; Joklik et al, pp 197–198; Ryan et al, pp 172–173,175)*

6. **(E)** The observation that the death curve is straight from time zero indicates that a single target is inactivated in *E. coli*. This target area should be the chromosome of a uninucleate cell, such as *E. coli*. If an enzyme or other cellular constituents of which *E. coli* has multiple copies were affected, the death curve would not be straight from time zero. That is, there would be a lag before the cell population began to die, because it would take time to destroy all the copies of the critical components or enzyme molecules required for cell survival. There are no known mutants of *E. coli* that lack nucleic acid. Thymine is part of cocarboxylase, which is involved in the decarboxylation of pyruvic and other keto acids. That *E. coli* can synthesize thymine does not explain why the death curve is straight from time zero following exposure to ultraviolet light. *(Jawetz et al, pp 43–44; Ryan et al, pp 172–173,175)*

7. **(D)** To obtain the number of bacteria per 1 mL of urine, the number of colonies that were counted (250) on the nutrient agar plate, on which 0.1 mL of a 10^{-3} dilution of urine sample was used, must be multiplied by 10 and then by 1,000. Multiplication by 10 converts the count to bacteria per milliliter instead of 0.1 mL, which represents one-tenth of 1 mL. Multiplication by 1,000 is also necessary because the urine sample has been diluted one thousand-fold (1:1000 or 10^{-3}) and there would have been one thousand times more bacteria if an undiluted sample of urine were used. Therefore, the calculation is as follows: $250 \times 10 \times 1000 = 2,500,000$, or 2.5×10^6 bacteria per 1 mL of urine.

8. **(D)** Chitin is a structural polysaccharide found in the exoskeletons of insects and crustaceans. Bacteria lack chitin. The cell walls of gram-positive and gram-negative bacteria contain peptidoglycan, which is a polymer of N-acetylglucosamine and N-acetylmuramic acid, as well as side and cross-linking chains of amino acids. Diaminopimelic acid has been found in the amino acid chains. Many gram-positive bacteria also contain teichoic acids, which are polymers of either ribitol or glycerol phosphate. Gram-negative bacteria may contain dideoxyhexoses such as colitose, abequose, tyvelose, or paratose in their cell walls. *(Joklik et al, pp 76–85; Ryan et al, pp 16–20,571)*

9. **(D)** The outer membranes of the cell walls of gram-negative bacteria are the cytologic sites of the bacterial cells where endotoxins are found. Chemically, endotoxins are lipopolysaccharides composed of a lipid A moiety, which is the toxic part of the endotoxin; a core that contains the unique component of endotoxins known as ketodeoxyoctulonic acid; and the O-specific polysaccharide region, which is a useful diagnostic marker of various gram-negative bacteria. Mesosomes are invaginations of the cytoplasmic membrane. Capsules are envelopes found outside the bacterial cell wall. Pili are proteinaceous spikes that play a role in the attachment of bacteria to human cells. *(Joklik et al, pp 82–87; Ryan et al, pp 157–158)*

10. **(C)** Bacterial spores have a highly dehydrated core (cytoplasm) which contains numerous ribosomes and one nucleus. The core is surrounded by the cortex and coats. Located in the core of bacterial spore are calcium dipicolinate and unique peptides which accounts for 10 to 20% of spore dry weight. Probably because of this unique structure and the compounds it contains, bacterial spores are highly resistant to heat, desiccation, and UV irradiation. *(Ryan et al, p 24)*

11. **(E)** The most common stain used in the clinical microbiology laboratory for detecting the presence of bacteria and assessing the quality of specimens is Gram stain. This stain yields valuable information that cannot be obtained from culture of the specimen alone. For ex-

ample, the Gram-stained smear is useful because it allows a presumptive etiologic diagnosis to be made within minutes. Gram stain may also indicate the relative abundance of different bacteria, whereas in culture the bacteria may grow at different rates, giving a false quantitative picture. The Gram-stained smear may indicate a need for laboratory procedures not routinely employed, such as anaerobic and fungal cultures or special staining techniques, and allow early clinical decisions concerning the appropriate antibiotic treatment. The auramine–rhodamine and Ziehl–Neelsen stains are used to detect acid-fast microorganisms such as *Mycobacterium tuberculosis* or other members belonging to genus *Mycobacterium*. Giemsa stain and Levaditi silver stain are used to stain spirochetes. *(Jawetz et al, pp 280,283; Ryan et al, pp 225–226)*

12. **(B)** Phase C in the bacterial growth curve represents the exponential or logarithmic phase of growth. There is a geometric progression in the increase of the number of cells produced. That is, the cell population proceeds from 1 cell to 2 to 4 to 8 to 16 to 32, and so forth. Similarly, the cellular DNA is synthesized exponentially during phase C of the bacterial growth. Penicillin inhibits cell wall synthesis, thus it would be expected to be detrimental at the phase of bacterial growth during which there is rapid synthesis of the cell wall. Thus, cells will be killed by penicillin most rapidly during phase C, and not during phases B or D where cell wall synthesis is not as rapid as in phase C. Finally, there is no increase in the number of cells per unit time during phase A or E. *(Jawetz et al, pp 39–43; Ryan et al, pp 35–36)*

13. **(D)** Phase C of the growth cycle represents the logarithmic phase of bacterial growth. During this phase there is an exponential rate of increase in the number of cells, of any macromolecular components such as protein and RNA, or of cell structures. Phase A represents the lag phase of bacterial curve. It is called lag because there is no increase in the number of cells. During this phase of growth, the cell increases in size as it prepares itself for division. The increase in cell size is associ-

ated with a good rate of metabolic activity. Synchronized growth occurs when all cells in a bacterial culture are induced to divide at the same time, giving rise to a stepwise increase in the cell population, not the type of curve shown for this question. Phase E represents the stationary phase of growth during which the number of viable cells produced equals the number of cells dying due to exhaustion of nutrients and accumulation of toxic products. The exponential (not the stationary) phase of growth is the phase during which the cells are most sensitive to antimicrobial agents. *(Jawetz et al, pp 39–43; Ryan et al, pp 36–35)*

14. **(A)** Phase A represents the lag phase of the bacterial growth curve. Phase A is required for the synthesis of required enzymes and necessary metabolic intermediates. The germination of spores could lead to a lag phase in the growth cycle of a spore-forming grampositive bacillus. Gram-negative bacilli are not known to produce spores. Use of a large inoculum, an excess of necessary intermediates, or an inoculum taken from the exponential phase of growth tends to eliminate the lag phase. Because the necessary enzymes or intermediates are already supplied to the cells, the cells are then ready to begin cell division. *(Jawetz et al, pp 39–43; Ryan et al, pp 35–36)*

15. **(E)** Currently, molecular biologic techniques are frequently used to detect various pathogens from clinical specimens. Thus, DNA probes directed at ribosomal RNA, which contains highly conserved regions characteristic for a given species, are now used to increase the sensitivity of pathogen detection (ribotyping). Utilization of duplicate specimens, nonradioactive probes, and frequent or prolonged assays are not likely to address adequately the problem of the occasional lack of sensitivity of DNA probes, which may contain common areas of homology in the base sequences of DNA among closely related bacterial species. *(Joklik et al, pp 8–14; Ryan et al, pp 244–245)*

16. **(B)** Since one fully viable cell (spore) is reproduced within one bacterial cell during

sporulation, the system provides an excellent model for studying differentiation. In recent years, this system has been exploited in *Bacillus subtilis* to elucidate the regulatory mechanisms that control the formation of one progeny cell within a competent mother cell. *(Ryan et al, p 24)*

17. **(C)** The PTS is an active transport system in which the sugar must be phosphorylated by the PTS prior to its entrance into the cell. The PTS requires phosphoenol pyruvate (PEP), which provides the phosphate for the phosphorylation of the sugar as well as energy for the transport. The PTS also requires enzyme I and the heat-stable protein HPr, both of which are nonspecific for the sugar that is transported. Finally, enzyme II and/or enzyme III, which are specific for the sugar that is transported, are needed for PTS. The PTS involves the following reactions:

$$PEP + enzyme\ I \rightarrow I\text{-}P + pyruvate$$

$$I\text{-}P + HPr \rightarrow HPr\text{-}P + I$$

$$HPr\text{-}P + enzyme\ II \rightarrow II\text{-}P$$

$$II\text{-}P + sugar \rightarrow sugar\text{-}P + enzyme\ II$$

(Joklik et al, pp 58–59; Ryan et al, p 27)

18. **(B)** The cell wall of gram-positive bacteria is a porous structure composed of peptidoglycan and teichoic acids, which allow the entrance of various types of compounds, including antibiotics that have a molecular weight of several thousands, into the cell. However, the cell wall of gram-negative bacteria is composed of peptidoglycan and an outer membrane with special channels called porins. These channels, consisting of proteins, allow sugars, amino acids, and certain ions with a molecular weight of 600 to 700 to pass into the cell by passive diffusion. Thus, the outer membrane of the cell wall of gram-negative bacteria confers considerable resistance to many antibiotics. *(Joklik et al, pp 76–84; Ryan et al, p 20)*

19. **(B)** Plate counts are used to determine the number of viable bacterial cells. Estimation of oxygen consumption measures viable bacterial cells of only aerobic bacteria. The Coulter counter or the Petroff–Hauser counting chamber is used to determine the total number of bacterial cells. Thus, these devices determine both the living and dead cells. *(Joklik et al, pp 62–63; Ryan et al, pp 34–35)*

20. **(D)** Bacteria divide by splitting into two equal parts (binary fission). The time required for bacteria to undergo binary fission is called the generation time. The given generation time for *P. aeruginosa* is 15 minutes. Thus, within 90 minutes, *P. aeruginosa* will have undergone six divisions. Therefore, the number of cells per milliliter if starting with 1×10^5 will proceed as follows: 2×10^5 in 15 minutes, 4×10^5 in 30 minutes, 8×10^5 in 45 minutes, 1.6×10^6 in 60 minutes, 3.2×10^6 in 75 minutes, and 6.4×10^6 in 90 minutes. *(Joklik et al, pp 66–69)*

21. **(C)** Bacteria reproduce by binary fission without the elaborate mitotic divisions observed in eukaryotic cells. Some fungi reproduce by spore formation. Yeasts may reproduce by budding. Viruses reproduce by host cell synthesis. *(Joklik et al, pp 52,66–69,719, 791–831,883–885,1071–1079)*

22. **(A)** Response to environmental change (such as osmotic shock, high or low pH, oxidation damages, restriction of nutrients, etc.) frequently involves phosphorylation of protein kinases. These responses involve teams of proteins that sense the environment, generate a signal, transmit that signal by protein–protein interactions, and activate the appropriate response regulon. In a number of cases, a response system includes a protein kinase that becomes phosphorylated by ATP on a particular conserved histidine residue in response to environmental stimulus. This kinase is coupled with a second protein called a phosphorylated response regulator.

23. **(B)** The word siderophore means an iron-bearing compound. Bacteria require iron for the synthesis of their cytochromes. Siderophores have been implicated in the virulence of *Neisseria meningitidis*, *Neisseria gonorrhoeae*, and other bacteria. The siderophores allow the bacteria to accumulate iron and transport it into the cell. Enzyme I, carboxydismutase,

nitrogenase, or HPr protein have not been shown to be involved with the uptake and transport of iron into the bacterial cell. *(Joklik et al, pp 60–61, Ryan et al, p 27)*

24. **(C)** When *E. coli* is exposed to high temperatures, some 20 genes are activated and produce a special class of proteins called heat-shock proteins. These heat-shock proteins are essential for survival of bacteria exposed to elevated temperatures or other stressful conditions. In the case of *E. coli,* heat-shock proteins are a subunit of RNA polymerase, sigma-31, which replaces the normal sigma-70 subunit, and locates the special promoters of the heat-shock genes. At least half of the heat-shock genes encode proteins that are proteases, or are protein chaperones that assist in the processing, maturation, or export of other proteins. *(Ryan et al, p 41)*

25. **(D)** The facultative anaerobic bacteria tend to have cytochrome C oxidase and peroxidase. However, their tolerance to superoxide radical (O_2^-) is not due to cytochrome C oxidase. Their tolerance to O_2^- is thought to be primarily due to the possession of superoxide dismutase and catalase. Obligate anaerobic bacteria do not possess these enzymes. Superoxide dismutase converts the potentially lethal O_2^- to hydrogen peroxide, which also possesses antibacterial properties in appropriate concentrations, while catalase breaks down H_2O_2 to H_2O and O_2 *(Joklik et al, p 46; Ryan et al, pp 295–296)*

26. **(D)** Invasions are proteins that are present in the outer membrane of certain intracellular pathogens such as *Yersinia, Salmonella,* and *Shigella.* These bacteria produce specialized adhesins, sometimes called invasions, that bind to host cell receptors that induce their uptake by host cells. When bacteria lose their ability to produce invasion due to genetic mutation, they can no longer invade the host cells. *(Ryan et al, pp 149,338)*

27. **(C)** There are various modes for the microbial reoxidation of the reduced form of nicotinamide–adenine dinucleotide (NADH) to nicotinamide–adenine dinucleotide (NAD),

allowing glycolysis to continue even in the absence of oxygen. Fermentation is a biologic oxidation in which the final electron acceptor is an organic compound rather than oxygen. The methods used for NADH reoxidation are characteristic for different microbes, yielding NAD and a reduced organic compound rather than oxygen. These methods include ethanol production in yeast, butyric acid production in clostridia, lactate production in streptococci and lactobacilli, and propionate production in the diphtheria bacillus and propionic acid bacteria. Since carbon dioxide reduction is not one of the modes that is directly coupled with NADH oxidation, choice C in the question is false and is thus the correct answer. *(Joklik et al, pp 33–49; Ryan et al, pp 29–30)*

28. **(A)** Bacteria grown with acetate, after conversion to acetyl-CoA, cannot readily yield pyruvate and phosphoenol pyruvate as they would when growing on glucose. Since the usual precursors for carbon dioxide fixation to C4 dicarboxylic acids are not readily available, some bacteria and plants, but not animal cells, provide extra C4 units by means of the glyoxylate cycle, a modification of the tricarboxylic acid (TCA) cycle with two additional enzymes: isocitrate lyase (isocitritase) and malate synthase. These two additional reactions modify the existing TCA cycle at isocitrate so that it effectively converts two acetyl-CoA molecules reductively to succinate. The TCA cycle must continue to function in order to produce oxalacetate and alpha-ketoglutarate for amino acid biosynthesis. *(Joklik et al, pp 34–41; Ryan et al, pp 28–29)*

29. **(C)** The Entner–Doudoroff glycolytic pathway is found in microbes, but not in animal cells. The reduced form of nicotinamide–adenine dinucleotide phosphate, rather than the reduced form of NADH, is the normal biosynthetic reducing agent. NADH is generally used to generate ATP via the respiratory chain to oxygen. For biosynthesis of glucose-6-phosphate from pyruvate via reversal of the Embden–Meyerhof pathway, the irreversible phosphofructokinase reaction needs

to be replaced by fructose bisphosphate phosphatase. The pyruvate kinase, which is reversible only to a slight extent, is replaced by phosphoenol pyruvate (PEP) synthase or by a combination of pyruvate carboxylase and PEP carboxykinase to form PEP. (*Jawetz et al, pp 74–76; Ryan et al, pp 29–30*)

30. **(A)** All of the statements except (A) are true. Fructose diphosphate (FDP) aldolase, although a key enzyme in glycolysis via the Embden–Meyerhof pathway, is not specific for that pathway. The FDP aldolase also functions as a portion of the hexose monophosphate (pentose phosphate) pathway. (*Joklik et al, pp 31–49; Ryan et al, pp 29–31*)

31. **(B)** All of the statements except (B) are true. The glyoxylate cycle is found in bacteria grown on two-carbon sources such as acetate. It also occurs in plants, but not in animal cells. (*Joklik et al, pp 31–52; Ryan et al, pp 28–30*)

32. **(E)** Since glutamate is not a methyl donor, statement (E) in the question is false and thus is the correct answer. S-adenosylmethionine is the correct methyl donor. All of the other statements about bacterial chemotaxis are correct. (*Joklik et al, pp 61–62; Ryan et al, pp 42–43*)

33. **(E)** The outer membranes of the cell walls of gram-negative bacteria are made of LPS, which has three major subunits: sugar side chain, core polysaccharide, and lipid A. This lipid-containing cell wall component is often referred to as endotoxin because it causes a febrile response, hypotension, and other adverse biologic reactions in humans and certain animals. Lipid A is the toxic moiety of LPS molecules. The sugar side chain determines the somatic or O antigenicity of each strain of bacteria. (*Joklik et al, pp 82–86; Ryan et al, pp 18–20*)

34. **(E)** The capsule, hyaluronidase, M protein, and lecithinase all are bacterial cell components or products that enhance the virulence or invasiveness of some microorganisms. The bacterial and fungal capsule is antiphagocytic. The capsules of *Streptococcus pneumo-*

niae and *Cryptococcus neoformans* are some of the typical examples. Similarly, M protein of group A beta-hemolytic streptococci is also antiphagocytic. Various hydrolytic enzymes, including hyaluronidase, collagenase, and lecithinase, help bacteria spread through the tissues. These enzymes are especially important in the pathogenicity of certain streptococci and *Clostridium perfringens* (gas gangrene organism). (*Joklik et al, pp 350,421–422,639; Ryan et al, pp 154–157*)

35. **(E)** The bacterial cytoplasmic membrane is a multifunctional organelle. Like the cell membrane of eukaryotic cells, it is the osmotic regulator for the cell. It is also an organelle equivalent to the eukaryotic mitochondrion in that essentially all the respiratory enzymes are located in the cytoplasmic membrane. Special proteins in the bacterial cytoplasmic membrane detect signals from the environment and regulate the chemotactic movement of the cell via flagellar motor proteins. (*Joklik et al, p 26; Ryan et al, pp 20–21*)

36. **(D)** There is a considerable difference in the cell wall structure between gram-positive and gram-negative bacteria. This difference in the wall structure is considered to be responsible for the different reaction of bacteria to the Gram stain. Once the walls are removed, all protoplasts react identically to the Gram stain; all bacterial protoplasts are gram-negative, and there is no way to differentiate whether they originated from *E. coli* or *Bacillus megaterium*. By the same token, all cell wall-defective organisms including mycoplasmas and L forms are gram-negative. All mycobacteria are gram-positive, and it is impossible to differentiate species based on reaction to the Gram stain. One cannot identify any species of bacteria or fungi based on the result of the Gram stain. (*Joklik et al, pp 16,498; Ryan et al, pp 16–20*)

37. **(E)** The consensus is that bacterial chromosome replication is a bidirectional process. It begins at a specific site of the bacterial chromosome known as the origin of replication. Replication occurs when a fixed amount of the initiator protein has been synthesized. Since

various enzymes are needed to form initiator protein and DNA, bacterial chromosome replication requires protein synthesis. *(Joklik et al, pp 99–104; Ryan et al, pp 30–31)*

38. (E) Phagocytosis is accompanied by a burst of oxygen and glucose consumption and increased hydrogen peroxide, lactate, and superoxide production, as well as a large increase in glucose metabolism via the hexose monophosphate (pentose phosphate) pathway. *(Joklik et al, p 351; Ryan et al, pp 151–153)*

39. (C) Flagellated bacteria swim (move forward) by counterclockwise rotation of their flagella. Clockwise rotation of the flagella cause bacteria to tumble. *(Ryan et al, p 21)*

40. (B) Many enzymes, called penicillin-binding proteins (PBPs) are involved in forging, breaking, and reforging the peptide cross-links between glycan chains. These proteins are so called because of their property of combining with penicillin. This dynamic process is necessary to permit expansion of the murein sac (peptidoglycan layer) during cellular growth, to shape the envelope, and to prepare for cell division. Heat-shock protein has nothing to do with the cell-wall formation. Although Braun's lipoprotein is an important component of gram-negative cell wall, it is not involved in murein (peptidoglycan) expansion, shaping, and septum formation. Porins are outer membrane proteins that play important roles in creating cell-surface charge, permeability barrier, etc. c-AMP binding protein plays no role in wall formation or wall expansion. *(Ryan et al, pp 19,33,192–193)*

41. (C) Strict or obligate anaerobes require low local oxidation reduction potential for growth. Some obligate anaerobes are killed by a brief exposure to air, although many can survive but cannot grow in the presence of air. The main reason that obligate anaerobes cannot survive or grow in the presence of oxygen is that these anaerobic bacteria lack one key enzyme (superoxide dismutase) that is essential for detoxication of superoxide molecule resulting from oxygen metabolism.

Obligate anaerobes can cause infections in humans without participation of other species of bacteria. Some obligate anaerobes such as *Clostridium tetani* form spore under certain conditions. *(Ryan et al, pp 29,295,301)*

42. (C) The frequency of initiation of chromosome replication (and, therefore, the number of growing points) varies with cell growth rate; the chain elongation rate is rather constant. *(Ryan et al, p 30)*

43. (C) The periplasmic space or periplasm is a narrow space between the cytoplasmic membrane and the thin peptidoglycan layer. This periplasm is filled with periplasmic gel that contains enzymes essential for transport of nutrients or cellular products. *(Ryan et al, p 18)*

44. (C) Complete killing of all forms of organisms (bacteria, viruses, fungi, parasites, etc.) is achieved only by sterilization. Disinfection is the destruction of pathogenic microorganisms. Pasteurization (heating at 74°C for 3 to 5 seconds or 62°C for 30 minutes) kills only important pathogens in liquids or milk. Boiling kills only vegetative forms of microorganisms and does not kill spores. *(Ryan et al, pp 171–172)*

45. (D) Solutions of 100% alcohol dehydrate rapidly but fail to kill because the lethal process requires water molecules. Ethanol (70 to 90%) and isopropyl alcohol (90 to 95%) are widely used as skin decontaminants before simple invasive procedures such as venipuncture. Any concentrations less than 70% are ineffective as disinfectants. *(Ryan et al, p 176)*

46. (D) In bacteria, the cell membrane serves to transport electron through a chain of carriers to ultimate acceptor. The passage of electrons through the carriers is accompanied by the secretion from the cell of protons, generating an H^+ differential between the external surface of the cell and the cell interior. This differential, called protonmotive force, can then be used in fueling several vital cell functions such as those listed above. *(Ryan et al, p 28)*

47. (D) Bacteria such as *Campylobacter jejuni* can grow best at low oxygen concentrations, but can also grow without oxygen. This type of microorganism is called a microaerophilic organism. In contrast to this, aerotolerant anaerobe (*Bacteroides fragilis,* for example) can survive but cannot grow well when oxygen is present in the environment. Strict anaerobe (*C. tetani*), of course, cannot survive or grow at all in the presence of oxygen. Aerobe (*Mycobacterium tuberculosis*) can grow only in the presence of oxygen. Facultative anaerobe (*E. coli*) grow well in both aerobic and anaerobic conditions. *(Ryan et al, p 29)*

48. (B) Lysozyme is a hydrolytic enzyme contained in phagocytes, serum, and tear. This enzyme cleaves the glycosidic bond between N-acetylmuramic acid and N-acetylglcosamine which makes the backbone of peptidoglycan. Lysozyme lyses many bacteria because their cell wall is susceptible to the lytic action of this enzyme. When exposed to lysozyme, many bacteria undergo lysis unless they are osmotically protected. Bacterial protoplasts are prepared by treating bacteria in the presence of osmotically protective media. *(Ryan et al, p 19)*

49. (A) The cell wall is responsible for the characteristic shape of a bacterium. When the cell wall is removed by enzymatic digestion, all bacteria become spherical, losing their original shape. *(Joklik et al, pp 24–25; Ryan et al, p 15)*

50. (D) The flagellum is a locomotive organelle of bacteria. It is made of a protein called flagellin. Immunologically, it is the source of H antigen (the organelle responsible for spreading on the soft agar surface). In contrast to this, nonflagellar antigens associated with the cell wall are called O, or somatic, antigens. *(Joklik et al, pp 21–23; Ryan et al, pp 15–24)*

51. (B) Protoplasts, formed by the complete removal of the cell wall, are surrounded only by the cytoplasmic membrane or cell membrane. In contrast, spheroplasts result from partial removal of the cell wall. In spheroplasts, some remnants of the cell wall, especially the outer cell membrane remnants, still remain attached to the cell surface. *(Joklik et al, p 25; Ryan et al, pp 20–21)*

52. (C) Lipopolysaccharide is the main component of the outer membrane of gram-negative bacteria. N-acetylmuramic acid is an amino sugar derivative constituting an essential structural unit of bacterial peptidoglycan. Lipid-P–P-muramic acid pentapeptide is an intermediate product formed in the cytoplasmic membrane during the biosynthesis of the peptidoglycan of *Staphylococcus aureus. (Joklik et al, pp 76–86; Ryan et al, p 19)*

53. (B) Teichoic acids are polysaccharides consisting of repeated units of glycerol or ribitol linked by phosphate occurring in the cell wall and cytoplasmic membrane of certain gram-positive bacteria. Teichoic acids complexed with lipid are called lipoteichoic acids. Teichoic acids are strong, negatively charged compounds, and are structurally linked to peptidoglycan. Teichoic acids are the principal antigenic components of the surface of gram-positive bacteria. Calcium dipicolinate occurs only in the cytoplasm of bacterial spores. *(Joklik et al, p 80; Ryan et al, p 24)*

54. (B) Thiamine is involved in the decarboxylation of pyruvic and other keto acids. *(Joklik et al, p 55)*

55. (D) Pyridoxal phosphate is involved in transamination and racemization of amino acids. Riboflavin plays a role in oxidation-reduction reactions, folic acid acts as a carrier of formyl groups, and pantothenic acid functions as a carrier of an acyl group. *(Joklik et al, p 55)*

56. (C) Isocitrate lyase (isocitrase) is one of the two additional enzymes of the glyoxylate cycle, the other being malate synthase. These enzymes modify the TCA cycle when bacteria are grown on two-carbon sources such as acetate. These two reactions convert two acetyl-CoA molecules reductively to succinate, thus generating additional C4 dicarboxylic acids to allow the TCA cycle to continue operating during growth. *(Jawetz et al, p 66; Joklik et al, p 41)*

57. **(B)** Transketolase is one of the enzymes of the nonoxidative portion of the hexose monophosphate (pentose phosphate) cycle, the other being transaldolase. These enzymes link this pathway to the Embden–Meyerhof glycolytic pathway. Transketolase requires thiamine pyrophosphate as a coenzyme. *(Jawetz, p 61)*

58. **(D)** In chronic granulomatous disease (CGD) of childhood, polymorphonuclear leukocytes alter the phagocyte's ability to kill phagocytosed bacteria, even though the leukocytes have responded correctly to the chemotactic stimuli and ingested the bacteria normally. Normally, when granulocyte membranes are stimulated during phagocytosis, there is a marked stimulation of the reduced form of nicotinamide–adenine dinucleotide phosphate (NADPH) oxidase. NADPH is formed as a result of increased activity of the oxidative portion of the hexose monophosphate (pentose phosphate) pathway. In the absence of NADPH, reoxidation to nicotinamide–adenine dinucleotide phosphate by NADPH oxidase, with concomitant formation of hydrogen peroxide (H_2O_2) and superoxide, the H_2O_2 required in the myeloperoxidase–halide bactericidal reaction is not completely effective; hence, the ingested bacteria are not readily killed. All of the other enzymes listed in the question are involved in some aspect of bacterial killing after phagocytosis, but only NADPH oxidase is specifically decreased in CGD. *(Joklik et al, pp 340–341)*

59. **(F)** Endotoxin is a toxic principle produced by gram-negative bacteria. It is firmly bound to their cell walls as a high-molecular complex composed of polysaccharide, lipid, and protein, called the endotoxic complex. Generally, endotoxin is released into the surrounding medium if the organism undergoes disintegration or lysis. Endotoxins are produced by a large variety of bacteria, predominantly Enterobacteriaceae, pathogenic or nonpathogenic for animal or man, such as *Salmonella, Shigella, Escherichia, Proteus, Pseudomonas, Klebsiella, Pasteurella,* and others. The toxic moiety of the endotoxin is lipid A, which has been shown experimentally to induce pyrexia, hypotension, tumor necrosis factor, and interleukin-1. *(Joklik et al, pp 80–87)*

60. **(I)** The lipid A of endotoxin is covalently bound to the polysaccharide component of endotoxin and consists of the core oligosaccharide and the O-specific chain. The O-specific chain contains up to six sugar residues. The nature sequence and architecture varies among species, strains, or serovars of gram-negative bacteria. Thus, the O-specific chain is used for the identification of gram-negative bacteria that may cause disseminated intravascular coagulation. The composition of the inner or outer core contains sugars, heptoses, phosphates, ethanolamine, and other components that do not vary sufficiently among gram-negative species, strains, or serovars. 3-Hydroxy-tetradecanoic acid and D-glucosamine are constituents of lipid A of endotoxins. *(Joklik et al, pp 80–87)*

REFERENCES

Jawetz E, Melnick JL, Adelberg EA, et al. *Review of Medical Microbiology,* 19th ed. Norwalk, CT: Appleton & Lange; 1991.

Joklik WK, Willett HP, Amos DB, Wilfert CM. *Zinsser Microbiology,* 20th ed. Norwalk, CT: Appleton & Lange; 1992.

Ryan KJ, Champoux JJ, Drew WL, Falkow S, Neithardt FC, Plorde JJ, Ray CD. *Sherris Medical Microbiology,* 3rd ed. Norwalk, CT: Appleton & Lange; 1994.

CHAPTER 2

Microbial Genetics
Questions

DIRECTIONS (Questions 61 through 74): Each of the questions or incomplete statements in this section is followed by five suggested answers or completions. Select the ONE lettered answer or completion that is BEST in each case.

61. The process of gene exchange in many bacteria is mediated by conjugation. All of the following statements about conjugation are true EXCEPT

    (A) a sex (fertility) factor must be present in the "male" bacterium
    (B) the "female" replicates the incoming DNA
    (C) sex pili are involved in conjugal exchange but their role is not absolutely known
    (D) conjugation can occur between different species of bacteria (eg, *Escherichia coli* and *Pseudomonas aeruginosa*)
    (E) the entire bacterial chromosome can be transferred during conjugation

62. The process in which DNA released by lysis of one bacterium is taken up by a second bacterium, leading to a change in phenotype of that second bacterium, is called

    (A) transduction
    (B) sexduction
    (C) conjugation
    (D) transformation
    (E) transfection

63. A prophage that contains phage genes as well as bacterial genes from the region of the bacterial chromosome adjacent to the attachment site is occasionally excised incorrectly. This DNA molecule can be packaged within a phage particle and transferred to a recipient bacterium by infection. This process is called

    (A) specialized transduction
    (B) sexduction
    (C) generalized transduction
    (D) transformation
    (E) complementation

64. The process by which any bacterial gene can be packaged inside a phage particle and then introduced into another bacterium by infection of that cell with the phage, leading to a change in the phenotype of the recipient cell, is called

    (A) generalized transformation
    (B) specialized transduction
    (C) generalized transfection
    (D) sexduction
    (E) generalized transduction

65. Damage of DNA by nitrogen mustard is due to

    (A) single-stranded breaks in DNA
    (B) double-stranded breaks in DNA
    (C) removal of amino group from adenine to form hypoxanthine
    (D) covalent bond formation between two bases on opposite strands of DNA
    (E) formation of thymine dimers

66. The SOS DNA repair pathway is

    (A) an induced pathway
    (B) not activated by ultraviolet irradiation
    (C) independent of the recA gene product in *Escherichia coli*
    (D) usually inoperative when a chemical mutagen causes DNA damage
    (E) not induced when DNA replication is inhibited

67. The role of the sigma factor is essentially regulatory in that it

    (A) stimulates DNA polymerase
    (B) inactivates adenyl cyclase
    (C) allows RNA polymerase to select nucleotide initiation sequences (promoters)
    (D) depresses the action of endonuclease
    (E) allows DNA polymerase to initiate DNA synthesis from the 5′ end

68. The lactose operon is correctly described as

    (A) containing five genes
    (B) constitutive
    (C) being controlled at the transcriptional level
    (D) an example of a positive control mechanism
    (E) independent of the lacI gene product

69. Which of the following statements about catabolite repression is true?

    (A) it does not require a controlling element for gene expression
    (B) it is an example of a negative cell-control mechanism
    (C) it is not applicable to the lactose operon
    (D) it can be encountered with bacteria growing in the presence of glucose and low intracellular levels of cyclic adenosine monophosphate (cAMP)
    (E) it does not depend on the cAMP activator protein

70. The rho protein is identified as

    (A) an effector for the production of C1 protein

    (B) the main repressor for lambda phage production
    (C) a subunit of DNA polymerase
    (D) being intimately involved with cell regulation at the RNA polymerase level
    (E) a subunit of the sigma factor

71. Which of the following statements about the nucleotide guanosine tetraphosphate ("magic spot") is true?

    (A) it stimulates operons for the utilization of agar
    (B) it inhibits a starvation-dependent protease
    (C) its accumulation is promoted by amino acid limitation
    (D) it is formed by a protein known as the "magic spot" enzyme
    (E) it does not play a key role in gene regulation during sporulation

72. When phage packages host DNA at random and can therefore transfer any bacterial gene during subsequent infection and expression, the process is called

    (A) generalized transformation
    (B) specialized transduction
    (C) generalized transduction
    (D) abortive transduction
    (E) generalized transfection

73. Bacteriophage may be involved in all of the following EXCEPT

    (A) transferring genetic information between different strains of bacteria
    (B) changing the properties of bacteria when they become lysogenized
    (C) transferring genetic information between male and female bacteria of the same species
    (D) causing all plasmids to replicate faster upon infection
    (E) expressing their genes in a temporally controlled fashion

74. All of the following are true statements about lysogens EXCEPT

(A) control of phage gene expression is usually at the transcriptional level

(B) lytic functions are not expressed

(C) phage DNA can exist in the bacterial cytoplasm

(D) phage repressor protects the bacteria from subsequent infections by all types of phage

(E) phage DNA can be covalently joined with the bacterial DNA

DIRECTIONS (Questions 75 through 77): Each group of items in this section consists of lettered headings followed by a set of numbered words or phrases. For each numbered word or phrase, select the ONE lettered heading that is most closely associated with it. Each lettered heading may be selected once, more than once, or not at all.

(A) enzyme repression

(B) feedback inhibition

(C) allosteric activation

(D) cooperativity

(E) sequential repression

75. Bacteria change their enzymatic biosynthetic activity so that the previously synthesized enzymes are used only to the extent needed

76. When microbes have an excess of glucose-6-phosphate, they may use some of this excess by making glycogen

77. Concerned primarily with economy in macromolecular synthesis

DIRECTIONS (Questions 78 through 107): Each of the questions or incomplete statements in this section is followed by five suggested answers or completions. Select the ONE lettered answer or completion that is BEST in each case.

78. Which of the following statements about bacterial transformation is true?

(A) it was first demonstrated in gram-positive pneumococcal encapsulation studies

(B) it cannot be used to study the effects of physical agents on the biologic activity of DNA

(C) it can result in the uptake of both DNA strands

(D) it involves transfer of DNA contained in a protein coat

(E) bacteria in a state that allows transformation are called incompetent

79. In order for the bacterial "recipient" of new information to stably express it, genetic recombination

(A) is not absolutely required for transformation with chromosomal DNA

(B) is absolutely required for conjugation with F′ cell

(C) may not be required for specialized transduction

(D) may not be required for generalized transduction

(E) requires abortive transduction

80. Essentially no free plasmid is present in

(A) an F⁺ cell

(B) high-frequency recombination (Hfr) cell or an F⁺ cell

(C) a cell with an F′ containing the chromosomal trpA gene

(D) conjugating cells

(E) a G⁺ cell

81. Bacteriophages are important in bacterial variation because they can carry bacterial DNA around in their capsids. Which of the following statements about transduction of bacteriophages is true?

(A) specialized transduction usually occurs with a lytic phage

(B) generalized transduction usually occurs with a lytic phage

(C) generalized transduction usually occurs with a lysogenic phage

(D) specialized transduction usually does not occur with a lysogenic phage

(E) incomplete transduction occurs only with zuzu phage

82. The process of sexual exchange in bacteria involves plasmids, about which it can be said that

    (A) sex factors are not conjugative plasmids
    (B) conjugative plasmids are all sex factors
    (C) F′ plasmids are sex factors with bacterial DNA
    (D) transfer genes (tra genes) are present only in conjugative plasmids but missing in sex factors
    (E) conjugal transfer is not a replicative process

83. Lysogenic phage conversion can change the properties of a bacterium since it

    (A) is usually due to a specialized transducing phage
    (B) is responsible for *Salmonella* flagellar antigenic switching (from H1 to H2)
    (C) usually requires phage lytic gene products
    (D) usually requires a phage lysogenic gene product
    (E) usually requires C factor

84. Which of the following statements is true concerning transformation in both gram-positive and gram-negative bacteria?

    (A) cells are normally competent all the time
    (B) specific DNA sequences are bound by specific receptor proteins on the cell surface
    (C) following binding of double-stranded DNA, one strand is degraded before uptake of the other single strand into the cell
    (D) following uptake, integration of the foreign DNA into the chromosome of the recipient cell requires regions of significant sequence homology between the foreign DNA and the DNA of the recipient
    (E) cells are never normally competent

85. Concerning a bacterial strain that harbors a free F plasmid, it can be said that

    (A) it is lysogenic
    (B) it will transfer bacterial genes at low frequency with a related strain lacking the F plasmid
    (C) it cannot simultaneously harbor a plasmid of another incompatibility group
    (D) it will never contain Hfr cells at a frequency of 101
    (E) the same drug resistance is never found on plasmids that are otherwise unrelated

86. Which of the following statements about bacterial transduction is true?

    (A) recipient F$^+$ cells cannot be transduced with DNA from F$^+$ donors
    (B) a defective phage, which was improperly excised from the bacterial chromosome, can mediate the reaction
    (C) under special conditions, a transducing particle can contain an entire bacterial chromosome
    (D) an entire plasmid can never be transferred
    (E) specialized transduction operates on a few genes with very slight efficiency

87. All of the following are true EXCEPT that plasmids are extrachromosomal self-replicating structures that

    (A) can acquire transposons and thus become R plasmids
    (B) are vehicles for the dissemination of antibiotic-resistance traits among bacteria
    (C) can, in some cases, mediate their own transfer between bacteria
    (D) have been found in virtually all medically important bacteria
    (E) are only infrequently transferred by conjugation

88. All of the following statements are true EXCEPT that R plasmids are accurately described as

    (A) having the ability to evolve from other plasmids by acquiring drug-resistance transposons

(B) found in both gram-positive and gram-negative bacteria

(C) usually transferable between bacteria of the same species able to undergo mutations as a result of antibiotic usage

(D) able to promote chromosomal transfer from diverse bacteria

(E) not existing before the modern era of antibiotic therapy

89. A plasmid that is not conjugal may be transferred to another cell by all of the following causes EXCEPT

(A) mobilization by a conjugal plasmid

(B) transformation of the original cell lyses and releases DNA into the medium

(C) transduction with a generalized transducing phage

(D) cell fusion following mating between male and female bacteria

(E) the combination of virulence and antibiotic resistance on single plasmids has no obvious medical consequence

90. Microbial mutations are due to all of the following causes EXCEPT

(A) substitutions (transversions)

(B) additions (insertions)

(C) deletions

(D) rearrangements

(E) inversions

91. Missense mutations can cause all of the following EXCEPT that they cannot

(A) alter the triplet code

(B) produce temperature-sensitive gene products

(C) alter the catalytic properties of an enzyme

(D) be silent mutations

(E) never be suppressed

92. The Ames test is correctly described by all of the following statements EXCEPT it

(A) is used to determine if a chemical is a mutagen

(B) uses strains of bacteria that are easy to mutate

(C) uses strains of *Salmonella* that can grow in a synthetic medium

(D) is an extremely quick method to detect mutagens that are presumable carcinogens

(E) requires the use of live animals

93. DNA repair in *E. coli* occurs by all of the following mechanisms EXCEPT

(A) excision repair

(B) SOS repair

(C) postreplication repair

(D) photoreactivation repair

(E) polymerization repair

94. Excision repair requires all of the following EXCEPT

(A) a DNA polymerase

(B) an endonuclease

(C) a DNA ligase

(D) a 5′-specific exonuclease

(E) a 3′-specific exonuclease

95. In response to certain forms of DNA damage, *E. coli* induces SOS repair reactions by proteins that affect all of the following diverse processes EXCEPT

(A) DNA repair

(B) respiration

(C) mutagenesis

(D) recombination

(E) cell division

96. All of the following statements about diphtheria toxin are true EXCEPT

(A) B fragment is the binding element, required for intercellular entry of A fragment

(B) A fragment gains entry into the cell and interferes with protein synthesis

(C) it consists of a single polypeptide chain that is later proteolytically cleaved into two fragments, A and B

(D) its effect is easily reversed before its entry into the cell by administration of a specific antibody

(E) both fragments are necessary for toxin activity

97. All of the following statements about plasmids are true EXCEPT that plasmids

(A) carrying resistance genes for antibiotics are called R plasmids

(B) are vehicles for the dissemination of antibiotic-resistant traits among bacteria

(C) are conjugative when they contain sufficient genetic information to enable them to mediate their own transfer by conjugation

(D) in vitro have their toxin production inhibited by high concentrations of iron

(E) never control genes regulating enzymes capable of destroying antimicrobial drugs

98. Phage conversion is responsible for the production of some toxins of all the following bacteria EXCEPT

(A) *Clostridium botulinum* (botulinum toxin)

(B) *Streptococcus pyogenes* (erythrogenic toxin)

(C) *Corynebacterium diphtheriae* (diphtheria toxin)

(D) *Bacteroides fragilis* (fragilinum toxin)

(E) *Staphylococcus aureus* (a food enterotoxin)

Questions 99 and 100 refer to the following figure, which shows the effect of nutrition-imposed growth rate on cell composition.

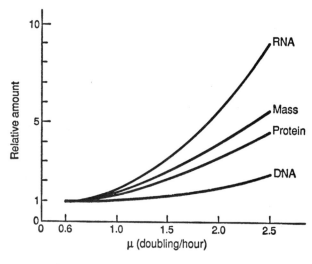

Figure 2–1

99. All of the following statements about the graph are true EXCEPT

(A) RNA, mass, protein, and DNA are exponential functions of growth rate

(B) as the cell grows faster, it becomes bigger

(C) as the cell grows faster, it contains more of each of its components

(D) RNA increases much faster than mass while protein increases somewhat slower

(E) the relative composition of a cell predictably stays the same, with all components increasing linearly, when growing in a good growth medium

100. All the following statements are true EXCEPT

(A) the average cell in a culture of *E. coli* B/r growing at 2.0 doublings per hour contains about five times as much RNA as do cells growing at 0.6 doubling per hour

(B) protein increases faster than DNA as the growth rate increases

(C) DNA increases faster than RNA as the growth rate increases

(D) cells from a rapidly growing culture are markedly enriched in RNA because they contain a higher proportion of ribosomes

(E) the average cell growing at 2.5 doublings per hour contains over twice the amount of DNA that a cell growing at 0.6 doubling per hour contains

101. During transcription, all of the following base-pairing rules for RNA polymerase are true EXCEPT

(A) the bacterial RNA polymerase is more complex than the eukaryotic RNA polymerase

(B) bacteria have only a single RNA polymerase

(C) in eukaryotic cells, messenger RNA (mRNA) is capped, spliced, and transported to the cytoplasm before it can be translated

(D) bacterial mRNA is usually translated as it is being transcribed

(E) the transcriptional start is relatively simple in bacteria as compared with that in eukaryotes

102. Which of the following statements about bacterial protein degradation is true?

(A) *E. coli* contains only one protease

(B) the lon protease is produced at low levels during normal growth of *E. coli*

(C) after heat-shock, the lon protease is no longer synthesized by bacteria

(D) the SOS response does not involve a protease

(E) the recA protein of bacterial cells is not a protease

103. All of the following statements about mutations that produce a defective gene product are true EXCEPT

(A) it can be counteracted if a second mutation is the exact reversal of the first

(B) a second mutation elsewhere in the genome, a suppressor, can nullify the effect of the original mutation in several ways

(C) a suppression of a missense mutation that causes an altered protein conformation cannot be reversed

(D) a suppression of frameshift mutations occurs by means of a second compensating mutation close to the site of the first mutation

(E) suppression of nonsense mutations due to the translational machinery encountering a nonsense codon occurs because there is no corresponding transfer RNA available

104. All of the following statements about conjugative transposons are true EXCEPT

(A) they are a mechanism for dispensing antibiotic resistance

(B) they can occur in gram-negative bacteria

(C) they are highly promiscuous

(D) recipient strains need not belong to the same species or genus

(E) strains need not have plasmids

105. All of the following statements about methylases and/or restriction endonucleases are true EXCEPT

(A) they provide bacteria a means of distinguishing between their own and foreign DNA

(B) restriction endonucleases hydrolyze DNA at restriction sites determined by specific DNA sequences

(C) they modify bases within restriction sites by methylation with methylases

(D) direct cleavage of donor DNA occurs before it can be established as part of a recombination replicon

(E) by methylation of bases, they provide the site with a chemical signal that protects the host DNA against cleavage

106. The bacterial cell uses as many as 1,000 to 2,000 chemical reactions to replicate itself. These reactions can all be categorized as belonging to one of the following types of reactions EXCEPT for

(A) assembly

(B) discombobulation

(C) polymerization

(D) biosynthesis

(E) fueling

107. Regulation of the extent of transcription, perhaps the most important level of control in bacterial systems, is correctly described by the following statements EXCEPT that there must be

(A) recognition and utilization of promoter sequences by DNA polymerase

(B) specific regulatory proteins that bind near or within the promoter sequence

(C) negative regulatory proteins that block promoter usage

(D) trans-acting elements in the gene that need not be near or even on the same control molecule

(E) cis-acting elements in the gene that must be located near or within the promoter that is being controlled

Microbial Genetics
Answers and Explanations

61. **(A)** Sex (fertility) factors are only a subclass of conjugative plasmids. A sex factor does not have to be present, a conjugative plasmid could be present. The point is that a conjugative plasmid in the male does do conjugation. The female receives the single-strand DNA and replicates it to make it double stranded. The exact role of pili is not known, but they are involved, either in bringing the bacteria together, letting DNA go through them, or both. Conjugation can, and does, occur between different bacteria. The entire bacterial chromosome can be transferred during conjugation, for example, when an Hfr (microbe that carries out high-frequency recombination) transfers the chromosome. It can happen, but only at low frequency. *(Joklik et al, p 139)*

62. **(D)** Transformation is the most primitive of the mechanisms for gene transfer among bacteria. Transformation has been demonstrated mainly in gram-positive bacteria such as *Bacillus subtilis* and the pneumonia streptococcus *Streptococcus pneumoniae*. Normally transformable bacteria develop competence only under certain specific growth conditions. Transformation can be induced artificially in some gram-negative microorganisms (*Escherichia coli*, for example) only when the cell is first rendered permeable to DNA by treatment with calcium chloride. Genetic transfer mediated by F' cells is known as sexduction. Transduction is described in the answer to question 3. *(Jawetz et al, p 89; Joklik et al, pp 136–138)*

63. **(A)** Transduction is based on the ability of a virus to transfer bacterial genes from one bacterial cell to another. Specialized transduction is based on the capability of bacteriophage DNA to integrate and be excised from the host chromosome. In specialized transduction, only specific bacterial genes can be transduced. For example, the bacterial virus lambda integrates on the host chromosome between the galactose and biotin genes. When the lysogenic cell is induced to initiate a lytic cycle, lambda (l) prophage is excised from the host genome and in the process the galactose gene is carried out with it (lgal). The excised lgal occasionally lacks certain genes essential for lytic growth. These defective particles are called ldgal. If ldgal particles are used to infect other bacteria, the transduced galactose gene can enter into a recombinational event with the galactose gene on the bacterial chromosome. *(Joklik et al, pp 138–139)*

64. **(E)** Generalized transduction is a mechanism that alters the phenotype of the host by transfer of any bacterial genes from one bacterial cell to another via bacteriophage. Bacteria infected with a lytic virus or a lysogenic cell is induced to produce lytic virus. During the maturation process, fragmented bacterial DNA may be packaged into the phage. Upon lysis of the cell, one or more of the phage particles will carry bacterial DN[...] [...]ing phage) instead of phage DN[...] ration of bacterial DNA int[...] is a random event, and an[...] could be transduced by th[...]

is no generalized transformation or generalized transfection. *(Jawetz et al, pp 87–89; Joklik et al, p 138)*

65. **(D)** Single- and double-stranded breaks in the DNA are due to x-rays. Nitrous acid deaminates adenine to form hypoxanthine. Formation of thymine dimers due to ultraviolet irradiation is the most common dimer formed but others can form from adjacent pyrimidines. *(Joklik et al, pp 129–130)*

66. **(A)** The SOS DNA repair pathway is induced (activated) by ultraviolet irradiation. In *E. coli*, it is dependent upon the recA gene product; it appears when DNA replication is inhibited, or when a chemical mutagen induces DNA lesions. *(Joklik et al, pp 131–132)*

67. **(C)** The role of the sigma factor is essentially a regulatory one in that it allows RNA polymerase to select initiation sequences from among all other nucleotide sequences on the chromosome. Initiation sequences, or promoters, are an integral part of all regions of DNA transcription. The sigma factor is not known to stimulate DNA polymerase, inactivate adenyl cyclase, or depress the action of endonuclease. *(Joklik et al, pp 72–73,105–106,117)*

68. **(C)** The lactose operon contains three genes: the genes for β-galactosidase (lacZ), the galactoside permease (lacY), and the galactoside acetylase gene (lacA). The enzymes are only present when lactose is present. Thus the lactose operon is inducible and not constitutive. It is an example of a negative control mechanism in that a controlling element, that is, a repressor protein, binds tightly to a site in the DNA in front of the lacZ gene. This site is called an operator. The presence of the bound repressor protein interferes with the initiation of DNA transcription by RNA polymerase. The addition of lactose combines with the repressor protein and thus allows RNA polymerase to function. The operon is influenced by the lacI gene product allolactose. *(Jawetz et al, pp 92–93; Joklik et al, pp 49,115)*

69. **(D)** This system involves positive regulation in that a controlling element is required be-

fore gene product can be expressed. That is, in the presence of a readily utilized compound such as glucose, resulting in low intracellular levels of cyclic adenosine monophosphate (cAMP), cAMP is required as an effector for the cAMP activator protein (CAP). The complex then binds at the lactose promoter to allow RNA polymerase to bind and begin DNA transcription. In the absence of CAP and cAMP, the RNA polymerase does not bind well. Thus CAP and cAMP are both positive regulators of the lactose operon. *(Joklik et al, pp 50,115–117)*

70. **(D)** As the RNA polymerase reads past the stop codon, the message will be devoid of ribosomes, allowing the rho protein to attach to messenger RNA (mRNA) and travel on it until it meets the RNA polymerase. When the rho-RNA polymerase complex reaches a termination site, synthesis of mRNA synthesis is inhibited. The effector for the lysogenic lambda phage is the CII protein. The rho protein is neither a subunit for DNA polymerase nor of the sigma factor, but it is involved in the control of transcription termination. *(Joklik et al, pp 118–119)*

71. **(C)** During starvation for an amino acid, the guanosine tetraphosphate (ppGpp) level in the cell is about ten times the basal level due to the stringent response. Thus, during the limitation of an amino acid, its accumulation is promoted. Activation of the operons for sugar utilization is not a factor. This is the function of cyclic adenosine monophosphate and not ppGpp. The ppGpp stimulates the "starvation-dependent" protease so that it can attack normal proteins and thus provide the amino acids. The ppGpp is formed by an enzyme called the stringent factor. The term "magic spot" comes from the fact that the ppGpp was first observed as an unusual spot on a chromatogram. The compound 3',5'-ppApp also appears to play a key role in gene regulation during bacterial sporulation. *(Joklik et al, pp 117–118)*

72. **(C)** In generalized transduction, bacteriophage are able to transfer genes derived from their bacterial host in a relatively indiscrimi-

nate manner; almost all host genes can be transferred. In specialized transduction, only certain genes from the previously infected bacterial host can be transferred. In abortive transduction, some generalized transductions lead to persistence, but not replication, due to failure of the exogenote to be integrated. Following zygote division, only one of the daughter cells receives the exogenote. The exogenote is maintained, but not replicated. Transfection and transformation do not involve phage particles directly. *(Jawetz et al, p 89; Joklik et al, pp 138–139)*

73. **(D)** Plasmids, small extrachromosomal genetic elements, share many properties with bacteriophages. They differ chiefly in their lack of an extracellular phase, hence they lack capsids. However, plasmids regulate their own replication, such that each one has a typical ratio of plasmid copies to host chromosome copies. This rate of plasmid replication is unaffected by infection of the host cell with a bacteriophage. *(Jawetz et al, p 83; Joklik et al, pp 115–119)*

74. **(D)** Phage repressor only protects the host bacteria from infections by closely related phages. Immunity is highly specific and lysogenic bacteria are only immune to the lysogenic phage and to closely related phages. Statement D mentions that phage repressor protects the bacteria from subsequent infections by all types of phages. D is an incorrect statement and is thus the correct answer. All other statements are true. *(Jawetz et al, p 89; Joklik et al, pp 914–916)*

75. **(B)** Feedback regulation of enzyme activity is an important mechanism for the fine regulation of metabolism, and biosynthesis in particular. Virtually every biochemical pathway is controlled, at least in part, by feedback regulation (allosteric inhibition) of the first step in previously synthesized enzymes. *(Jawetz et al, pp 78–80; Joklik et al, pp 119–120)*

76. **(C)** Sometimes it is an advantage for a cell undergoing accumulation of an intermediate or end product to activate rather than inhibit a specific enzyme to relieve that excess. For example, the enzyme that can make glycogen from accumulated glucose-6-phosphate via glucose-1-phosphate would relieve this intermediate accumulation. Cooperativity produces an exponential increase in catalytic activity in response to an arithmetic increase in substrate. *(Jawetz et al, pp 78–80; Joklik et al, pp 116–120)*

77. **(A)** It is not economical for a cell to make an enzyme and not use it. It is better, and cheaper, to adjust the enzyme level by modulating enzyme synthesis. For a cell with a generation time of 20 minutes, the level of a stable protein can be reduced eight-fold in an hour simply by completely repressing its enzyme synthesis. There is no sequential repression. *(Jawetz et al, pp 78–80; Neidhardt et al, pp 304–307)*

78. **(A)** Transformation has been demonstrated in both gram-positive and gram-negative bacteria (see the explanation to Question 62). During transformation, DNA is taken up by the cell and converted into a deoxyribonuclease-resistant form. Double-stranded DNA is broken into shorter lengths, averaging 9×10^6 daltons before uptake. The bound double-stranded DNA fragments are converted to single-stranded DNA, which is then taken up. The single strand physically displaces a homologous strand of the recipient chromosome. *(Joklik et al, pp 136–137)*

79. **(C)** As explained previously, genetic recombination is required for successful completion of transformation. In case of specialized transduction, the formation of a stable transduction is dependent on either recombination of the DNA sequence into the bacterial chromosome or formation of a lysogen by the transducing particle. Thus, genetic recombination may not be required for specialized transduction. In generalized transduction, the outcome of the transduction depends on what happens to the bacterial DNA. If it is recombined into the recipient bacterial DNA, it is a stable transduction. If it remains in the cytoplasm, it will be segregated out and will lead to an abortive transduction. *(Jawetz et al, p 89; Joklik et al, pp 136–139)*

80. **(B)** The sex or fertility (F) factor is double-stranded DNA that is about 2% the size of *E. coli* chromosomal DNA. It replicates autonomously. The plasmid carrying the F factor and other genes related to conjugation is called a conjugal plasmid and remains F+, although converting an F− cell to an F+. The donor remains F+ because of replacement synthesis of the transferred strand. An F′ plasmid containing chromosomal trpA gene can be present in the cytoplasm of F′ cells. Cells that bear the F′ factor are capable of not only transferring the conjoined genes (trpA) at a high frequency, but also of conferring maleness to female cells at an equally high frequency. *(Jawetz et al, p 88; Joklik et al, pp 138–139)*

81. **(B)** Specialized transduction is limited to genes that are adjacent to the site of prophage integration. This limitation is due to the mechanism whereby specialized transducing phages are formed. Specialized transducing phage particles can only be generated by starting with a bacterial culture that has been infected with lysogenic phages. When treated with small doses of ultraviolet light, such a lysogenic culture will lose the active viral repressor protein and begin to enter the lytic cycle. Generalized transducing phages are formed when host DNA rather than phage DNA is packaged into the phage capsid when a culture is infected with a lytic phage. When a bacterial culture is infected with temperate phages under conditions of low multiplicity of infection, several lytic cycles of phage reproduction occur before most of the cells have been infected and lysed. It is during this lytic cycle that occasional mistakes take place and host DNA of the same size is put into the phage head. There is no zuzu phage. *(Jawetz et al, p 89; Joklik et al, pp 138–139)*

82. **(C)** The sex factor or fertility factor (F factor) possesses several genes that code for the formation of sex pili and tra (a transfer operon) and aid the donor in attaching to a recipient cell. Therefore, the sex factors are conjugative plasmids. However, conjugative plasmids may not contain the F factor, although they contain genes for pilus formation and permit transmission of copies of themselves. Some large conjugative plasmids, called R factors, carry genes associated with antibiotic resistance. F′ is a piece of DNA containing F factor and neighboring host chromosomal sequences. *(Joklik et al, pp 139–140)*

83. **(D)** Some bacteriophages have evolved mechanisms that control their replication, allowing them to maintain a stable relationship with the host bacterial cells. This stable relationship between phages and host cells is called lysogeny. The bacterial cell containing the phage is called a lysogen, and the phage is called a temperate phage. Temperate phage DNA that enters the cell (prophage) may integrate into the host chromosome, or it may remain physically independent of the host genome. Once integrated, phage DNA and its replication mechanisms are regulated by the system that controls replication of the bacterial chromosome. Some prophages are capable of changing the cell's phenotype via its gene product, and this process is called phage conversion or lysogenic conversion. It requires temperate phages, not phage lytic gene products. The phages involved in the conversion do not have to be specialized transducing phages. For example, *Corynebacterium diphtheriae* is virulent (toxigenic) only when it carries the temperate phage beta. *Salmonella* flagellar antigenic switching mechanism (phage variation) does not involve lysogenic phages. *(Joklik et al, pp 145–148,927–928)*

84. **(D)** The state of competence naturally appears only at a certain stage in the division cycle or in a culture. Specific DNA sequences (8 to 12 base pairs long) are recognized by cell surface receptor proteins only in gram-negative bacteria (*Hemophilus influenzae*). DNA molecules containing the recognition sequence are taken up into the cytoplasm in the duplex form. In gram-positive bacteria, one strand is degraded before uptake of the other strand into the cell. *(Jawetz et al, p 89; Joklik et al, pp 139–140)*

85. **(B)** Lysogenic cells evolve from the introduction of temperate phage DNA, not of the F

factor. Both the F factor and the DNA of temperate corynephages are extrachromosomal genetic units that are capable of replicating either autonomously or as integral parts of the host chromosome. In this sense, both the F factor and temperate phage DNA may be called episomes. Plasmids are most frequently transferred by conjugation and are unable to integrate into the host chromosome. Plasmids can be classified into a number of compatibility groups. Two members of the same group cannot coexist in the same cell. The cell containing a plasmid of one type can accommodate a plasmid of another incompatibility group. For example, *E. coli* K12 may carry an F factor and one each of several groups of R factors. (*Jawetz et al, p 87*)

86. **(B)** In transduction, a fragment of donor chromosome is carried to the recipient by a phage produced in the donor cell. Although conjugation is gene transfer that occurs between sexually different bacteria, a transducing phage particle can contain an entire bacterial chromosome. An entire bacterial chromosome is too large to be contained in a bacteriophage capsid. (*Jawetz et al, p 89; Joklik et al, p 138*)

87. **(E)** Bacteria (virtually all medically important bacteria) are hosts to small, extrachromosomal DNA molecules called plasmids, which are most frequently transferred by conjugation. Plasmids can be divided into two classes, conjugative and nonconjugative, based on their ability or inability to initiate or mediate a conjugal act that allows the transfer of a plasmid copy from one bacterial cell to another. The best-known groups of plasmids are the sex factors, Col factors, R factors, and penicillinase plasmids. Transposons are accessory DNA elements consisting of insertion sequences (IS elements) that are joined to other genes (multiple antibiotic resistance genes, for example). IS elements possess inverted repeat sequences at the ends. Transposons can move from one plasmid to another and from plasmid DNA to chromosomal DNA and vice versa. Both transposons and IS elements are not capable of autonomous replication but nevertheless play

an important role in genetic variability and the virulence of the bacteria. (*Jawetz et al, pp 89–90; Joklik et al, pp 145–149*)

88. **(A)** Plasmids can acquire transposons that contain specific antibiotic-resistant determinants to become R plasmids. R plasmids consist of two components: the resistance transfer factor (RTF), which is analogous to the F factor, and the resistance (R) determinants. These two components of the R factors are connected by IS elements on both sides of the R determinant to give a single, closed, double-stranded, circular DNA molecule. R factors can be grouped by incompatibility or compatibility with each other and with the F factor. R factors do promote chromosomal transfer from diverse bacteria, including *Pseudomonas* species. Indications are that R plasmids existed before the modern era of antibiotic therapy. (*Jawetz et al, pp 89–90; Joklik et al, pp 145–149*)

89. **(A)** In bacteria, no fusion of cells occurs following mating between male and female cells. Each plasmid also encodes an immunity protein so that the cell producing a colicin does not commit suicide. (*Jawetz et al, pp 88–89; Joklik et al, pp 146–147*)

90. **(E)** The frequency of microbial mutations is usually very low, one in a million or less. Mutations are due to changes in the sequence of purine and pyrimidine bases of DNA or RNA. Therefore substitutions, additions, deletions, or rearrangements (not inversions) of the nucleic acid bases are likely to induce microbial mutations. (*Joklik et al, pp 126–130*)

91. **(E)** A missense mutation is one in which the triplet code is altered so as to specify an amino acid different from that normally located at a given locus in an enzyme (or protein). This situation may lead to the production of temperature-sensitive gene products and modifications in the catalytic properties of an enzyme (ie, the enzyme-substrate apparent Michaelis constant, K_m, or the maximum catalytic activity, V_{max}). Finally, a missense mutation may modify the internal bonding of a protein in such a way that its

secondary or tertiary structure may be functional at a low, but not at a high, temperature. These missense mutations are often suppressed, and because of code redundancy, some have no consequence and are silent mutations. *(Joklik et al, pp 126–127)*

92. **(E)** One of the simplest and yet most effective tests to determine if a chemical is a mutagen, without using animals, is the Ames test. It uses known strains of *Salmonella* that cannot synthesize histidine (his–) and that are especially easy to mutate. The rate at which his+ revertants occur in the presence of the chemical is an indicator of its mutagenic ability. A strong indication that cancer often arises as a result of a mutational event is that most carcinogens are also mutagens. *(Joklik et al, p 130)*

93. **(E)** In *E. coli*, when DNA is damaged by spontaneous error, chemicals, or radiation, DNA damage is usually corrected by four known pathways. These pathways include excision repair, SOS repair, photoreactivation, and postreplication repair. Pathway means a complex series of enzymatic reactions that act on a DNA lesion to restore the function of the DNA. This restoration may be done by the removal of a damaged DNA base. There is nothing in microbial genetics called polymerization repair. *(Joklik et al, pp 130–133)*

94. **(E)** Excision repair requires an endonuclease to cut the thymine dimer. Then a 5'-specific exonuclease will degrade the damaged DNA strand but a 3'-specific exonuclease is not needed. A DNA polymerase is subsequently required to fill in the gap by synthesizing new DNA from the 3' end. Finally, the enzyme DNA ligase is needed to form a covalent bond between the newly synthesized DNA and the old DNA. Error-prone repair pathways are not limited to bacteria. *(Joklik et al, pp 131–132)*

95. **(B)** A special set of repair reactions is carried out by proteins that are specifically induced in response to certain forms of DNA damage. The proteins induced by the SOS system re-

pair reactions that affect diverse processes including DNA repair, mutagenesis, recombination, and cell division (but not respiration). These processes enhance survival in extreme environmental conditions. The SOS response is induced both by mutagens and by some nonmutagens that block replication. Some of the proteins are involved in excision repair, recombinational repair, and error-prone repair. Error-prone repair pathways are not limited to bacteria and their mechanism is not known for certain. Creating frequent mutations may increase genetic variability in the face of environmental pressure. Error-free DNA repair is usually encountered in excision repair, photoreactivation repair, and postreplication repair. The inhibition of cell division presumably gives the cell a chance to correct lesions before it attempts to propagate. *(Jawetz et al, p 90; Joklik et al, pp 132–133)*

96. **(D)** Diphtheria toxin loses its toxigenicity but not its immunogenicity when it is converted to a toxoid. Phage genes sometimes determine new host properties as a result of phage infection, a process called phage conversion. This process is what happens when *C. diphtheriae* becomes lysogenic with the beta phage. Phage conversion is different from transduction in that the new genes controlling diphtheria toxin production are derived entirely from the phage DNA, rather than from the host bacterial DNA. The A fragment contains an enzyme that specifically adenosine diphosphate ribosylates the mammalian cell elongation factor EF-2, blocking protein biosynthesis. Both the A and B fragments of the toxin after cleavage are required for toxin activity. *(Jawetz et al, pp 133,189; Joklik et al, pp 488–492)*

97. **(E)** R plasmids may carry resistance to one antibiotic, or to as many as ten or more distinct antimicrobial agents. Plasmid-mediated resistance is not the same as that which one would expect from mutational events. The conjugative transfer mechanism is specified by a group of plasmid genes that encode for a complex set of enzymatic and structural genes. Plasmids lacking this transfer mechanism are called nonconjugative plasmids.

When a bacterial cell contains both a conjugative and a nonconjugative plasmid, the nonconjugative plasmid may accompany the conjugative plasmid during its transfer. Not only are plasmids transferable, but many of their genes, including most of the antibiotic-resistant genes, have the ability to move from one DNA element to another; from plasmid to plasmid, from plasmid to chromosome, or from chromosome to plasmid. These subplasmid elements are transposons. Plasmids may control genes regulating enzymes capable of destroying antimicrobial drugs. *(Jawetz et al, pp 88–89,149,153; Joklik et al, pp 147–148)*

98. **(D)** Phage genes, but not genes from the bacterial host cell, introduced into a new bacterial cell as a result of phage infection (transduction) may introduce new properties, such as the ability to make specific toxins. This process is called phage conversion and is involved in the production of botulinum toxin by *C. botulinum*, streptococcal erythrogenic toxin (associated with scarlet fever) by *S. pyogenes*, diphtheria toxin by *C. diphtheriae*, and many other toxins. When the bacteria are "cured" of the responsible lysogenic phage, the ability to produce the toxin is lost. There is no such toxin as fragilinum toxin. *(Jawetz et al, pp 86,188–189; Joklik et al, pp 927–928)*

99. **(E)** All bacteria grow faster when transferred from a poor to a good growth medium. The growth rate can vary over a tenfold range, depending on the richness of the medium, and so forth. To accomplish this remarkable feat, the composition and size of the microbe changes. If a microbe is to grow faster, it needs more, but not excessive, protein-synthesizing machinery. Unused enzymes are disadvantageous metabolic expenses. *(Neidhardt et al, pp 418–442)*

100. **(C)** DNA always increases more slowly than RNA, mass, or protein as the growth rate increases. The ribosomes contain the cellular protein synthesizing machinery, the ribosomal RNA, and the transfer RNA, containing relatively stable RNA as compared to the fast turnover of messenger RNA. The important observation was that fast-growing cells of many microbes are rich in ribosomes and thus in RNA. *(Neidhardt et al, pp 421–422)*

101. **(A)** Bacterial RNA synthesis is much simpler than that in eukaryotes. Bacteria contain only one RNA polymerase, whereas eukaryotes have at least three specialized enzymes for that purpose. Eukaryotic messenger RNA (mRNA) is capped, spliced, and then transported to the cytoplasm before it may be translated. In bacterial mRNA synthesis, it is usually translated as it is being transcribed, and the start signal is much simpler in bacteria than in eukaryotes. *(Joklik et al, p 104)*

102. **(B)** Intracellular proteases contribute to post-translational protein control. *E. coli* contains at least eight different proteases. It was first examined in detail as an increased induction of protease activity following heat-shock response. Degradation of the denatured or abnormal proteins formed as a result of the heat-shock response may be an important function of this response. The lon protease, which is produced in low amounts during normal growth, is markedly increased following heat shock. The recA bacterial protein is a specific protease that is part of the SOS response and is active only when the cells have sustained DNA damage. *(Joklik et al, p 121)*

103. **(C)** Many mutations resulting in production of a defective gene product can be counteracted by a second mutation. If this second mutation is an exact reversal of the first, the normal wild type is present again, although very often the second mutation is not a simple reversal of the first one. A second mutation that is elsewhere in the genome, a suppressor, can nullify the original mutation by several different mechanisms. If the primary mutation caused an altered protein structure, there are several ways that the altered protein conformation can be restored. For one example, a second amino acid substitution elsewhere in the protein can sometimes result in a conformation that is quite close to the wild-type protein. The suppression of a frameshift mutation occurs through a second compensating frameshift mutation. The suppression of nonsense mutations is an important form of suppression. The translational machinery encounters a nonsense codon, such as UAG, for which no corresponding transfer RNA (tRNA) is available. However, nonsense suppressors are mutations that do allow a particular tRNA to recognize one of the nonsense codons, and the inserted amino acid may make a protein that is not perfect, but acceptable. *(Joklik et al, pp 126–127)*

104. **(B)** Very little is known about the mechanism of DNA transfer in any gram-positive mating system. Conjugative transposons, however, provide a mechanism for dispersing antibiotic-resistance determinants among pathogenic bacteria and are thus of great medical importance. They have an involvement in the spread of antibiotic resistance among clinically important strains of gram-positive bacteria. Conjugative transposons are highly promiscuous; the donor and recipient strains need not even belong to the same species or even the same genus. Many of the strains involved carry no detectable plasmids. *(Joklik et al, pp 124–125)*

105. **(D)** Gene transfer in bacteria is not completely random since several significant barriers reduce, but do not completely prevent, transfer of genes between different species. Most broad host-range plasmids can only survive in a few species, and conjugal acts between species are probably very inefficient. The restriction-modification systems generally destroy incoming DNA, reducing (but not eliminating) it about a thousand-fold. Most bacterial cells contain a two-enzyme system, an endonuclease and a DNA methylase, that recognizes the same short sequence in DNA. The methylase enzyme protects the endogenous DNA of a cell against self-digestion. Foreign DNA entering the cell will not contain the specific methyl groups added by the methylase; therefore, it is generally cleaved and degraded. Restriction enzymes possess great selectivity that allows them to recognize very specific regions for DNA cleavage. Restriction systems are not completely efficient, and some incoming DNA molecules may escape restriction (par-

ticularly when there are many millions of bacteria per milliliter present). *(Jawetz et al, p 95; Joklik et al, p 149)*

106. **(B)** About 2,000 distinct metabolic reactions are involved in the replication of an ordinary microbial cell. These reactions may be grouped according to their metabolic products. Biosynthetic pathways for sugars such as glucose lead from 12 metabolic precursor metabolites (such as glucose-6-phosphate and fructose-6-phosphate, phosphoenol pyruvate, α-ketoglutarate, and acetyl-CoA), to 75 to 100 building blocks. All organisms require essentially the same set of building blocks, but those microbes that lose the pathway to produce any of them must obtain them preformed in the medium. Biosynthetic pathways, not the more conventional classification as catabolic and anabolic pathways, lead to production of amino acids, nucleotides, sugars, fatty acids, coenzymes, etc. Bacteria display their superb metabolic versatility and diversity in their fueling pathways, from the ingredients of the external medium to the metabolic needs. In addition to precursor metabolites, biosynthetic pathways require large quantities of reduced pyridine nucleotides, energy (as adenosine triphosphate), and nitrogen, and lesser quantities of reduced sulfur. Virtually all biosynthetic pathways, polymerizations, and assembly processes are essentially the same in all bacteria. The dozen required precursor metabolites are drawn off at various places in the fueling pathways: the Embden–Meyerhof pathway produces six of the precursor metabolites, the tricarboxylic acid cycle produces three, the pentose phosphate cycle produces two more, and to complete the dozen, acetyl-CoA is produced by a reaction linked to the tricarboxylic acid cycle. Polymerization reactions consist of directed linkage of activated molecules into long, sometimes branched, domains. All the macromolecules are formed from building blocks that include 20 amino acids, 8 nucleotides, numerous sugars, and fatty acids. Assembly reactions involve the chemical modifications of macromolecules, their transport to specific cellular locations, and their association to form cell structures such as envelope, appendages, nucleoid polysomes, inclusions, and complexes of enzymes. Sometimes these structures form spontaneously by self-assembly, although in some cases other macromolecules must aid this directed assembly. *(Neidhardt et al, pp 62–64,120–121, 133–136)*

107. **(A)** Regulation of bacterial transcription is probably the most important level of control in bacterial systems. The extent of transcription is dependent on the recognition and utilization of promoter sequences by RNA polymerase, not DNA polymerase. Specific regulatory proteins bind near or within the promoter sequence. There are both negative and positive regulatory proteins that either block or enhance promoter usage. Two specific elements in the genome are required for these mechanisms. First, there must be a gene coding for the regulatory proteins. It is said to be trans-acting when the gene need not be near the promoter it actually controls. Also, when the specific nucleotide sequence to which the regulatory protein binds is in a location near or within the promoter that is being controlled, it is said to be a cis-acting element. *(Joklik et al, p 114)*

REFERENCES

Jawetz E, Melnick JL, Adelberg EA, et al. *Review of Medical Microbiology,* 19th ed. Norwalk, CT: Appleton & Lange; 1991.

Joklik WK, Willett HP, Amos DB, Wilfert CM. *Zinsser Microbiology,* 20th ed. Norwalk, CT: Appleton & Lange; 1992.

Neidhardt FC, Ingraham JL, Shaechter M. *Physiology of the Bacterial Cell.* Sunderland, MA: Sinauer Associates; 1990.

Immunology
Questions

108. Monoclonal antibodies can be produced by cell fusion or somatic cell hybridization between myeloma tumor cells with

(A) erythrocytes

(B) activated macrophages

(C) sensitized splenic T cells

(D) mast cells

(E) normal antibody-producing B cells

109. The most likely cells to be lysed when treated with anti-CD4 antibody and complement are

(A) cytotoxic T cells

(B) macrophages

(C) T helper cells

(D) B cells

(E) erythrocytes

110. Cytotoxic T cells are best characterized by which of the following cell-surface markers?

(A) CD4

(B) CD3

(C) CD8

(D) surface IgM

(E) CD2

111. A 4-year-old child with X-linked agammaglobulinemia is brought to the emergency room because of a laceration sustained in a minor traffic accident. Immunologically, this child is best treated with

(A) active immunization with tetanus toxin

(B) active immunization with tetanus toxoid

(C) active immunization with heat-killed *Clostridium tetani*

(D) passive immunization with human immune globulin (antitetanus toxin)

(E) passive immunization with horse immune globulin (antitetanus toxin)

112. Immune unresponsiveness is caused by

    (A) receptor blockage by free antigen
    (B) suppression by T cells
    (C) absence of lymphocytes with the appropriate receptors
    (D) presence of blocking antibody
    (E) all of the above

113. A mixed lymphocyte reaction that results in marked cellular differentiation and a very good induction of cytotoxic T lymphocytes is a result of

    (A) similarity at major histocompatibility complex (MHC) class I and MHC class II loci
    (B) disparity at MHC class I and MHC class II loci
    (C) disparity at MHC class I loci and similarity at MHC class II loci
    (D) disparity at MHC class II loci and similarity at MHC class I loci
    (E) none of the above

114. Cytotoxic T cells are involved in all of the following functions EXCEPT

    (A) lysis of cells infected with viruses
    (B) autoimmune diseases
    (C) graft rejection
    (D) tumor destruction
    (E) antigen presentation

115. T-helper lymphocytes are important in augmentation of

    (A) antibody production
    (B) delayed-type hypersensitivity reactions
    (C) mixed lymphocyte reaction
    (D) A, B, and C
    (E) A and C only

116. The chance of successful transplantation between donor and recipient is minimum when the donor and recipient have

    (A) different MHC class II molecules
    (B) similar MHC class I and MHC class II molecules

    (C) different MHC class I molecules
    (D) different MHC class I and MHC class II molecules
    (E) none of the above

117. One difference that distinguishes the genetics of heavy chains from that of light chains is the

    (A) presence of V genes
    (B) presence of J genes
    (C) presence of C genes
    (D) processing of nuclear messenger RNA by splicing out intervening sequences
    (E) ability to translocate variable-region gene clusters to different C genes

118. Which of the following is NOT a characteristic of the antigen-specific T-cell receptor (TCR)?

    (A) involvement in major histocompatibility complex antigen recognition
    (B) it is composed of two identical subunit chains
    (C) the presence of a hydrophobic transmembrane region
    (D) the gene region encoding T-cell receptor alpha chains is analogous to Ig light-chain genes
    (E) the beta chains are encoded by a group of genes analogous to Ig heavy chains

119. Natural killer cells do NOT

    (A) recognize and destroy certain tumor cells
    (B) lyse virus-infected cells
    (C) require antibody for their cytotoxic activity
    (D) occur in humans
    (E) overtly display either T- or B-lymphocyte cell-surface markers

120. All of the following are correct statements concerning immunoglobulin genetics EXCEPT

    (A) immunoglobulins are encoded by genes located on more than one chromosome

(B) the immunoglobulin combining site for antigen is contributed by the hypervariable regions within each of the heavy- and light-chain variable regions

(C) myeloma proteins are homogeneous and result from one B cell becoming malignant

(D) IgG and IgM molecules are distinguished by the difference in their heavy-chain constant region sequences

(E) two types (lambda and kappa) of light chains can occur within one immunoglobulin molecule

121. A 24-year-old woman with non-X-linked agammaglobulinemia is 8 months pregnant. Her child will be at risk for infection by which of the following agents?

(A) encapsulated *Streptococcus pneumoniae*

(B) *Leishmania donovani*

(C) *Mycobacterium tuberculosis*

(D) *Histoplasma capsulatum*

(E) none of the above

122. Human leukocyte antigen complex

(A) stimulates mixed lymphocyte reactions

(B) stimulates antibody production

(C) restricts immune responses

(D) elicits vigorous graft rejection

(E) all of the above

123. A patient suffering from bacterial infection received a penicillin injection and almost immediately experienced respiratory distress and fell into unconsciousness. This reaction is most likely to be mediated by

(A) T cells

(B) IgG and IgM

(C) IgE

(D) IgA

(E) IgG and complement

124. The role of MHC class II in graft rejection is to

(A) enhance the function of suppressor T cells

(B) serve as a recognition element for helper T cells, thus promoting cytotoxic T-cell response

(C) protect the graft by inducing blocking antibody production

(D) serve as the recognition element for cytotoxic T cells

(E) promote the migration of activated macrophages

125. Acquired immunodeficiency syndrome (AIDS) patients infected with tuberculosis are likely to react less vigorously to the tuberculin test because of the deficiency in the function of

(A) platelets

(B) CD8$^+$ T cells

(C) CD4$^+$ T cells

(D) stem cells

(E) B cells

126. The immunologic abnormalities found in AIDS are those of severe and profound cellular immunodeficiency. These deficiencies include

(A) an absence of or impaired delayed hypersensitivity

(B) lymphopenia caused by an absolute deficiency of CD4$^+$ T cells

(C) reversal of the usual 2:1 ratio of CD4$^+$/CD8$^+$ blood lymphocytes

(D) depressed lymphocyte response to mitogens

(E) all of the above

127. Infection with *M. tuberculosis* will usually provoke which of the following cytokine profile that drives T_H-0 to the T_H-1 subsets?

(A) IL-4 and IL-10

(B) IL-2, INF-γ, and IL-12

(C) IL-5 and IL-6

(D) IL-1, 4, and INF-γ

(E) IL-1 and IL-13

128. Patients with schistosomiasis often develop T lymphocyte-mediated eosinophilic granulomas in the liver as a result of reaction to

   (A) soluble antigens excreted by the parasite's eggs
   (B) surface antigens of the parasite
   (C) surface antigens of the damaged liver cells
   (D) toxin elaborated by the parasite
   (E) antiparasitic drugs

129. The immunity to infectious agents that is provided by serum lysozyme is

   (A) acquired and T-cell mediated
   (B) acquired and B-cell mediated
   (C) innate and IgG mediated
   (D) innate and nonspecific
   (E) acquired and IgE mediated

130. A quantitative precipitation reaction between an antigen and antiserum was performed. No precipitate was formed between the reactants. The absence of precipitate may be because

   (A) the serum does not contain antibodies to the antigen
   (B) the antigen is monovalent
   (C) the proportion of the reactants is such that there is a great excess of antigen
   (D) A, B, and C
   (E) none of the above

131. During differentiation, antibody of a particular B cell

   (A) may switch from one idiotype to another
   (B) may switch from one isotype to another
   (C) may switch from one κ-chain marker allotype to another
   (D) is induced by interaction with antigen
   (E) all of the above

132. Cells or cell clones can switch classes of antibody, eg, from IgM to IgG. Such switches involve change in

   (A) variable regions of heavy and light chains
   (B) constant regions of heavy chain
   (C) constant regions of light chain
   (D) constant and variable regions of heavy chain
   (E) constant and variable regions of heavy and light chains

133. Interleukin-2

   (A) is produced by T-helper cells
   (B) promotes T-cell division
   (C) potentiates B-cell division
   (D) activates natural killer cells
   (E) all of the above

134. An AB, Rh-positive mother and an O, Rh-negative father (wife and husband) come to you for advice to prevent possible hemolytic disease of their newborn. You will advise

   (A) to administer RhoGAM to the mother after birth of her first child
   (B) not to administer RhoGAM because none of their children are in danger of hemolytic disease of the newborn
   (C) to administer RhoGAM to the mother after the birth of each child
   (D) to administer RhoGAM to the newborn and to the mother after birth of A, Rh-positive and B, Rh-positive children
   (E) to administer RhoGAM to all newborns except for the first child

135. Mice depleted of T cells by neonatal thymectomy failed to produce antibody to most antigens tested. The capacity of these animals to form antibody will be restored if

   (A) mature B cells are injected into the mice
   (B) normal bone marrow cells are transplanted
   (C) thymus cells are injected into the mice
   (D) interleukin-2 is injected into the mice
   (E) the mice are irradiated

136. An AIDS patient who received a tuberculin test 48 hours earlier showed a weak erythematous skin reaction (6 mm in diameter) at the site of injection. The proper interpretation of this observation is that this patient

(A) has never been exposed to tubercle bacilli

(B) has active tuberculosis

(C) has been exposed to tubercle bacilli

(D) needs bacillus Calmette–Guérin (BCG) vaccination

(E) is infected with multidrug-resistant tubercle bacilli

137. Immunoglobulin allotypes are

(A) confined to the variable region

(B) determined by major histocompatibility complex genes

(C) found only on heavy chains

(D) caused by limited substitution of different amino acid residues of the constant region in kappa chain or gamma-1 heavy chain

(E) not found in mice

138. The ability of T cells to discriminate between self and nonself is learned in the

(A) liver

(B) spleen

(C) lymph nodes

(D) thymus

(E) bone marrow

139. The variable regions of heavy chains and the variable regions of light chains in a given immunoglobulin molecule

(A) define the molecular size

(B) are encoded on the same chromosome

(C) contain different amino acid sequences

(D) have the same amino acid sequences

(E) occur only in IgG

140. All of the following statements are true EXCEPT

(A) the variable regions of various kappa chains differ from each other but the constant regions of various kappa chains are nearly identical

(B) the variable regions of heavy chains of different Ig classes can be identical but the constant regions differ

(C) the variable regions of heavy chains of IgE antibodies directed against different antigens are different but the constant regions are identical

(D) heavy chains of IgG have three constant domains and one variable domain

(E) heavy chains of IgM have only one constant domain

141. IgG-1 human antistaphylococcal and IgG-1 human antistreptococcal antibodies from a given individual will most likely have

(A) kappa chains with identical hypervariable segments

(B) identical idiotypic specificities

(C) identical variable regions in heavy chains

(D) identical isotypic specificities

(E) different Fc fragments

142. An individual who is heterozygous for Gm allotypes contains two allelic forms of the protein in serum, but individual lymphocytes form only one of the two forms. This is due to

(A) a rearrangement of a heavy-chain gene on only one chromosome

(B) rearrangements of heavy-chain genes on both chromosomes

(C) a rearrangement of a light-chain gene on only one chromosome

(D) rearrangements of light-chain genes on both chromosomes

(E) all of the above

143. Immature B lymphocytes

(A) produce only μ chain

(B) are progenitors of T as well as B lymphocytes

(C) express IgM on their cell surface

(D) secrete immunoglobulin (Ig) but do not express cell-surface Ig

(E) must go through the thymus to mature

144. A patient with asplenia shows a defect in

    (A) complement activation
    (B) acute-phase protein production
    (C) opsonization and production of IgG-2
    (D) phagocytic activity
    (E) detoxication

145. Cytotoxic T cells of an individual infected with influenza virus will destroy target cells

    (A) from another host infected with poliovirus
    (B) infected with the influenza virus and identical at MHC class I loci of the cytotoxic cells
    (C) infected with the influenza virus and identical at MHC class II loci of the cytotoxic cells
    (D) infected with poliovirus and identical at MHC class I loci of the cytotoxic cells
    (E) infected with poliovirus and identical at MHC class II loci of the cytotoxic cells

146. In order for the precipitin reaction to occur

    (A) the antigen may be univalent but the antibody must be multivalent
    (B) the antibody may be univalent but the antigen must be multivalent
    (C) both antigen and antibody must be univalent
    (D) both antigen and antibody must be multivalent
    (E) valence is irrelevant since only affinity is important

147. A monoclonal antibody

    (A) has antibody-combining sites that are identical
    (B) may belong to the IgM, IgA, IgE, IgD, or IgG classes
    (C) may be present in the serum of patients with multiple myeloma
    (D) can be obtained by the hybridoma fusion technique
    (E) all of the above

148. The diversity of antibody-binding sites of immunoglobulin molecules has been ascribed to

    (A) multiple germ-line variable-region genes
    (B) somatic mutation
    (C) V-J joining in light chains and V-D-J joining in heavy chains with recombination taking place between different nucleotides within a single codon
    (D) random assortment of light and heavy chains
    (E) all of the above

149. Passive immunization

    (A) provides long-lasting protection
    (B) provides protection without hypersensitivity
    (C) is the only way to treat humans exposed to rabies
    (D) provides immediate protection
    (E) employs sensitized T cells

150. Factors influencing the immune response include

    (A) the route of administration
    (B) the physical state of the immunogen
    (C) adjuvants that increase the response
    (D) the chemical nature of the immunogen
    (E) all of the above

151. The secondary humoral response is characterized by

    (A) longer lag phase
    (B) longer persistence of IgM synthesis
    (C) longer persistence of IgG synthesis
    (D) lower rate of IgG synthesis
    (E) none of the above

152. A vaccine antigen that primarily induces opsonizing antibody is

    (A) influenza virus
    (B) BCG
    (C) poliovirus
    (D) *Hemophilus influenzae* type b vaccine
    (E) diphtheria toxoid

153. A 9-year-old male child is brought to an emergency room with a 2-day history of fever, blood in the urine, and a puffy face. He complained of a sore throat some 13 days earlier but received no medical attention. On examination, he is febrile, has periorbital and ankle edema, and slightly elevated blood pressure. Laboratory tests showed erythrocytes and granular casts in the urine, reduced glomerular filtration rate, reduced C3 level, and elevated anti-streptolysin O titer. Throat culture yielded *Streptococcus pyogenes*. The most likely diagnosis of this patient is

(A) kidney cancer
(B) urinary tract infection
(C) scarlet fever
(D) infectious mononucleosis
(E) acute glomerulonephritis

154. Children with chronic granulomatous disease are often infected by

(A) *Streptococcus pyogenes*
(B) *Staphylococcus aureus*
(C) tubercle bacilli
(D) *Streptococcus pneumoniae*
(E) all of the above

155. The molecule that does not participate in adhesive interactions in the immune response is

(A) Mac-1
(B) immunoglobulin superfamily molecules
(C) selectin family molecules
(D) cholesterols
(E) leukocyte functional antigen (LFA-1)

156. All of the following contribute to the development of a compromised state of the host defense EXCEPT

(A) radiation therapy
(B) extended use of broad-spectrum antibiotics
(C) human immunodeficiency virus (HIV) infection
(D) malnutrition
(E) toxoid vaccination

157. Opsonization of microbial cells by complement is prevented by

(A) flagellin
(B) adhesin
(C) capsule
(D) peptidoglycan
(E) teichoic acid

158. All of the following statements are true EXCEPT

(A) toxoids are used as immunogen
(B) exotoxins are highly toxic at very low doses
(C) exotoxins may cause diseases without the presence of the organisms that produce them
(D) some gram-negative bacteria produce exotoxins
(E) all exotoxins consist of two subunits, A and B

159. Which of the following contributes to the killing of phagocytosed facultative intracellular pathogens?

(A) rapid phagosome–lysosome fusion
(B) the inability of the pathogens to escape from the phagosomes into the cytoplasmic space where microbicidal systems are absent
(C) rapid acidification of intracellular pH
(D) the absence of protective layers resistant to lysosomal enzymes
(E) all of the above

160. A product involved in intracellular killing of phagocytosed microbial cells via an oxygen-independent mechanism includes

(A) hydrogen peroxide
(B) superoxide radical
(C) singlet oxygen
(D) OH radical
(E) hydrolytic enzyme

161. An effector microbicidal molecule generated by the myeloperoxidase-H_2O_2-halide system is

    (A) chlorine gas
    (B) hydrochloric acid
    (C) sodium chloride
    (D) hypochlorite (ClO^-)
    (E) superoxide radical

162. The human leukocyte antigen (HLA) complex

    (A) induces complement activation
    (B) controls T-cell recognition and elicits allograft reaction
    (C) is involved in the adherence to endothelial cell surface
    (D) is involved in platelet aggregation
    (E) consists of HLA-A and HLA-B gene clusters

163. Antigen-presenting cells

    (A) are all phagocytic cells
    (B) are DR-negative
    (C) are capable of presenting antigens to plasma cells
    (D) include B cells, dendritic cells, Langerhans' cells, and macrophages
    (E) all of the above

164. B-cell receptor for antigen

    (A) is also present in pre-B cells
    (B) is encoded for by the genes that encode the T-cell receptor
    (C) cannot recognize antigen alone
    (D) is a surface-bound immunoglobulin
    (E) also functions as a lymphokine receptor

165. Antigen is initially presented to T lymphocytes by

    (A) macrophages
    (B) neutrophils
    (C) plasma cells
    (D) platelets
    (E) erythrocytes

166. All of the following statements concerning neutrophils are true EXCEPT

    (A) they constitute the first line of nonspecific cellular defense for the host
    (B) they, together with monocytes and macrophages, are the principal phagocytic cells
    (C) they are relatively short-lived cells that do not divide after leaving the bone marrow
    (D) they cannot present antigen
    (E) they can differentiate into B cells upon activation

167. In the primary immune response, as opposed to the secondary response, there is

    (A) production of antibodies with a lower affinity for antigen
    (B) a higher antibody titer of IgG at the peak of the response
    (C) a synthesis of IgG that precedes the synthesis of IgM
    (D) a shorter lag period
    (E) all of the above

168. Which of the following statements correctly describes T-dependent responses?

    (A) the switch from IgM to IgG production by B cells is dependent on T cells
    (B) the switch from production of IgM of low affinity to IgG of high affinity depends on T-helper lymphocytes
    (C) activated T-helper cells stimulate the proliferation of antigen-bearing B cells, some of whose daughter cells become memory B cells
    (D) T-helper cells are activated by reacting with both antigen and MHC class II antigen on the macrophages
    (E) all of the above

169. Hapten-carrier complexes, in T-dependent antibody responses, are known to

    (A) respond in the same way as haptens alone
    (B) induce the T cells to produce antibody

(C) induce new receptors on the B-cell surface

(D) allow the T cells to react with hapten determinants

(E) allow the B cells to react with hapten determinants

170. Papain digestion of an IgG molecule produces

(A) F(ab')$_2$

(B) kappa chains

(C) lambda chains

(D) Fab

(E) all of the above

171. In Ouchterlony double-diffusion agar analysis, the size, shape, intensity, and position of a precipitin line with respect to antigen and antiserum wells is affected by all of the following EXCEPT the

(A) concentration of the antibody

(B) molecular size of the antigen

(C) concentration of the antigen

(D) temperature

(E) isotype of the antibody in the antiserum

172. Biologic activities associated with the Fc fragment of an IgG molecule include all of the following EXCEPT

(A) placental transport

(B) complement binding

(C) binding to phagocytes

(D) binding to K cells

(E) antigen binding

173. At the equivalence zone of the quantitative precipitin curve, the supernatant will

(A) produce a precipitate with additional antigen

(B) produce a precipitate with additional antibody

(C) contain a high concentration of soluble immune complex

(D) contain neither detectable antigen nor antibody

(E) none of the above

174. IgA antibodies are secretory immunoglobulin molecules that

(A) cross the placental barrier when coupled to the transport piece

(B) bind C1q in the activation of the classic complement pathway

(C) are the predominant immunoglobulin of serum

(D) mainly exist in a monomeric form

(E) are the predominant immunoglobulin of saliva

175. Which of the following is the most frequently employed diagnostic laboratory technique for the microscopic detection of antigens in tissue sections, in cell suspensions, or on cell monolayers?

(A) agglutination

(B) radioimmunoassay

(C) mixed lymphocyte reaction

(D) immunofluorescence

(E) precipitation

176. Which of the following may be employed to detect the presence of antitetanus toxin antibodies in a patient's serum?

(A) enzyme-linked immunosorbent assay using antigen-sensitized plates

(B) counterimmunoelectrophoresis

(C) agglutination methods with an antigen-sensitized particle

(D) immunodiffusion in agar

(E) all of the above

177. All of the following forces or bonds are involved in the interaction between an antigen and an antibody EXCEPT

(A) hydrogen bonds

(B) van der Waals force

(C) ionic bonds

(D) covalent bonds

(E) electrostatic bonds

178. An antiserum directed against human IgG will react with

    (A) mu Fc fragment
    (B) J chain
    (C) alpha Fc fragment
    (D) gamma Fc fragment
    (E) rabbit kappa chain

179. An antiserum prepared against IgG would react with

    (A) idiotypic determinants
    (B) allotypic determinants
    (C) isotypic determinants
    (D) kappa chain
    (E) all of the above

180. Circulating immune complexes can

    (A) be cleared by the mononuclear phagocyte system (reticuloendothelial system)
    (B) be bound to glomerular receptors
    (C) be located in synovial Fc-bearing cells
    (D) suppress the phagocytic splenic clearance rate
    (E) all of the above

181. The Fc portion of the immunoglobulin molecule

    (A) defines the antibody specificity
    (B) is involved in idiotypic characterization of the molecule
    (C) is produced by pepsin digestion
    (D) is located in the light chain
    (E) is produced by papain digestion

182. All of the following cells belong to monocyte–macrophage lineage EXCEPT

    (A) blood monocytes
    (B) histocytes in tissues
    (C) Kupffer cells in liver
    (D) dendritic reticulum cells of lymph nodes
    (E) T lymphocytes

183. IgE is produced by

    (A) basophils
    (B) plasma cells
    (C) T lymphocytes
    (D) eosinophils
    (E) mast cells

184. Immune complexes that contain C3b or C4b adhere to cells that possess

    (A) MHC class I antigens
    (B) MHC class II antigens
    (C) complement receptors
    (D) viral antigens
    (E) all of the above

185. Helper T lymphocytes recognize which of the following on a presenting cell?

    (A) HLA class I and class II antigens
    (B) HLA class I antigen
    (C) HLA class II antigen
    (D) HLA class I antigen and surface immunoglobulin
    (E) all of the above

186. Lysis of bacteria by specific antibody is accurately described as

    (A) requiring only late complement components (C5 to C9)
    (B) being seen most frequently with gram-positive organisms containing thick capsules
    (C) being seen more frequently with bacilli than with cocci
    (D) requiring both early and late complement components
    (E) none of the above

187. Anaphylotoxins

    (A) cause enhanced capillary permeability
    (B) produce edema
    (C) induce smooth muscle contraction
    (D) cause hypotension
    (E) all of the above

188. C1 is correctly characterized as

(A) a constituent of the classic complement pathway

(B) composed of three proteins: C1q, C1r, and C1s

(C) having an activated subunit that cleaves C4 and C2

(D) requiring calcium for biologic activity

(E) all of the above

189. Biologic consequences of complement activation include

(A) chemotaxis of phagocytes

(B) immune adherence and opsonization

(C) anaphylotoxin activity

(D) membrane damage

(E) all of the above

190. Defects in the complement system could result in

(A) marked increase in bleeding time

(B) impaired elimination of microbial antigen and circulating immune complexes

(C) increased resistance to viral infections

(D) failure to produce complement-fixing antibody

(E) all of the above

191. Alternative (properdin) pathway of complement activation is triggered by

(A) antigen–antibody complex

(B) endotoxin and cobra venom

(C) C1q

(D) proteases

(E) Mg^{2+}

192. In a typical complement fixation test, complement is bound to

(A) free hemolysin

(B) erythrocytes

(C) antigen–antibody complex

(D) free antigen

(E) free antibody

193. Initiation of T-cell proliferation involves

(A) antigen recognition

(B) production of interleukin-1 by the antigen-presenting cell

(C) release of interleukin-2 by T cells

(D) interaction between a major histocompatibility complex molecule and T-cell receptor

(E) all of the above

194. The most desirable matching in tissue transplant is "six-antigen match," namely

(A) HLA-A, HLA-B, and HLA-DR on donor and recipient

(B) HLA-A, HLA-B, and HLA-DQ on donor and recipient

(C) HLA-A, HLA-B, and HLA-C on donor and recipient

(D) HLA-DR, HLA-DQ, and HLA-DP on donor and recipient

(E) HLA-C, HLA-DR, and HLA-DQ on donor and recipient

195. The antimicrobial compounds associated with activated macrophages are

(A) hydrogen peroxide and singlet oxygen

(B) superoxide and hydroxyl radicals

(C) lysozyme and hydrolytic enzymes

(D) nitric oxide and reactive nitrogen metabolites

(E) all of the above

196. Which of the following statements concerning rheumatic fever is true?

(A) it usually affects elderly adults aged 50 to 70 years

(B) it is a complication of β-hemolytic streptococcal infection

(C) it is caused by immediate hypersensitivity to streptococci

(D) it occurs as a complication of viral pharyngitis

(E) all of the above

197. Noncellular mediators of antibody-dependent cellular cytotoxicity include

(A) C5a

(B) C5b67

(C) C1q

(D) eosinophilic chemotactic factor

(E) all of the above

198. A man with blood group phenotype AB

(A) is classified as a universal donor

(B) may be given blood type AB, A, or B, but not type O

(C) has anti-A and anti-B in his serum

(D) has A and B antigen in his red blood cells

(E) may donate his blood to individuals with blood group phenotype O

199. All of the following predispose to *Candida albicans* infection EXCEPT

(A) pregnancy

(B) broad-spectrum antibiotics

(C) drug addiction

(D) malignancy

(E) all of the above

200. The development of immune complex disease depends on the ability of

(A) an immune complex to form or deposit at a fixed tissue site, and then activate the complement system

(B) neutrophils to release abundant interleukin-1

(C) phagocytes to rapidly clear circulating immune complex

(D) macrophages to produce excessive hydrolytic enzymes

(E) T cells to release a large quantity of tissue necrosis factor

201. Features of human systemic lupus erythematosus include

(A) formation of anti-DNA antibodies

(B) circulating immune complexes

(C) immune-complex deposits in the glomeruli

(D) proteinuria due to altered membrane permeability

(E) all of the above

202. Immunologic suppression for transplantation may be induced by

(A) lymphoid irradiation

(B) antilymphocyte globulin

(C) cyclosporin

(D) steroids

(E) all of the above

203. Helper T cells can mediate graft damage by

(A) fixing cytotoxic antibodies

(B) promoting production of lytic complement

(C) producing tissue necrosis factor

(D) expressing interleukin-2 receptor

(E) helping cytotoxic T cells and releasing lymphokines that activate macrophages

204. Immunologic tolerance may be induced by

(A) natural exposure to an antigen in embryonic life

(B) high doses of antigen in adult life

(C) artificial exposure to an antigen in embryonic life

(D) all of the above

(E) none of the above

205. Stem cells from bone marrow possess all of the following characteristics EXCEPT they

(A) are immunocompetent

(B) may differentiate into T or B cells

(C) may enter but not exit the thymus

(D) contain genetic material to become antigen-recognizing cells

(E) may become monocytes and macrophages

206. For successful receptor-ligand signal transduction, B cells are required to have

(A) the cell membrane

(B) antigen-specific immunoglobulin (IgM and IgD)

(C) guanosine triphosphate-binding protein (G protein)

(D) antigen

(E) all of the above

207. The fully developed plasma cells

(A) can divide actively

(B) retain the same cell-surface marker proteins as their ancestral B cells

(C) enter the bloodstream

(D) excrete many thousands of immunoglobulin molecules

(E) are surface IgM-negative

208. When a B cell undergoes class switch from IgM production to IgA

(A) the cell-surface immunoglobulin is completely replaced with another class of immunoglobulin

(B) the cell-surface immunoglobulin disappears

(C) the specificity of IgA changes from that of IgM

(D) the specificity of IgA has the same specificity as that of IgM

(E) none of the above

209. The maturation of T cells is accompanied by changes in

(A) cell size

(B) cell-surface markers

(C) DNA content

(D) surface immunoglobulin class

(E) type of T-cell receptor (alpha, beta to gamma, delta)

210. The reason that corneal grafts may be performed without human leukocyte antigen matching or immunosuppression is that

(A) the cornea lacks antigens

(B) the anterior chamber of the eye is an immunologically "privileged" site lacking lymphatic drainage

(C) the cornea secretes immunosuppressive compounds

(D) the cornea is highly vascularized

(E) none of the above

211. Which of the following organs is NOT regarded as an immunologically "privileged-site" (shielded from antigen under normal conditions)?

(A) testes

(B) spleen

(C) thymus

(D) brain

(E) anterior chamber of the eye

212. The most frequently diagnosed specific primary immunodeficiency among Caucasians is

(A) selective IgA deficiency

(B) severe combined immunodeficiency

(C) DiGeorge syndrome (thymic aplasia)

(D) infantile X-linked hypogammaglobulinemia

(E) chronic granulomatous disease of children

213. In order to find a suitable donor for kidney transplant, a series of tissue typings was performed on four potential donors. The test results are summarized as follows:

Recipient: A3, A33, B12, B35, DR2, DR4

Donor 1: A1, A2, B12, B17, DR2, DR4

Donor 2: A3, B35, DR2, DR4

Donor 3: A2, A23, B12, B35, DR2, DR4

Donor 4: A3, A23, B12, B35, DR4, DR6

Based on these data, the most suitable kidney donor is

(A) donor 1

(B) donor 2

(C) donor 3

(D) donor 4

(E) all of the above

214. Tissue transplant from one monozygotic twin to the other is highly successful because

(A) the donor and the recipient have the same class I and class II molecules

(B) the donor and the recipient have the same class I molecules

(C) the donor and the recipient have the same class II molecules

(D) identical twins have higher suppressor cell activity

(E) the donor and the recipient have the same class III molecules

215. The leukocytes from a potential kidney transplant recipient (R) were tested in five separate mixed leukocyte reaction cultures with irradiated leukocytes from five potential donors (1, 2, 3, 4, and 5). The results of the test (counts per minutes of 3H-thymidine incorporated into each culture) are summarized below:

Donor + Recipient	Count per Minutes
1 + R	16,750
2 + R	28,830
3 + R	85,000
4 + R	2,500
5 + R	42,000

The best kidney donor would be

(A) donor 1

(B) donor 2

(C) donor 3

(D) donor 4

(E) donor 5

216. Selective IgA deficiency may manifest

(A) pulmonary infections

(B) gastrointestinal infections

(C) no symptoms

(D) immune complex diseases

(E) all of the above

217. A 7-year-old patient has profound cellular immunodeficiency and is at risk of exposure to measles. The most appropriate prophylactic measure for this patient is

(A) administration of a high dose of complement prepared from a measles-immune donor

(B) transfusion of blood

(C) a thymus graft

(D) administration of gamma globulin with high titers of antimeasles antibodies

(E) administration of fresh plasma from a healthy individual

218. Both cytotoxic T lymphocytes (CTLs) and natural killer (NK) cells kill tumor cells, but they differ in that

(A) CTLs require MHC class II antigen for target-cell recognition while NK cells do not

(B) NK cells require MHC class II antigen for target recognition while CTLs do not

(C) CTLs require MHC class I antigen for the recognition of target cells while NK cells do not

(D) NK cells require MHC class I antigen for the recognition of target cells while CTLs do not

(E) CTLs do not have large azurophilic granules while NK cells do

219. A 13-year-old orphan who has no record of tetanus toxoid immunization is involved in an automobile accident. The accident caused multiple lacerations and wounds that are contaminated with soil. This patient must be

(A) given human tetanus globulin

(B) given tetanus toxoid

(C) given human immune globulin and tetanus toxoid

(D) given full blood transfusion

(E) released after penicillin injection

220. Which of the following immunologic functions remains intact in a patient who has no C3 component of complement?

(A) opsonization of microbial cells

(B) bacteriolysis

(C) generation of chemotactic factors

(D) generation of anaphylotoxins

(E) none of the above

221. Symptoms associated with immediate hypersensitivity reaction are caused by

(A) IgG-mediated activation of the classic complement pathway

(B) activation of the alternative complement pathway by enteric bacteria

(C) IgA-mediated activation of bronchial inflammatory response

(D) IgE-mediated discharge of histamine and other pharmacologically active compounds from mast cells

(E) IgM-mediated release of granules from granulocytes

222. Heat-shock proteins

(A) differ distinctly from stress proteins

(B) rarely occur in prokaryotic organisms

(C) are implicated as important targets in autoimmune responses

(D) are recognized mainly by alpha, beta T-cell receptor

(E) are produced only by eukaryotic cells

223. All of the following are examples of antigenic mimicry responsible for autoimmune responses EXCEPT

(A) immune reactions to heart muscle after infection with certain streptococci

(B) structural similarities between measles virus antigens and myelin basic protein

(C) structural similarities between various bacterial antigens and acetylcholine receptors

(D) structural similarities between coxsackie B virus and heart muscle

(E) structural similarities between bacterial endotoxin and plasma membrane lipids

224. All of the following are implicated in lysis of target cells by cytotoxic T cells EXCEPT

(A) pore-forming protein (perforin)

(B) serine esterase

(C) lymphotoxin (tissue necrosis factor beta)

(D) all of the above

(E) none of the above

225. Events that occur in phagocytes during phagocytosis of bacteria include all of the following EXCEPT

(A) polymerization of actin

(B) respiratory burst

(C) formation of phagolysosome

(D) adenosine triphosphatase-dependent contraction

(E) release of interleukin-2

226. Extracellular matrix proteins that are important in cell–cell interaction and cell adherence include all of the following EXCEPT

(A) proteoglycans

(B) collagen and elastin

(C) laminin

(D) keratin

(E) fibronectin

227. LFA-1

(A) belongs to the beta-1 integrin family

(B) is expressed only in neutrophils and macrophages

(C) belongs to the beta-4 integrin family

(D) is expressed only in T cells

(E) is essential for adhesion of leukocytes to endothelial cells

228. *Hemophilus influenzae, Streptococcus pneumoniae,* and *Neisseria meningitidis* are the most common bacteria that infect normal children less than 2 years old. This is due to

(A) the inability of their immune systems to produce antibodies against polysaccharides

(B) the inability of their immune systems to produce antibodies against proteins

(C) their undeveloped cell-mediated immune systems

(D) the transient neutropenia occurring during this stage of development

(E) the lack of certain complement components at this stage of development

229. All of the following statements are true about immunology EXCEPT

    (A) passive immunity results when pre-formed antibodies against a microbe, formed in another host, are administered
    (B) the slow perfusion of antigen provided by adjuvants improves the antibody response to that antigen
    (C) T cells proliferate and differentiate to become antibody-secreting plasma cells
    (D) the specificity of the antibody molecule is determined by the hypervariable domain of the Fab fragment
    (E) vaccination results in an acquired, artificial, active immunity

230. All of the following are nonspecific soluble circulating defense factors that contribute to innate immunity EXCEPT

    (A) complement components
    (B) opsonic antibodies
    (C) lysozymes
    (D) acute phase proteins
    (E) interferons

231. All of the following are characteristics of both macrophages and neutrophils EXCEPT

    (A) phagocytosis
    (B) chemotactic movement
    (C) lysosomal granules containing hydrolytic enzymes
    (D) receptor for Fc portion of IgG
    (E) antigen presentation to T cells

232. An example of naturally acquired passive immunity is

    (A) maternally derived antibody in the fetus
    (B) previous infection by a microorganism
    (C) protection due to normal bacterial flora
    (D) ability of the phagocytic cells to engulf and kill microorganisms
    (E) injections of pooled hyperimmune gamma globulins

233. Agammaglobulinemia should be treated with

    (A) IgA
    (B) IgG
    (C) IgD
    (D) IgM
    (E) IgE

234. Patients with chronic granulomatous disease are defective in

    (A) neutrophil production in the bone marrow
    (B) neutrophil chemotaxis
    (C) metabolic generation of hydrogen peroxide
    (D) opsonization
    (E) phagocytic activity

235. HIV-1 is transmitted via

    (A) infected body fluid such as blood and semen
    (B) swimming pools
    (C) shared bathroom facilities
    (D) dusts
    (E) all of the above

236. All of the following are involved in the intracellular killing of phagocytosed microbes EXCEPT

    (A) lysosomal enzymes such as lysozyme and proteases
    (B) oxygen metabolites such as superoxide, hydrogen peroxide, singlet oxygen, and hydroxyl radicals
    (C) low pH
    (D) cytochromes
    (E) cationic proteins and defensins

237. Phagocytes of children suffering from chronic granulomatous disease are deficient in

    (A) nicotinamide adenine dinucleotide phosphate (NADPH) oxidase
    (B) myeloperoxidase
    (C) phagosome–lysosome fusion

(D) lysosomal enzymes

(E) chloride ion uptake

238. The major mechanism of host resistance to tuberculosis is

(A) humoral antibodies

(B) delayed hypersensitivity

(C) high level of calcium in serum

(D) increased microbicidal activity of activated macrophages

(E) massive proliferation of polymorphonuclear leukocytes

239. Secondary immunodeficiency is caused by all of the following EXCEPT

(A) malnutrition

(B) Hodgkin's lymphoma

(C) multiple myeloma

(D) HIV infection

(E) all of the above

240. Bence Jones proteins are

(A) fragments of lactoferrin

(B) denatured acute phase proteins

(C) prostaglandin E2

(D) DNA binding proteins

(E) monoclonal free light chains

241. A vaccine produced from an extracellular toxic bacterial product that is made nontoxic, but maintains antigenicity, is known as a(n)

(A) mycotoxin

(B) antitoxin

(C) endotoxin

(D) exotoxin

(E) toxoid

242. Molecules of the MHC class II locus

(A) are lipoproteins

(B) are encoded in the HLA-B gene locus

(C) are found on all nucleated cells

(D) include complement components

(E) are encoded in the HLA-D gene locus

243. European Caucasian individuals possessing the HLA-B27 antigens have an 88% relative risk, compared to individuals without the antigen, of having

(A) rheumatoid arthritis

(B) myasthenia gravis

(C) ankylosing spondylitis

(D) multiple sclerosis

(E) psoriasis

244. Antigen receptors of B lymphocytes are

(A) MHC class I loci molecules

(B) MHC class II loci molecules

(C) MHC class III loci molecules

(D) immunoglobulin molecules

(E) Fc-receptor molecules

245. All of the following statements about monocytes are true EXCEPT that they

(A) can become macrophages

(B) are actively phagocytic

(C) function best in MHC-compatible environments

(D) can present antigen

(E) only populate lymph nodes

246. An antigen

(A) is always an immunogen

(B) is always smaller than 100 daltons

(C) is usually a homopolymer

(D) has one or more epitopes

(E) cannot be created from a hapten

247. Freund's complete adjuvant is used to

(A) suppress overproduction of antibody

(B) enhance antibody responses

(C) treat tuberculosis

(D) reduce blood pressure

(E) activate complement

248. All of the following statements about B-cell development are true EXCEPT

(A) B lymphocytes arise from pluripotential hematopoietic stem cells

(B) in embryogenesis, the first recognized cells of B lineage make only a mu heavy chain

(C) B cells continue to arise from stem cells throughout life

(D) pre-B cells yield immature B cells that have surface IgM

(E) immature B cells yield mature B cells only after antigen stimulation

249. All of the following statements about B-cell antigen-specific receptors are true EXCEPT

(A) surface immunoglobulin synthesized by a given B-cell clone serves as the antigen receptor for that clone

(B) surface immunoglobulin is dimeric and contains only two heavy chains

(C) it is likely that different receptor isotypes have different functions on the same cell

(D) differentiation of immunoglobulin (Ig) secretion requires further interaction with T cells of T-cell–derived lymphokines

(E) the surface form of the heavy chain of Ig is larger than the secreted form of heavy chains of IgG, IgD, or IgA

250. All of the following are T-independent antigens EXCEPT

(A) bacterial lipopolysaccharide

(B) polymerized flagellin

(C) pneumococcal polysaccharide

(D) serum albumin

(E) poly-D amino acids

251. Lethal infection may result if AIDS patients receive

(A) diphtheria toxoid

(B) heat-killed bacterial vaccine

(C) tetanus toxoid

(D) BCG

(E) acellular pertussis vaccine

252. The fragment required for an IgG molecule to cross the placenta is

(A) Fab

(B) Fd

(C) $F(ab')_2$

(D) Fc

(E) none of the above

253. The antibody residues that predominantly make up the antigen-combining site, as the "contact" amino acids, are located within the

(A) heavy chains

(B) framework regions

(C) hypervariable regions

(D) constant domains

(E) disulfide bonds

254. All of the following statements concerning the hypervariable regions of an immunoglobulin molecule are true EXCEPT that they are

(A) located at the carboxyl terminal end

(B) also called the complementarily determined regions

(C) the antigen-contacting amino acid areas

(D) defined as the idiotype of the antibody

(E) located within the $F(ab')_2$ piece of the molecule

255. All of the following statements concerning a monoclonal antibody are correct EXCEPT it

(A) has antibody-combining sites that are identical

(B) may belong to the IgM, IgA, IgE, IgD, or IgG classes

(C) may be present in the serum of patients with multiple myeloma

(D) can be obtained by the hybridoma technique

(E) has not been found to have diagnostic or therapeutic use

256. Antigen-antibody interactions are stabilized by

(A) covalent bonds

(B) the formation of disulfide bonds at the combining site

(C) the generation of hydrophilic zones due to a conformational change in the antibody molecule

(D) noncovalent charge neutralization and hydrogen bonding leading to hydrophobic sites

(E) complement binding at the CH2 domain, thereby stabilizing the complex

257. The number of combining sites on an antibody molecule or a fragment such as Fab is best determined by

(A) radial immunodiffusion

(B) immunoelectrophoresis

(C) the quantitative precipitin curve

(D) complement fixation test

(E) equilibrium dialysis

258. Radial immunodiffusion is used to

(A) establish the heterogeneity of an antigen

(B) demonstrate cross-reactions between antigens

(C) demonstrate the homogeneity (purity) of an antigen

(D) quantitate an antigen

(E) identify the isotype of an antibody

259. A small molecule that can react with preformed antibodies but cannot, by itself, induce their formation is referred to as a(n)

(A) complete antigen

(B) antigenic determinant

(C) hapten

(D) helper factor

(E) suppressor factor

260. Mechanisms of antibacterial immunity include all of the following EXCEPT

(A) antibody- and complement-mediated bacteriolysis

(B) antibody- and complement-mediated opsonization for enhanced phagocytosis

(C) antibody neutralization of toxins

(D) intracellular destruction by activated macrophages

(E) cytotoxic T-cell–mediated bacteriolysis

261. Opsonin-treated bacteria are more readily engulfed by phagocytes than are untreated bacteria because

(A) the capsule is removed by opsonin

(B) opsonin digests the wall component

(C) opsonin induces lysosomal enzymes

(D) the surface of a phagocyte contains receptors for the Fc portion of an antibody

(E) opsonin facilitates adenosine–triphosphate generation

262. The generation of antibody diversity is best explained by

(A) somatic mutation

(B) germ-line diversity (multiple genes)

(C) combinative amplification of germ-line diversity

(D) a combination of germ-line diversity, recombination events, and somatic mutations

(E) adaptations to the environment

263. Somatic mutations can account for some degree of antibody diversity. These mutations

(A) occur randomly in the different loci that control immunoglobulin synthesis

(B) predominantly affect the kappa chains

(C) scramble the order of genes and gene fragments

(D) tend to involve only the V genes

(E) account for the C-gene switch during differentiation

264. The most likely clinical consequence of a genetic deficiency of complement component C3 is increased

(A) susceptibility to viral infections
(B) incidence of malignancy
(C) susceptibility to the damaging effects of endotoxins on blood vessels
(D) susceptibility to bacterial infections
(E) susceptibility to fungal infections

265. The following statement that BEST describes the function of properdin in the alternative complement pathway is that

(A) it is the recognition protein of the alternative complement pathway
(B) it interacts directly with cell membranes
(C) it stabilizes the C3 convertase of the alternative pathway
(D) one of its cleavage fragments is chemotactic
(E) it is opsonic

266. All of the following agents are immunosuppressive EXCEPT

(A) corticosteroids
(B) cyclosporin A
(C) lymphoid irradiation
(D) alkylating agents
(E) vitamin C

267. The immunoglobulin fragment that binds C1q is

(A) Fab
(B) Fd
(C) F(ab')$_2$
(D) Fc
(E) Fv

268. A carboxypeptidase that inactivates C3a and C5a is

(A) C1 inactivator
(B) factor I
(C) factor H
(D) S protein
(E) anaphylotoxin inhibitor

269. The final step in both the classical and alternative complement pathways, which leads to the subsequent membrane attack mechanism, is

(A) deposition of C4b2a
(B) cleavage of C5
(C) construction of C3 convertase
(D) construction of C5 convertase
(E) deposition of C6

270. The diagnosis of poststreptococcal glomerulonephritis rests on

(A) a low C3 level
(B) increasing titers of antistreptolysin O (ASO)
(C) the preceding history of a sore throat
(D) linear deposition of IgG along the glomerular basement membrane in a renal biopsy
(E) all of the above

271. Natural killer cells

(A) are large granular lymphocytes
(B) do not express markers (OKT3, OKT4, OKT8) found in human T lymphocytes
(C) lack Fc receptors
(D) do not vary in their sensitivity to regulatory actions of interferon or interleukins
(E) do not vary in the range of targets they will lyse

272. The pathogenic antibody in Graves' disease has specificity for

(A) nuclei
(B) adrenal cell
(C) thyroglobulin
(D) thyroid-stimulating hormone (TSH) receptor
(E) acetylcholine receptor

273. Children with insulin-dependent diabetes mellitus usually have serum antibodies against

(A) pancreatic islet cells
(B) gastric parietal cells

(C) nuclei

(D) IgG molecules

(E) thyroid microsomes

274. The method of choice for measuring total IgE in serum is

(A) radial immunodiffusion

(B) radioimmunoassay

(C) indirect immunofluorescence

(D) serum protein immunoelectrophoresis

(E) countercurrent electrophoresis

275. The first line of defense against viruses is

(A) antibody directed to internal viral antigens

(B) antibody directed to external viral antigens

(C) interferon

(D) IgM directed to an external antigen

(E) IgG directed to an external antigen

276. Surface membrane immunoglobulin is a marker of which of the following cell type?

(A) monocytes

(B) neutrophils

(C) T lymphocytes in blood

(D) B lymphocytes in blood

(E) bone marrow stem cells

277. Immune interferon (IFN-γ)

(A) acts on virus-infected cells

(B) is produced by leukocytes

(C) is produced by fibroblasts

(D) activates macrophages

(E) blocks viral replication

278. Antibody to *Streptococcus pyogenes* M proteins

(A) promotes attachment of the bacterium to host-cell membrane

(B) triggers complement-mediated damage to outer lipid bilayers

(C) enhances the antibacterial activity of the natural killer cells

(D) kills the bacterium

(E) opsonizes *S. pyogenes* by the Fc and C3b receptors for phagocytosis

279. Patients with the Chediak–Higashi syndrome have phagocytes that

(A) produce proteins that interfere with chemotaxis

(B) lack C3b receptors, which are needed for attachment to bacteria

(C) show a reduced ability of their lysosomes to fuse with phagosomes to release microbicidal substances

(D) produce limited amounts of myeloperoxidase

(E) show defects for the engulfment of microbes

280. Type I hypersensitivity

(A) is also known as delayed-type hypersensitivity

(B) occurs when an IgE response is directed against pollens

(C) does not require IgE-sensitized mast cells

(D) involves degranulation of polymorphonuclear eosinophils

(E) is independent of pharmacologic mediators

281. Type II hypersensitivity

(A) is antibody-independent

(B) is complement-independent

(C) does not involve killer cells

(D) requires immune-complex formation

(E) is antibody-dependent cytotoxic hypersensitive

282. Passive cutaneous anaphylaxis

    (A) measures antigen-specific IgE by intra-dermal injection
    (B) is used to determine type IV hypersensitivity
    (C) is mediated by the C5 component of complement
    (D) cannot be performed in atopic individuals
    (E) can be performed with IgE that has been heated at 56°C for 30 minutes

283. Arthus hypersensitivity

    (A) occurs 2 to 4 days after antigen challenge
    (B) is not mediated by complement-fixing IgG
    (C) produces cell death and extensive local destruction
    (D) cannot be manifested in the absence of high levels of IgE
    (E) does not require the intervention of natural killer cells

284. Grossly elevated serum levels of IgE can be found in

    (A) tuberculosis
    (B) leprosy
    (C) brucellosis
    (D) parasitic infestations
    (E) Arthus hypersensitivity

285. T cells

    (A) have IgG receptors
    (B) do not have CD3 antigen
    (C) are involved in antibody-dependent cellular cytotoxicity
    (D) are not important in phagocytosis
    (E) account for 8 to 15% of leukocytes in peripheral blood

286. MHC class I molecules are normally expressed on

    (A) B cells only
    (B) antigen-presenting cells only
    (C) most nucleated cells
    (D) T cells only
    (E) erythrocytes and platelets only

287. MHC class II molecules are expressed on all of the following cells EXCEPT

    (A) B cells
    (B) macrophages
    (C) monocytes
    (D) vascular endothelial cells
    (E) erythrocytes

288. Rheumatoid factor

    (A) is a synonym for autoanti-IgG antibodies
    (B) cannot combine with anti-DNA
    (C) is not involved in immune-complex formations
    (D) is a protease found in the synovial fluid
    (E) is primarily a macrophage product

289. Peptides that bind to MHC class I molecules

    (A) are derived from endocytosed exogenous molecules
    (B) are synthesized in the cytoplasm
    (C) cannot be recognized by a specific T-cell receptor
    (D) are always of microbial origin
    (E) are never processed by the immune system

290. Removal of immune complexes

    (A) is independent of C3 for particulate complexes
    (B) does not require IgG
    (C) occurs primarily in the liver
    (D) is independent of the size of the immune complex
    (E) has not been associated with the Kupffer cells

291. Formation of small immune complexes is due to

    (A) insufficient levels of antibody
    (B) an excess of C5a

(C) insufficient amounts of rheumatoid factor

(D) production of IgM

(E) low-affinity antibody

292. The maximal reaction time for tuberculin-type hypersensitivity is

(A) 2 to 5 hours

(B) 6 to 10 hours

(C) 12 to 20 hours

(D) 48 to 72 hours

(E) at least 4 days

293. Type IV hypersensitivity

(A) cannot be transferred from one individual to another by serum

(B) runs parallel with protective immunity

(C) involves only T_H cell types at the reaction site

(D) can be divided into two types of delayed hypersensitivity reactions

(E) cannot be elicited without histamine

294. Cytokine that favors T_H-1 type responses and counteracts the action of IL-10 is

(A) IL-1

(B) IL-2

(C) IL-4

(D) IL-6

(E) IL-12

295. Granulomatous hypersensitivity

(A) is not clinically important

(B) has not been encountered in schistosomiasis

(C) results from the presence of persistent microorganisms within macrophages

(D) causes few pathologic effects in diseases associated with T-cell–mediated immunity

(E) cannot be diagnosed by the lymphocyte transformation test

296. Clonal abortion is associated with

(A) immature B cells

(B) repeated antigenic challenge

(C) high doses of T-dependent antigens

(D) elimination of T_H cells

(E) overproduction of T_H cells

297. Clonal exhaustion can be induced by

(A) single challenge with a T-independent antigen

(B) repeated challenge with a T-independent antigen

(C) single challenge with a T-dependent antigen

(D) repeated challenge with a T-dependent antigen

(E) single challenge with either a T-dependent or a T-independent antigen

298. The isolation of different cell populations with different surface antigens stained with different fluorescent antibodies can be achieved by

(A) fluorescent spectrophotometer

(B) sucrose gradient centrifugation

(C) fluorescent microscopy

(D) immunoelectrophoresis

(E) fluorescence-activated cell sorter

DIRECTIONS (Questions 299 through 357): Each group of items in this section consists of lettered headings followed by a set of numbered words or phrases. For each numbered word or phrase, select the ONE lettered heading that is most closely associated with it. Each lettered heading may be selected once, more than once, or not at all.

Questions 299 and 300

(A) lymphocytes

(B) macrophages

(C) eosinophils

(D) basophils

(E) polymorphonuclear leukocytes

299. Memory cells

300. First white blood cells to be mobilized in acute pyogenic infection

Questions 301 and 302

 (A) natural killer cells

 (B) T cells

 (C) dendritic macrophages

 (D) pre-B cells

 (E) eosinophils

301. Antigen presenter

302. Helminth infections

Questions 303 and 304

 (A) radial immunodiffusion

 (B) immunoelectrophoresis

 (C) double diffusion in agar (Ouchterlony technique)

 (D) complement fixation

 (E) quantitative precipitin curve

303. A method that employs antibody-coated red cells as the indicator system

304. A method used to identify the light- and heavy-chain isotypes of a multiple myeloma protein

Questions 305 and 306

 (A) C1 and C2

 (B) C3a and C5a

 (C) C3b and C4b

 (D) C5a, Bb, and C5b,6,7

 (E) C8 and C9

305. Immune adherence and opsonization

306. Membrane damage

Question 307

 (A) C1 and C2

 (B) C3a and C5a

 (C) C4b and C4b

 (D) C5a, C5b,6,7, and Bb

 (E) C8 and C9

307. Anaphylotoxins

Questions 308 through 310

 (A) lytic antibody (IgG)

 (B) neutralizing antibody (IgG)

 (C) neutralizing and adhesion-blocking antibody

 (D) opsonizing antibody

 (E) macrophage activation by T cells

308. Protection against poliovirus

309. Major host defense against *Mycobacterium tuberculosis*

310. Key immunologic protection for *Clostridium tetani*

Questions 311 through 313

 (A) tryptase

 (B) leukotriene B4

 (C) prostaglandin DX2

 (D) heparin sulfate

 (E) eosinophil chemotactic factor of anaphylaxis

311. Binds histamine

312. Activates C3

313. Causes constriction of bronchial smooth muscle

Questions 314 through 316

 (A) toxoid

 (B) toxin

 (C) living attenuated microorganisms

 (D) killed virulent microorganisms

 (E) none of the above

314. Rubeola vaccine

315. Whooping cough vaccine

316. Tetanus vaccine

Questions 317 and 318

For each subset of T helper cell type described, select the lymphokines produced.

    (A) IL-12 and INF-γ
    (B) IL-4 and IL-10
    (C) IL-3, GM-CSF, and TNF-α
    (D) IL-1, IL-2, IL4, and IL-10
    (E) IL-10 and IL-12

317. T$_H$-1 cells

318. T$_H$-2 cells

Questions 319 and 320

    (A) T cells
    (B) B cells
    (C) macrophages
    (D) dendritic cells
    (E) T cells, B cells, macrophages, and dendritic cells

319. Express MHC class I antigens

320. Express surface immunoglobulin

Questions 321 through 323

    (A) variable regions of light chains
    (B) variable regions of light and heavy chains
    (C) variable regions of heavy chains
    (D) constant regions of heavy chains
    (E) constant regions of light and heavy chains

321. Determine allotype

322. Determine idiotypes

323. Determine immunoglobulin class

Questions 324 through 328

    (A) IgG
    (B) IgA
    (C) IgM
    (D) IgD
    (E) IgE

324. Involvement in allergic hypersensitivities

325. Predominant antibody induced in primary response

326. Predominant antibody induced in secondary response

327. Predominant antibody in external secretions

328. Found mainly on surface of B cells

Questions 329 through 332

    (A) immediate hypersensitivity
    (B) cytotoxic antibody
    (C) immune complex diseases
    (D) delayed-type hypersensitivity
    (E) none of the above

329. Autoimmune hemolytic anemia and Goodpasture syndrome

330. Atopy, urticaria, and asthma

331. Contact dermatitis, tuberculosis, and sarcoidosis

332. Tetanus, botulism, and diphtheria

Questions 333 through 336

    (A) rheumatoid arthritis
    (B) Hashimoto's thyroiditis
    (C) Graves' disease
    (D) systemic lupus erythematosus
    (E) myasthenia gravis

333. Mediated by antibody directed against thyroglobulin

334. Mediated by antibody directed against rheumatoid factors

335. Mediated by antibody directed against DNA

336. Mediated by antibody directed against acetylcholine receptor

Questions 337 through 339

    (A) chronic granulomatous disease

    (B) DiGeorge syndrome

    (C) X-linked agammaglobulinemia

    (D) severe combined immunodeficiency syndromes

    (E) AIDS

337. Virtual absence of both B and T cells

338. Thymic hypoplasia

339. Defect in intracellular microbicidal mechanisms

Questions 340 and 341

    (A) RNA processing

    (B) alternative RNA splicing

    (C) hypermutation

    (D) DNA rearrangement

    (E) post-transcriptional modification

340. D to J joining

341. Joining of V-D-J to constant regions of heavy chains

Questions 342 and 343

    (A) interferon-β

    (B) interferon-γ

    (C) interleukin-3

    (D) interleukin-4

    (E) tumor necrosis factor

342. Inhibits viral replication

343. Induces fever

Questions 344 through 346

    (A) IgA

    (B) IgM

    (C) IgG

    (D) IgD

    (E) IgE

344. Binds to rheumatoid factor

345. May contain a peptide chain not synthesized by B cells

346. Found in the milk of lactating women

Questions 347 through 350

For each cellular activity indicated, select the cell type most likely to have such activity.

    (A) macrophages

    (B) T helper cells

    (C) cytotoxic T cells

    (D) suppressor T cells

    (E) B cells

    (F) neutrophils

    (G) eosinophils

    (H) basophils

    (I) mast cells

    (J) plasma cells

    (K) stem cells

    (L) natural killer cells

347. Produce and secrete IgA, IgG, and IgE

348. Phagocytic antigen-presenting cells

349. Markedly increase during *Ascaris* infections

350. MHC-unrestricted, nonphagocytic, and tumoricidal

Questions 351 through 354

For each patient, select the disease from which he or she is most likely to be suffering.

    (A) chronic granulomatous disease

    (B) Chediak–Higashi syndrome

    (C) acquired immunodeficiency syndrome

    (D) X-linked agammaglobulinemia

    (E) DiGeorge syndrome

(F) systemic lupus erythematosus

(G) Wiskott–Aldrich syndrome

(H) severe combined immunodeficiency disorder (SCID)

(I) selective IgA deficiency

(J) neutropenia

351. This 23-year-old male has developed severe systemic candidiasis. Laboratory tests show the following:

Nitroblue tetrazolium reduction test: Normal
Anti-HIV test: Negative
T4:T8 ratio: Normal
Serum complement level: Normal
Granulocyte count: 1100/mm³
Serum IgG level: 1500 mg/dL
Serum IgA level: 280 mg/dL

352. A 6-month-old infant has been suffering from repeated pneumonia, otitis media, and cutaneous infections. The patient has profound lymphopenia and her lymphocytes do not respond to mitogens. Serum immunoglobulin levels are abnormally diminished. T-cell and B-cell functions are severely impaired

353. Neutrophils from this patient, who has been suffering from repeated staphylococcal and *Candida* infections, show normal phagocytotic activity. However, intracellular killing of certain bacteria such as staphylococci is severely impaired and nitroblue tetrazolium reduction test is negative. Myeloperoxidase activity of neutrophils is normal. The patient, however, has no history of streptococcal infection

354. A kidney biopsy taken from a young woman complaining of fever, rash, and arthritis shows marked deposits of immunoglobulin, complement (C3), and fibrinogen in the basement membrane. High titers of anti-DNA antibody is also detected in her serum

Questions 355 through 357

For each statement listed below, select the lymphokine or cytokine most likely to have the specified activities.

(A) interleukin-1

(B) interleukin-2

(C) interleukin-3

(D) interleukin-4

(E) interleukin-5

(F) interleukin-6

(G) interleukin-7

(H) interleukin-8

(I) interferon-γ

(J) tissue necrosis factor beta

(K) prostaglandin E2

(L) leukotrienes

(M) granulocyte-macrophage colony-stimulating factor

355. T-cell and natural-killer-cell product that activates macrophages for microbicidal and tumoricidal activity

356. Macrophage product that enhances vascular permeability, increases sensitivity to pain, and produces fever

357. T-cell product that stimulates growth of pluripotent hematopoietic stem cells

Immunology
Answers and Explanations

108. (E) The myeloma cell used for fusion is usually a doubly deficient mutant unable to secrete myeloma protein and lacking thymidine kinase. Normal B lymphocytes do not proliferate in vitro but can supply thymidine kinase to the thymidine–kinase-negative fusion partner, ie, myeloma cell. Thus, the specificity of antibody and the ability to survive in the absence of thymidine are controlled by the B-cell partner of the fusion, and the myeloma partner contributes an unlimited capacity to proliferate. Since no other cells listed in the question are immunoglobulin producers, they cannot be used for making fusion-derived immortalized antibody-producing hybridomas. (*Joklik et al, p 206; Roitt et al, pp 28.8–28.10*)

109. (C) Most animal cells undergo lysis when treated with antibodies specific to the cell-surface protein in the presence of complement. CD4 is a cell-surface antigen (marker) characteristically associated with T-helper cells. No other cells listed in the question have this surface marker protein in their cell membrane. Thus, when treated with anti-CD4 antibody and complement, the cells most likely to undergo cytolysis are T helper cells. (*Joklik et al, pp 250–254,291–292*)

110. (C) CD8 antigen is the most characteristic surface marker found in all cytotoxic T cells. This surface marker also occurs in suppressor T cells. CD4 is a surface marker for T-helper cells. CD2 (sheep erythrocyte receptor) and CD3 also occur in T cells other than cytotoxic T cells. Surface IgM (with or without IgD) is the hallmark of B cells. CD3 is an integral part of the T-cell receptor (TCR) complex. (*Joklik et al, pp 250–254; Roitt et al, pp 2.7–2.8*)

111. (D) Although antitoxin prepared in a horse can be used for the prophylactic purpose at the time of injury, the risk of anaphylaxis and serum sickness makes it more preferable to use human immune globulin instead. Since the patient is unable to produce immune globulin because of the underlying genetic defect, active immunization with tetanus toxoid is not the choice in this case even if the patient had a previous record of immunization with tetanus toxoid. For active immunization against tetanus, toxoid (nontoxic), not toxin (extremely toxic), is used. Since tetanus is an exotoxin-associated disease, immunization with heat-killed *Clostridium tetani* cells would not elicit tetanus immunity at all. (*Joklik et al, p 646, Roitt et al, pp 21.1–21.4*)

112. (E) All of the events listed in the question can cause immune unresponsiveness. Animals treated repeatedly with very high or very low doses of antigen fail to make an immune response to an optimal immunization challenge with the same antigen due to receptor blockage. The presence of blocking antibody prevents immune response due to masking of antigenic determinants. Suppressor T cells produce factors that can interfere with a variety of immunologic activities such as T-cell helper activity, IgE response, delayed hypersensitivity, or even T-independent triggering of B cells. If lymphocytes with appropriate receptors are absent, no immune response would result. *(Joklik et al, pp 259–263)*

113. **(B)** In a mixed lymphocyte culture, leukocytes from two unrelated (allogeneic) individuals are mixed in vitro. After 5 to 7 days, substantial proliferation (primarily T-helper and some cytotoxic cells) can be measured because of the recognition of foreign major histocompatibility antigens on the leukocytes. Antigens of class I regions react preferentially with precursors of cytotoxic T-effector cells (CD8) and antigens of class II regions react preferentially with helper T cells (CD4). Thus, for a maximum response, disparity at both class I and II loci is needed. No proliferation occurs if class I and II loci are similar. A fair cytotoxic T-lymphocyte response can be seen when disparity is only at class I determinants and a strong (but not maximum) cell proliferation is seen when disparity is only at class II determinants. *(Joklik et al, pp 259,266–268,274–275)*

114. **(E)** Cytotoxic T cells perform all of the functions listed in the question except E. Macrophages and B cells are antigen-presenting cells. *(Joklik et al, pp 258–259; Roitt et al, pp 9.4–9.7)*

115. **(D)** T-helper cells are central to the development of immune responses. They help B cells to make antibody and modulate the actions of a variety of cells belonging to the immune system. Such cells include cytotoxic T cells, natural killer cells, macrophages, granulocytes, and antibody-dependent cytotoxic cells. Both cytotoxic T cells and T-helper cells are involved in mixed lymphocyte reactions, and macrophages are involved in delayed-type hypersensitivity reactions. *(Joklik et al, pp 256–257; Roitt et al, pp 9.2–9.4,22.3–22.4)*

116. **(D)** As explained previously (question 113), a maximum cellular proliferation (T helper cells) and induction of cytotoxic T lymphocytes are seen in mixed lymphocyte reactions when disparity occurs at MHC class I and class II loci. Since these cells play primary roles in transplanted tissue rejection, the

chance of successful transplant between donor and recipient is minimal when the donor and recipient have different MHC class I and II molecules. *(Joklik et al pp 274–275,282–283; Roitt et al, pp 26.1–26.6)*

117. **(E)** V, J, and C genes are present in both heavy- and light-chain genes. Processing of nuclear messenger RNA (mRNA) (primary RNA transcript) by splicing out intervening sequences (introns) to produce mRNA takes place during gene recombination of both heavy and light chains. In both mouse and man, the kappa light-chain locus has a single C gene and the genes for heavy-chain constant regions (CH) of different isotypes are arranged in a tandem array. The newly assembled heavy-chain V-D-J gene set can be translocated to a position immediately 5' to any of the heavy-chain C-region genes. However, in a given light chain (kappa or lambda), the newly assembled V-J gene set (light chain lacks D segment) is always combined with the same C-region gene (C kappa or C lambda). *(Joklik et al, pp 230–235; Roitt et al, pp 6.4–6.7)*

118. **(B)** T-cell receptor (TCR) recognizes a complex of foreign antigen peptide bound in the peptide-binding cleft of a major histocompatibility complex molecule. TCR consists of two integral membrane glycoprotein subunits (alpha, beta or gamma, delta), covalently linked by a disulfide bond. Each subunit has a similar domain structure, remarkably reminiscent of the structure of immunoglobulin. The gene region encoding alpha chains is analogous to immunoglobulin (Ig) light-chain genes. The beta chains are encoded by a group of genes analogous to Ig heavy chains. Thus, the two subunits are not identical (heterodimeric). They differ in size (in humans) and amino acid composition, which are responsible for the antigenic specificity of the receptor. Each chain contains a hydrophobic transmembrane region. *(Joklik et al, pp 235–236; Roitt et al, pp 5.1–5.3)*

119. **(E)** Natural killer (NK) cells are a special subpopulation of lymphocytes, which without prior sensitization can recognize, attack,

and kill certain tumor and virally infected cells. For these cytotoxic activities, NK cells do not require antibody. In humans, NK cells comprise 1 to 2% of the total lymphocyte pool. Characteristically, NK cells do not overtly display either T- or B-lymphocyte markers. *(Joklik et al, pp 375–377; Roitt et al, pp 2.7–2.8,8.8,16.2–16.3)*

120. **(E)** All the statements described in A through D are true. Each of the immunoglobulin (Ig) chains are coded for on separate chromosomes. For example, the genes coded for the heavy chain of human Ig are located on chromosome 14, alpha chain on chromosome 22, and kappa chain on chromosome 2. In a given immunoglobulin molecule, either lambda or kappa light chain, not both, can occur. *(Joklik et al, pp 223–235; Roitt et al, pp 6.1–6.14)*

121. **(A)** *Streptococcus pneumoniae* is one of the bacterial agents most frequently responsible for acute ear infection and meningitis in infants. The host defense against this encapsulated bacteria relies heavily on phagocytes, which can engulf and kill the bacteria only when the target cells are covered with opsonin (immune globulin, complement). In a patient with agammaglobulinemia, this opsonization may not occur optimally. Consequently, encapsulated *S. pneumoniae* may not be killed, resulting in infection. The resistance to other microorganisms listed in the question depends predominantly on cell-mediated immunity, which is not affected in this patient. *(Roitt et al, pp 17.1–17.11,18.1–18.6)*

122. **(E)** Human leukocyte antigen complex is involved in all the functions described in A through D. *(Joklik et al, pp 259,264–285)*

123. **(C)** Anaphylaxis triggered by penicillin injection is an immediate hypersensitivity reaction (type 1 immunologic reaction), which is typically mediated by IgE antibodies. IgE antibodies bind via characteristic Fc domains with very high affinity to specific Fc receptors on the surface of mast cells and basophils. On cross-linking of such antibodies by multivalent antigen, the effector cell is

stimulated to release almost immediately (within 1 minute in vitro) preformed, pharmacologically active shock mediators (histamine, chemotactic factors, proteolytic enzymes, heparin, etc.). All other immunoglobulin molecules, complement, and T cells do not mediate type 1 immunologic reaction. *(Joklik et al, p 319; Roitt et al, pp 22.1–22.6)*

124. **(B)** Two ways in which T cells may mediate graft-cell destruction are known. Foreign MHC class II antigens on the graft stimulate host T-helper cells to help cytotoxic T cells, which, in turn, destroy the target graft cell. Cytotoxic T cells recognize the graft via the foreign MHC class I antigens. Foreign MHC class II antigens on the graft stimulate host T-helper cells, causing release of lymphokines, which stimulate macrophages. Activated macrophages enter the graft and destroy it. MHC class II antigen neither enhances the function of suppressor T cells nor promotes macrophage migration. MHC class II molecules do not induce blocking antibody production. *(Joklik et al, pp 210,274–275, 282–283; Roitt et al, p 26.3)*

125. **(C)** One of the characteristics of AIDS is lymphopenia caused by an absolute deficiency of CD4+ T (T-helper) cells. Since T-helper cells are central to the immune system, AIDS patients are expected to have a severe and profound deficiency in the cell-mediated immune system. Tuberculin reaction is a typical cell-mediated delayed-type hypersensitivity reaction. Thus, AIDS patients who are infected with *Mycobacterium tuberculosis* are likely to react less vigorously to injected tuberculin when compared with normal individuals suffering from tuberculosis. CD8+ T cells, stem cells, and platelets are not the major target cells of human immunodeficiency viruses. *(Joklik et al, pp 322–323,337–338)*

126. **(E)** All of the deficiencies listed in the question occur in AIDS patients. *(Joklik et al, pp 337–338; Roitt et al, pp 21.6–21.7)*

127. **(B)** When *Mycobacterium tuberculosis* triggers release of IL-2 from T cells, and IL-12 and

INF-γ from monocytes, macrophages and NK cells, the T_H subset that develops will be biased toward T_H-1. Activation of macrophages which results from the action of these lymphokines is critically important in the host resistance to *M. tuberculosis*. In contrast to this, release of IL-4 and IL-10 will bias toward T_H IL-10. IL-4 inhibits the production of INF-γ. IL-13 blocks IL-12 production and its (IL-13) production is not triggered by tubercle bacilli. IL-5 and -6 act on B cells, stimulating their growth and differentiation. IL-1 is made by many cells that include macrophages, B cells, endothelial cells, and fibroblasts. It stimulates T and B cells and induces inflammatory responses. IL-1 travels to the brain where it induces fever. *(Roitt et al, pp 8.9,9.3)*

128. **(A)** Soluble antigens excreted by the eggs stimulate the formation of T lymphocyte-mediated eosinophilic granuloma. This type of granuloma has nothing to do with antiparasitic drugs, surface antigens of the parasite itself, or damaged liver cells. No specific toxins are known to be produced by blood flukes (*Schistosoma*). *(Roitt et al, pp 25.10–25.11; Ryan et al, pp 724–725)*

129 **(D)** Lysozyme is a hydrolytic enzyme that is capable of digesting bacterial cell walls containing peptidoglycan. The enzyme is present in serum, tear, and phagocytic cells protecting the host from invading microorganisms nonspecifically. *(Roitt et al, 17.6–17.7)*

130. **(D)** All of the conditions listed in A through C may result in no precipitate formation. Precipitation follows the reaction of divalent IgG antibody with multivalent (not monovalent) antigen. With antigen excess, the amount of antibody precipitated usually falls since adequate crosslinking for the formation of large complexes no longer occurs. *(Joklik et al, p 238)*

131. **(B)** Some progeny of activated B cells undergo heavy-chain class (isotype) switching and begin to express immunoglobulin heavy-chain class other than mu and delta (eg, gamma, alpha, or epsilon). Since only one V-D-J rearrangement occurs per cell and the V-D-J portion of the heavy chain remains unchanged during differentiation, idiotype switch is unlikely to occur. Antibody produced by B cells during differentiation is not induced by any specific antigen. Class switching is a unique property of the heavy-chain gene cluster that is not shared by the light-chain system. *(Joklik et al, pp 206,232–233; Roitt et al, pp 2.9,10.10–10.14)*

132. **(B)** All other regions of heavy and light chains are not involved in such a switch. For further explanation, see the comment given in the answer to question 131. *(Joklik et al, pp 206,232–233; Roitt et al, pp 10.10–10.14)*

133. **(E)** Interleukin-2 (IL-2) is a lymphokine produced by T-helper cells and plays a major role in enhancing the immune system of the host. All of the activities listed in A through D are known functions of IL-2. Cytotoxic T cells, T-helper cells, B cells, natural killer cells, and macrophages have receptors for IL-2. *(Joklik et al, pp 255,312–316; Roitt et al, pp 8.8–8.13)*

134. **(B)** Under the circumstance described (Rh-positive mother and Rh-negative father), none of their children is in danger of developing hemolytic disease of the newborn. Therefore, no prophylactic use of RhoGAM is necessary. Hemolytic diseases of the newborn occurs (except for the first child) when the mother is Rh-negative and the father is Rh-positive. In such instances, the mother is sensitized to Rh antigens on the infant's erythrocytes and makes IgG antibodies to these antigens. These antibodies cross the placenta and react with the fetal erythrocytes, causing their destruction. Rhesus D (RhD) is the most commonly involved antigen. RhoGAM (anti-RhD antibodies) is aimed at destroying fetal Rh-positive erythrocytes that enter the mother's circulation before they sensitize the Rh-negative mother. Even if the mother is Rh negative and the father is Rh positive, RhoGAM is not indicated for the first child. *(Roitt et al, pp 23.5–23.6)*

135. **(C)** B cells generally require the presence of T cells for stimulation by antigen toward antibody formation. In animals, the thymus is

regarded as a central lymphoid organ and plays a critical role in the differentiation process from bone marrow stem cells to T lymphocytes. In thymectomized mice, transplantation of normal bone marrow, mature B cells, injection of interleukin-2, or other treatments such as irradiation cannot restore the ability to form antibody. *(Joklik et al, pp 208,256)*

136. **(C)** Because of deficiency in the cellular immune system, AIDS patients show decreased delayed-type hypersensitivity to various antigens, including purified protein derivative of tuberculin. In normal individuals, a skin reaction (erythema) that exceeds 10 mm in diameter is considered positive. In the case of AIDS patients, this criterion does not apply because their cell-mediated hypersensitivity is weakened by human immunodeficiency virus infection. It is recommended in the new guideline that this size (6 mm) of skin reaction should be considered tuberculin test positive. As in normal individuals, the presence of active infection cannot be confirmed by the tuberculin test only. Whether tubercle bacilli causing infection are multidrug resistant or not can only be determined by drug susceptibility tests, not by the tuberculin test. In the United States, BCG vaccination is not used for prophylaxis of tuberculosis. *(Joklik et al, pp 322–323,337–338; Roitt et al, p 25.5; Morbidity and Mortality Weekly Report, pp 27–31)*

137. **(D)** Although there is great homology between the constant (C) regions of all immunoglobulins, certain amino acid sequences in the C region are characteristic of each major class (delta, mu, and alpha). Limited substitutions characterize subclasses or isotypes (eg, gamma-1, alpha-2) of the heavy chain of IgG and IgA of all members of a species. Other limited substitutions of different amino acid residues of the constant region occur only in the kappa chains or the gamma-1 heavy chains of an individual. These individual-specific markings are called allotypes: Km and Gm allotypes. *(Joklik et al, p 205; Roitt et al, p 4.8)*

138. **(D)** The ability of T cells to discriminate between self and nonself is learned in the thymus. This process is dependent on the elimination of T cells in which T-cell receptor gene rearrangements are nonproductive, as well as on the elimination of T cells with productive rearrangements that recognize self-MHC or self-MHC–peptide complexes. The thymus processes only T cells. All other organs listed in this question play important roles in the development or function of the immune system but not in training of T cells so that they can discriminate between self and nonself. *(Joklik et al, pp 250–252,276; Roitt et al, pp 10.4–10.8)*

139. **(C)** Extensive amino acid substitution is a special feature of the peptides adjacent to the amino terminus of the heavy and light chains of all classes of immunoglobulins (not limited to IgG). This part of the heavy (H) and light (L) chain is called the variable (V) region. Short sequences within the V region, called hypervariable sequences, bind with specific antigen. The genes encoding for H and L chains of immunoglobulin molecules are located on separate chromosomes (see the explanation for Question 120). The function of the constant regions, especially of the H chains, is to confer different biologic properties on the immunoglobulin molecules. It is not the V region that defines the molecular size of immunoglobulin molecules. The molecular size of an immunoglobulin molecule is determined by the number of four-chain units per antibody molecule. *(Joklik et al, pp 205,224–227; Roitt et al, pp 6.1–6.14)*

140. **(E)** Heavy chains of IgM have four constant (C) domains in contrast to three in those of IgG. Light chains have only one C domain. In both heavy and light chains, there is only one variable domain. All statements listed in A through D are correct. *(Joklik et al, pp 224–227; Roitt et al, pp 4.1–4.7)*

141. **(D)** Immunoglobulin class and subclass depend on the structure of the heavy chain. IgG-1 is a heavy-chain subclass of IgG. The constant regions of all IgG-1 heavy chains from one individual possess the same amino acid composition and thus share the identical

isotypic specificities. Since the specificity and idiotype of each IgG-1 molecule is determined by the amino acid sequence of hypervariable segments of heavy and light chains, IgG-1 human antistaphylococcal and IgG-1 human antistreptococcal antibodies from one individual do not share the same amino acid sequences at variable regions. Therefore, the statements listed in A through C are incorrect. Fc fragment is a product of papain digestion of IgG with the constant regions of two heavy chains and no combining sites for antigen. So IgG-1 molecules with different specificity obtained from the same individual are most likely to share the same Fc fragment. (*Joklik et al, pp 225–227,262; Roitt et al, pp 4.2–4.8*)

142. **(A)** Gm allotypes are determined by minor differences (a few amino acids) in the constant region of heavy chains. These differences reflect alleles (alternate forms of a gene for a particular locus). If an individual is heterozygous for Gm allotypes, he/she inherited one allele from his/her mother and a different allele from his/her father. Both alleles are expressed in that individual; they are codominant. This codominance is why this individual contains two allelic forms of the protein. The reason that individual lymphocytes form only one of the two forms is that, once a functional rearrangement has taken place in the DNA of a given cell, no further rearrangement takes place in DNA in that particular cell. Only one of the two homologous chromosomes has a functional rearrangement (called allelic exclusion), and a given chromosome has only one functional rearrangement of immunoglobulin heavy-chain DNA. (*Joklik et al, pp 206,223–227*)

143. **(C)** By definition, immature B cells assemble IgM molecules and insert them into membrane. In other words, immature B cells are surface IgM positive. Pre-B cells have mu chains in the cytoplasm. Immature B cells cannot differentiate into T cells. Only plasma cells excrete IgG. Mature B cells express immunoglobulin on the cell surface. Only T cells, not B cells, enter the thymus to mature. B cells develop in the microenvironment of the bone marrow or fetal liver, and on other lymphoid organs such as the spleen, tonsils, and Peyer's patches of the gut. (*Joklik et al, p 251; Roitt et al, pp 10.10–10.11*)

144. **(C)** The spleen is responsive to blood-borne antigens. Responses to blood-borne antigens result in secretion of antibodies into the circulation and in local, cell-mediated responses. The spleen also serves as a reservoir for platelets, erythrocytes, and granulocytes. Patients who have undergone splenectomy are much more susceptible to blood-borne infections. The spleen has no significant role in complement activation and detoxication. Detoxication and acute phase protein production are the functions associated with the liver. (*Roitt, pp 3.3–3.4*)

145. **(B)** Cytotoxic T cells recognize a foreign antigen in association with a MHC class I antigen. CD8 molecules enhance the binding interactions with common MHC class I determinants. To lyse virally infected cells, the target cells (infected cells) and effector cells (cytotoxic T cells) must share the identical MHC class I antigens. Since polio and influenza viruses do not share antigens, cytotoxic T cells from an individual infected with influenza virus cannot recognize cells infected with poliovirus, because polio antigens are not expressed on the surface of such polio-infected cells. Therefore, the T-cytotoxic cells that can recognize and lyse cells infected with influenza virus cannot detect and lyse cells infected with poliovirus even if such infected cells share the identical MHC class I or class II loci with effector cells. MHC class II antigens are involved in recognition of foreign antigens by helper T cells, not cytotoxic T cells. (*Joklik et al, pp 274–275,354–355; Roitt et al, pp 16.4–16.5*)

146. **(D)** In precipitation reaction, valence of antigen and antibody is important. The precipitation reaction depends on formation of an insoluble antigen–antibody complex upon mixing soluble antibody and soluble antigen. Since a lattice-like conglomeration of antigen molecules connected by antibody molecules is the basis of precipitation reaction, both

antigen and antibody need to be divalent or multivalent. This requirement is why no precipitation occurs with haptens, which are monovalent antigens. Antibodies are at least divalent. *(Joklik et al, pp 236–239; Roitt et al, pp 28.1–28.3)*

147. (E) All of the statements listed in this question are correct. *(Joklik et al, pp 206,243–244)*

148. (E) All of the statements listed in this question are correct. *(Joklik et al, pp 227–228,230–233)*

149. (D) Passive immunization supplies preformed specific antibodies against an infectious agent or its product (toxin). Consequently, it does provide immediate post-exposure protection, whereas vaccination might take 1 to 2 weeks before specific antibodies arise in protective amounts in the vaccinated individuals. Specific serum therapy (for tetanus and botulism) is a form of passive immunization. Since the foreign antibodies are rapidly decaying, the protection is not long lasting. Since the antibodies are usually produced in a different species, the foreign protein antiserum may develop hypersensitivity to the foreign protein. This hypersensitivity is what occurs in serum sickness, which may develop 4 to 18 days later. Passive transfer of specific cellular immune effectors such as sensitized T cells is not technically feasible in humans because of the need for complete human lymphocyte antigen (HLA) matching to avoid rejection. Both passive and active immunization is used to treat humans exposed to rabies. *(Joklik et al, pp 365,1029–1030; Roitt et al, p 19.9)*

150. (E) All of the factors listed in the question influence the immune response. Adjuvants can result in increased immunogenicity for a weak immunogen. Some of the adjuvants used are water-in-oil emulsions (eg, Freund's complete adjuvant), finely particulate suspensions (eg, alum precipitates), and silica or bentonite particles. *(Joklik et al, pp 219–220; Roitt et al, 11.1–11.2)*

151. (C) The secondary response, after a second exposure to the same immunogen as in the primary response, is characterized by a substantially shorter lag phase and a higher antibody level for a longer period of time. IgM antibody synthesis may initially be the same as during the primary response, but it does not persist as long. IgG antibody synthesis rate is more rapid, reaches higher levels, and persists for a longer time. *(Joklik et al, pp 248–249; Roitt et al, pp 8.13–8.16)*

152. (D) *Hemophilus influenzae* type b vaccine is composed of a polysaccharide capsule with repeating antigenic determinants that behave as T-independent (ie, it activates B cells independently of T cells). The anticapsular antibody is an opsonizing antibody. *H. influenzae* coated with the anticapsular antibody can be readily phagocytosed because phagocytes have receptors for the Fc portion of the antibody. The antibody that binds to the capsular antigen fixes complement. Complement fixation facilitates phagocytosis because phagocytes have receptor for certain component (C3b) of complement. Influenza virus and poliovirus both elicit neutralizing antibodies. Toxoids elicit antitoxin antibody, which is a neutralizing antibody. BCG immunization elicits cell-mediated immunity, not humoral immunity. *(Joklik et al, pp 214,340,1140; Roitt et al, pp 19.1–19.10)*

153. (E) The clinical and laboratory finding clearly suggests that the patient is suffering from poststreptococcal glomerulonephritis. Immunoglobulin, complement, and antigens that react with antibodies against group A streptococci have been identified in the glomerulus. The M proteins of some nephriogenic strains have been shown to share antigenic determinants with glomeruli, which suggests an autoimmune mechanism similar to rheumatic fever. The disease can occur at any age, but is most common in male children. Griffiths types 1, 4, 12, 25, and 49 have been noted to be nephrogenic. No increase in anti-streptolysin O occurs in case of kidney cancer, urinary tract infection, and infectious mononucleosis. A diffuse red "sandpaper" rash appears from the upper chest to the trunk and extremities. *(Ryan et al, pp 273–276; Roitt et al, pp 24.1–24.2)*

154. (B) Patients with chronic granulomatous disease are repeatedly infected with catalase-positive microorganisms such as staphylococci. In contrast to this, the patients are rarely infected with catalase-negative bacteria such as streptococci. This is because catalase-negative bacteria accumulate hydrogen peroxide, activating the defective myeloperoxide–hydrogen peroxide–halide system of the host neutrophils. Chronic granulomatous disease patients cannot generate hydrogen peroxide metabolically because of their genetic defect in NADPH oxidase. *(Ryan et al, p 817)*

155. (D) The molecules that participate in adhesive interactions in the immune response belong to at least three identified families of molecules: the integrin family, the immunoglobulin superfamily, and the selectin family. The integrin family includes the three leukocyte cell adhesion molecules: Leu-CAM-LFA-1, Mac-1, and p150,95. The immunoglobulin superfamily includes, in addition to immunoglobulin and the antigen-specific T-cell receptor, the T-cell coreceptor molecules CD4 and CD8, the T-cell activation antigen, and others. The selectin family includes the MEL14/LAM-1 and ELAM-1. *(Joklik et al, p 297)*

156. (E) Radiation therapy, human immunodeficiency virus infections, and malnutrition all weaken the immune system. The use of broad-spectrum antibiotics for an extended period of time promotes opportunistic infections by drug-resistant organisms by eliminating the normal microbial flora that are sensitive to the antibiotics. *(Joklik et al, pp 394–400)*

157. (C) The capsule protects bacteria from phagocytosis in two different ways. Encapsulated bacteria are not readily phagocytosed because the slimy capsules make it difficult for phagocytes to hold firmly on the bacterial surface. Some of the microbial cell wall components (complement receptors, for example) are masked by the capsule making it difficult or impossible for complement to bind. Encapsulated bacteria, therefore, cannot bind complement directly. The plasma membrane of phagocytes possess receptors for C3b, C3d, C3bi, or mannose. However, these receptors of phagocytes cannot function efficiently in such encapsulated bacteria unless they are first coated with specific anticapsular antibodies and complement. All other bacterial components do not mask the complement receptors or opsonin receptors of the bacterial cell surface. *(Joklik et al, pp 350,390)*

158. (E) All of the statements listed in A through D are correct. Exotoxins are those toxins that are released extracellularly by bacteria. They are produced by both gram-positive and gram-negative bacteria. Diphtheria toxin is produced by *Corynebacterium diphtheriae*, which is a gram-positive bacterium. Cholera toxin is produced by *Vibrio cholerae*, which is a gram-negative bacterium. In contrast to exotoxins, endotoxin is a toxin associated with the cell wall of gram-negative bacteria. Diphtheria and tetanus toxoids are used as vaccines to immunize children, and in some cases, adults. Ingestion of foods contaminated with botulinum toxin or staphylococcal enterotoxin can cause severe diseases even if viable bacteria that produce these toxins are absent in the foods. Although many microbial exotoxins consist of A and B subunits (B subunit binds to cell-surface receptors and A subunit mediates toxic activity), some others do not have such A-B structure. *(Joklik et al, pp 390–391)*

159. (E) All conditions listed in A through D facilitate intracellular killing of phagocytosed pathogens. *(Joklik et al, pp 350–351; Roitt et al, pp 17.9–17.10)*

160. (E) All compounds listed in A to D are products of oxygen metabolism and participate in microbicidal activity of phagocytes via oxygen-dependent mechanisms. Hydrolytic enzymes, such as lysozyme, can kill phagocytosed bacteria even in the absence of oxygen. *(Joklik et al, p 350)*

161. (D) Neutrophils contain myeloperoxidase, which utilizes hydrogen peroxide and halide ions to produce hypohalite ions such as hypochlorite. Hypochlorite is highly microbicidal. Although all of the compounds listed in this question are microbicidal under certain conditions, they are not the effector molecules generated by the myeloperoxidase system. *(Joklik et al, p 351)*

162. **(B)** Human leukocyte antigen (HLA) is the major histocompatibility complex in man. HLA-A, HLA-B, HLA-DP, HLA-DQ, and HLA-DR are the main components. The complex is a remarkable cluster of genes that control T-cell recognition of self and nonself. HLA complex plays no role in platelet aggregation, adherence to endothelial cell surface, or activation of complement. *(Joklik et al, pp 214,265–270)*

163. **(D)** Antigen-presenting cells (APCs) do not present antigens to plasma cells, but rather to mature B cells, with the help of T-helper cells. The stimulated B cells then proliferate into plasma cells, which are the antibody-forming cells. APC are DR (class II gene product)-positive. Although B cells can present antigens, they are not phagocytic cells. *(Joklik et al, pp 209–210; Roitt et al, pp 8.3–8.8)*

164. **(D)** The B-cell receptor for antigen is a surface-bound immunoglobulin (mostly IgM and IgD) and can directly recognize antigen, without the necessity of MHC class II determinants. The B-cell receptor is not encoded for the genes that encode the T-cell receptor. The gene encoding for antibodies are rearranged in the course of progenitor cell development. Pre-B cells have μ (mu) heavy chain in their cytoplasm, not on the cell surface. The B-cell receptor for antigen can recognize antigen alone, and it does not function as a lymphokine receptor. *(Joklik et al, pp 233–235,252; Roitt et al, pp 2.7,10.10)*

165. **(A)** Among the cell types listed, only macrophages can present antigens to T cells. In addition to macrophages, Kupffer cells, interdigitating dendritic cells, B cells, and certain other cells (astrocytes of the brain, follicular cells of the thyroid, endothelium of vascular tissues, and some fibroblast) can also present antigens to T cells. *(Roitt et al, p 8.3)*

166. **(E)** All of the statements listed in A through D of this question are correct. Neutrophils can be activated, but they do not further differentiate to any other types of cells. Pro-B and pre-B cells differentiate into B cells. *(Roitt et al, pp 2.14–2.15; Roitt et al, pp 2.15,10.10)*

167. **(A)** The secondary immune response produces much higher antibody titer of IgG at the peak of the response. The secondary response has a shorter lag period. In both the primary and secondary immune response, the synthesis of IgM precedes that of IgG. *(Joklik et al, pp 247–249; Roitt et al, pp 8.13–8.15)*

168. **(E)** All of the statements listed in A through D of this question are correct. With most antigens, the maturation and differentiation of B cells and the switch from IgM to IgG production is dependent upon T cells. More specifically, the switch from production of IgM to IgG depends upon a subpopulation of T cells designated T helper (T_H) lymphocytes. *(Joklik et al, pp 220,256–258; Roitt et al, pp 9.1–9.4)*

169. **(E)** Haptens without carriers are not immunogenic and therefore cannot elicit antibody formation in T-dependent antibody responses. Hapten-carrier complexes can neither induce antibody production in T cells themselves nor induce new receptors on T cells. *(Joklik et al, pp 207,219; Roitt et al, pp 8.6,25.2)*

170. **(D)** The enzyme papain cleaves the heavy chains on the amino-terminal side of the single interheavy chain disulfide bond. Thus papain digestion of an IgG molecule would produce one Fc fragment and two Fab fragments. Reduction of the light chain–heavy chain disulfide bonds in the presence of denaturants results in the separation of light chains (kappa or lambda) and heavy chains or heavy-chain fragments. $F(ab')_2$ and small peptides are produced when IgG molecules are digested by pepsin. Bence Jones proteins are either kappa or lambda type of light chains. *(Joklik et al, pp 225–227; Roitt et al, p 4.10)*

171. **(E)** Ouchterlony analysis is a powerful yet simple technique that allows qualitative detection of antigens in solution and permits

the determination of antigenic relationship between different antigens. Although the result of analysis is affected by a number of factors (see A through D), it is not affected by isotypes of the antibody in the antiserum. Isotype refers to class or subclass of an immunoglobulin common to all members of that species. (*Joklik et al, pp 238–239; Roitt et al, p 28.2*)

172. **(E)** Antigen binding occurs at the variable region located in Fab, not Fc, fragments. The surface of phagocytes (macrophages and neutrophils), K cells, and placental syncytiotrophoblast cells is equipped with the receptor for the Fc fragment of an IgG molecule. The C1q component of complement interacts with a portion of the Fc fragment. (*Joklik et al, pp 225–230; Roitt et al, pp 4.10–4.12*)

173. **(D)** Both antigen and antibody are completely precipitated at the equivalent zone, and no uncombined (free) antigen, antibody, or immune complex is found in the supernatant. Maximum complement is fixed at this zone. Additional antibody or antigen is found in the supernatant at the zone of antibody excess or antigen excess, respectively. (*Joklik et al, pp 238–239; Roitt et al, p 28.1*)

174. **(E)** IgA antibodies are secretory immunoglobulin molecules occurring most commonly in seromucous secretions such as saliva, colostrum, milk, and tracheobronchial and genitourinary secretions. IgA molecules contain one unique component (secretory component) not found in other immunoglobulin molecules. IgA molecules held in dimeric form are coupled to the transport (secretory) piece in the epithelium as they traverse epithelial cell layers. IgA cannot cross the placental barrier. IgG molecules can cross the barrier. The classic pathway of the complement system is activated by antigen–antibody complexes or by aggregated immunoglobulins. Human immunoglobulins belonging to the IgM class or the IgG1, IgG2, or IgG3 subclasses are capable of initiating the classic pathway, whereas the IgA, IgD, IgE classes, and IgG4 subclass are not. (*Joklik et al, pp 223–227; Roitt et al, pp 4.5–4.8*)

175. **(D)** Although all of the techniques listed in this question may allow the detection of antigen for certain purposes, immunofluorescence is by far the most suitable and frequently used technique for the visual microscopic detection of antigens in tissue sections or on the cell surface. Agglutination, radioimmunoassay, and mixed lymphocyte reaction are not suitable for visual microscopic detection of antigen in the diagnostic laboratory. (*Joklik et al, pp 238–244; Roitt et al, pp 28.1–28.7*)

176. **(E)** All of the techniques listed in the question can be used for the detection of antitetanus toxin antibodies in a patient's serum. However, enzyme-linked immunosorbent assay is by far the most sensitive of all. The counterimmunoelectrophoresis and immunodiffusion methods are the least sensitive techniques. (*Joklik et al, pp 238–244; Roitt et al, pp 28.1–28.7*)

177. **(D)** The interaction between an antigen and an antibody is noncovalent. Under proper conditions, most antigen–antibody complexes can be dissociated. (*Joklik et al, pp 236–237; Roitt et al, p 7.2*)

178. **(D)** Each of the five immunoglobulin classes has an antigenically distinct set of heavy chains. It is called gamma in IgG. Antiserum directed against human IgG, therefore, reacts with gamma Fc fragment (a portion of gamma heavy chain that contains Fc at its C end). Since mu fragment and J chain are components of IgM, an antiserum directed against IgG does not react with the IgM components. By the same token, an antiserum directed against IgG does not react with alpha Fc fragment because alpha chain is the heavy chain of IgA molecules. Since human and rabbit immunoglobulins are antigenically distinct, an antiserum directed against human IgG will not react with rabbit kappa chain. (*Joklik et al, pp 223–227; Roitt et al, pp 4.1–4.12*)

179. **(E)** Isotypic variation of IgG refers to the different heavy- and light-chain classes and subclasses. The variants produced are present in

all healthy individuals within a given species. Allotype variation occurs predominantly in the constant region; not all variants are found in all normal individuals. Occurrence of idiotypic variation is limited to the variable region only, and idiotypes are specific to each antibody molecule. In a given individual, light chains of IgG exist in two antigenically distinct forms, kappa and lambda. In man, antibodies with kappa and lambda light chains are present in about an equal number. Therefore, an antiserum prepared against the whole molecules of IgG would react with all of the determinants or components of IgG molecules listed in the question. *(Joklik et al, pp 205,223–227; Roitt et al, pp 4.1–4.12)*

180. **(E)** All of the statements (A through D) listed in the question are correct. Immune complexes formed in vivo are usually cleared by the mononuclear phagocytic cells of different tissues (previously known as the reticuloendothelial system). The spleen represents one of such tissues. Immune complexes containing low-affinity antibody tend to persist in circulation and are bound to glomerular receptors or localized in synovial Fc-bearing cells, causing immune complex diseases (glomerulonephritis and rheumatoid arthritis). *(Joklik et al, pp 321–322; Roitt et al, pp 2.11–2.13,10.3)*

181. **(E)** Idiotypic determinants and antibody specificity of the immunoglobulin molecule are located in the variable region only. Fc is located in heavy chains, not in light chains. Pepsin digestion gives rise to pFc fragment, which corresponds to the constant gamma-3 domain of heavy chain. Papain cleaves the IgG molecule in the hinge region between the constant gamma-1 and constant gamma-2 domains to give two identical Fab fragments and one Fc fragment. *(Joklik et al, pp 225–226; Roitt et al, pp 4.1–4.10)*

182. **(E)** This particular group of cells is previously termed "the reticuloendothelial system" (RES). The cells belonging to this group have two main functions: phagocytosis and

antigen presentation. T lymphocytes cannot present antigen and cannot phagocytose. *(Roitt et al, pp 2.11–2.13)*

183. **(B)** B cells produce antibodies of five major classes: IgM, IgD, IgG, IgA, and IgE. There are four subclasses of IgG and two of IgA. Each terminally differentiated plasma cell is derived from a specific B cell and produces antibodies of just one class or subclass. *(Roitt et al, p 10.12)*

184. **(C)** A variety of cells—phagocytes, lymphocytes (subsets of both B and T cells), other blood cells (erythrocytes, nonprimate platelets, endothelium), and other tissue cells (glomerular cells)—possess receptors for the complement components. These receptors are called complement receptors. The other cell-surface proteins (classes I and II MHC antigens and viral antigens) do not function as complement receptors. Complement receptors are also present on the surface of many microbial cells *(Joklik et al, pp 292–293; Roitt et al, pp 13.10–13.12)*

185. **(C)** Class I restricted T cells (cytotoxic T cells) recognize endogenous antigens synthesized within the target cell, whereas class II restricted T cells (helper T cells) recognize exogenous antigens. The presentation of antigen by B cells to helper T cells is restricted by MHC class II molecules. Although multiple cell surface molecules interact during antigen presentation to T cells, the presentation is restricted either by class I or class II molecules, never by both. *(Roitt et al, pp 7.1–13,8.1–8.8)*

186. **(D)** Lysis of bacteria with opsonin requires the complement system activated by the classic pathway. In this system, both early and late complement components are required. *(Joklik et al, pp 291–292; Roitt et al, pp 13.13–13.14)*

187. **(E)** All of the activities listed in this question are associated with anaphylotoxins (C3a and C5a). C3b, not C3a, promotes immune adherence (cytoadherence) by phagocytes bearing complement receptors. *(Joklik et al, p 293)*

188. (E) All of the statements listed in A through D are correct. *(Joklik et al, pp 286–293; Roitt et al, pp 13.1–13.5)*

189. (E) All of the activities listed in this question are biologic consequences of complement activation. *(Joklik et al, pp 286–293; Roitt et al, pp 13.12–13.16)*

190. (B) Complement is not directly involved in plasma coagulation. Complement is not involved in antibody formation. Thus its defect does not affect the production of complement-fixing antibody. Complement defect does not enhance resistance to viral infections. *(Joklik et al, pp 293–294)*

191. (B) Antigen–antibody complex triggers activation of complement via the classic pathway. Other compounds listed in the question play roles in complement activation but do not trigger its activation. *(Joklik et al, p 290)*

192. (C) Hemolysin and erythrocytes are used in a complement-fixation test to detect the presence of "unused" or "unfixed" complement in the test system. An antibody itself does not bind to complement unless it first binds to an antigen. In rare instances, however, some antigens can fix complement. *(Joklik et al, pp 241–242; Roitt et al, pp 28.4)*

193. (E) All of the statements are associated with T-cell proliferation. *(Joklik et al, p 156; Roitt et al, pp 8.9–8.14)*

194. (A) Many tissue transplant and typing centers aim at a "six-antigen match," listed in A, which is an ideal match. All others are considered to be less than ideal. *(Joklik et al, pp 276–279,282; Roitt et al, pp 26.2–26.3)*

195. (E) All of the compounds listed in the question are involved in intracellular killing of microbes by activated macrophages. Nitric oxide is a newly added member of antimicrobial effector molecules metabolically produced from L-arginine in activated macrophages. *(Joklik et al, pp 314–318; Roitt et al, pp 17.6–17.8)*

196. (B) Rheumatic fever develops in a small group of individuals several weeks after a streptococcal infection of the throat. It is a form of autoimmune disease because "autoantibodies" to heart valve antigens can be detected in the patients. However, these antibodies are not autoantibodies in a strict sense of the word. These "autoantibodies" are produced in response to streptococcal antigens (M proteins), and heart valve antigens happen to cross-react with these antistreptococcal antibodies. Rheumatic fever usually occurs between the ages of 5 and 15 years, and affects connective tissues and endocardium. Recurrences lead to permanent damage to the heart valve and polyarthritis. No immediate hypersensitivity reaction is involved in this disease. *(Roitt, p 27.9; Ryan et al, p 273)*

197. (E) Antibody binds to target-cell membrane and activated C1q. This binding activates the classic complement pathway, depositing C3a and C4b2b3b (C5 convertase) on the target cell. The C5 convertase can activate the lytic pathway, causing membrane damage by C5 to C9 complement components. Eosinophilic chemotactic factor produced by T cells, mast cells, and basophils attracts eosinophils. Eosinophils bind certain parasites coated with IgG or IgE, and release cytotoxic proteins. *(Joklik et al, pp 291–292; Roitt et al, pp 9.5–9.7)*

198. (D) Individuals with type AB blood do not have antibody to the A and B antigens. If they did have they would agglutinate their own red blood cells. Such individuals cannot be classified as universal donors because their blood would be agglutinated by individuals with blood type A or B who have anti-B and anti-A in their serum respectively. Since individuals whose blood type is O have anti-A and anti-B antibodies in their serum, they cannot receive blood from individuals with blood type AB. *(Joklik et al, pp 212,283–284; Roitt et al, 23.3–23.5)*

199. (E) *Candida albicans* is one of the most common opportunistic pathogens. All of the conditions listed here create a "compromised state" in the host. Malignancy tends to suppress the normal immune functions. Hormonal and physiological changes associated with pregnancy increase the incidence of vaginal candidiasis. The use of broad-spectrum antibiotics (such as tetracycline) for extended periods of time eliminates the normal microbial flora allowing *C. albicans* to grow without competition. The use of nonsterile needle or repeated punctures of the skin allows *C. albicans* and *Candida parapsilosis* to colonize in the wound. *(Roitt et al, pp 21.1,21–10)*

200. **(A)** Antigen–antibody complexes are commonly formed in response to a wide range of microbial and other foreign antigens, and usually are cleared by phagocytic cells without any host damage. Under certain conditions, however, antigen–antibody or antibody–antibody (eg, rheumatoid factor, cryoglobulin) complexes may lead to localized tissue inflammation. Whether they do depends largely on the ability of an immune complex to form or deposit at fixed-tissue sites and then activate the complement complex. The size of the complex, charge, solubility, tissue affinity, etc. would influence the development of immune-complex diseases. All others are not the major mechanism of the development of immune-complex diseases. *(Joklik et al, pp 321–322)*

201. **(E)** Human systemic lupus erythematosus is a type III hypersensitivity. It is characterized by the production of autoantinuclear antibodies, circulating immune complexes, immune complex deposits in the glomeruli, positive lupus cell tests, and positive Coombs' tests. Proteinuria is usually present in the patients due to altered membrane permeability in the kidney. *(Joklik et al, pp 211,321–322; Roitt et al, p 27.2)*

202. **(E)** The destruction of the effector B and T cells by lymphoid irradiation and antilymphocyte globulin injection or the use of immune suppressants such as cyclosporin and steroids would suppress rejection of transplanted tissues. Cyclosporin is thought to in-

hibit, among other effects, interleukin-2, which drives antigen-activated cells into proliferation. *(Joklik et al, pp 282–283; Roitt et al, pp 26.8–26.12)*

203. **(E)** T-helper cells are activated by antigen presenting cells to release lymphokines. IL-2 and INF-γ are required for Tc cell activation. IL-2, IL-4, and IL-5 are involved in B-cell activation. INF-γ acts as a macrophage-activating factor. T-helper cells neither promote complement production nor mediate graft damage by expressing IL-2 receptors. T-helper cells do not mediate graft damage directly by producing tissue necrosis factor. T-helper cells do not fix cytotoxic antibodies. *(Joklik et al, pp 283–284,378–379; Roitt et al, pp 26.5–26.7)*

204. **(D)** All of the three events (A through C) listed in the question induce immunologic tolerance. High doses of such antigens as the diphtheria toxoid or the pneumococcal polysaccharide saturate the B- and T-cell receptors and thus suppress the normal immunologic response of the lymphoid cells. Either natural or artificial exposure to an antigen during embryonic life when the B and T cells are immature will not allow these cells to respond to the antigen during the adult life of the host into which the antigen was injected. *(Joklik et al, pp 258–262; Roitt et al, pp 12.2–12.10)*

205. **(A)** Stem cells are not immunocompetent. All of the statements listed in B through E are correct. *(Joklik et al, p 250; Roitt et al, pp 10.1–10.2)*

206. **(E)** To successfully transduce receptor-ligand signal, B cells must have all of the components listed in the question. *(Joklik et al, pp 234–235, Roitt et al, p 2.9)*

207. **(D)** The fully developed plasma cells no longer divide or enter the bloodstream. The plasma cells carry very little surface immunoglobulin. They also develop some new cell-surface glycoproteins and lose some, but the cell-surface IgM specificity remains unchanged. *(Joklik et al, p 206; Roitt et al, pp 2.9,4.1)*

208. **(D)** When a B cell undergoes class switch from IgM to IgA, the cell possesses both IgM and IgA on the cell surface. The specificity of IgA remains the same as that of IgM. *(Joklik et al, p 206; Roitt et al, pp 6.9–6.12,8.14–8.15, 10.12–10.13)*

209. (B) The maturation of T cells can be followed through changes in surface markers. Unlike B cells, mature T cells do not carry surface immunoglobulin, but they do express T-cell receptors with idiotypes that can be recognized through binding studies with appropriate monoclonal antibodies. No significant changes in cell size and DNA content occur during T-cell maturation. There is no change in the type of T-cell receptor during T-cell maturation. *(Joklik et al, pp 208,235–236; Roitt et al, pp 10.5–10.7)*

210. (B) The cornea is not a highly vascularized tissue. Primary corneal grafts are usually performed without HLA matching or immunosuppression, not because the cornea lacks antigens, but rather because the anterior chamber of the eye is one of a limited number of what are known as immunologically privileged sites. Privileged sites lack lymphatic drainage, and the small amount of antigen released into the bloodstream from grafts in these sites is not sufficient to trigger a cellular response. When the recipient cornea is moderately vasculated or inflamed, it could be rejected. *(Joklik et al, p 283)*

211. (B) All of the organs or tissues (except the spleen) listed in the question are immunologically privileged sites, which are shielded from antigen under normal conditions. *(Joklik et al, p 209)*

212. (A) IgA deficiency is the most common immunodeficiency. One in 700 Caucasians have the defect, but it is not found in other ethnic groups. *(Roitt et al, 21.2)*

213. (B) In an ideal match, a six-antigen match (HLA-A, HLA-B, and HLA-DR) on donor and recipient should be the same. Among the four donors listed, donor 2 has the tissue type closest to that of the recipient. *(Joklik et al, pp 282–283; Roitt et al, pp 26.3–26.9)*

214. (A) Both MHC class I and class II antigens are critically important in the self and nonself recognition in the immune system. In humans, class I antigens are coded for by HLA-A, HLA-B, and HLA-C genes, and MHC class II antigens are coded for by DR, DQ, and DP genes. In an identical twin brother or sister, these key class I and class II antigens are identical; thus, the recipient recognizes the donor's tissues as "self," not as "nonself." *(Joklik et al, pp 282–283; Roitt et al, p 26.3)*

215. (D) The results of the mixed lymphocyte reaction correlate with the degree of dissimilarity of histocompatibility. Higher counts indicate more stimulation suggesting immunologic unrelatedness of tissues tested. Human leukocyte–antigen-identical sibs do not stimulate mixed leukocyte reaction, indicating that their tissues are mutually transplantable. *(Joklik et al, p 269; Roitt et al, pp 26.8–26.10)*

216. (E) Selective IgA deficiency has been observed in apparently healthy individuals. As expected, however, IgA deficient individuals suffer from the respiratory, gastrointestinal, and urogenital tract infections. People with IgA deficiency also tend to develop immune complex diseases (type III hypersensitivity). About 20% of IgA-deficient individuals also lack IgG2, IgG4, and are very susceptible to pyogenic infections. In humans, most antibodies to the capsular polysaccharides of pyogenic bacteria are in the IgG2 subclass. *(Joklik et al, p 331; Roitt et al, p 21.2)*

217. (D) Passive immunization using gamma globulin with high titers of antimeasles antibodies is the best prophylactic measure that one could take in this situation. Other measures are either inappropriate or ineffective for preventing measles in this patient. *(Joklik et al, pp 204,341–342,1013; Roitt et al, p 16.3)*

218. (C) Cytotoxic T cells require MHC class I, not class II antigen. Natural killer (NK) cells are not MHC restricted. Both cytotoxic T cells and NK cells have large azurophilic granules. *(Roitt et al, pp 1.4,2.7–2.8,9.5–9.7)*

219. (C) If there is no record of prior tetanus toxoid immunization in this patient, one should assume that he/she has no antitetanus toxin antibody. This finding indicates that the chance of developing tetanus is very high in this patient. Administration of human immune globulin will prevent the immediate threat of tetanus, and toxoid immunization will prevent future incidence of the disease. All other measures are inappropriate. *(Joklik et al, pp 365,647–648; Roitt et al, p 19.9)*

220. (E) Individuals with defects of C3 suffer from severe recurrent bacterial infections. Sera from these patients generate less chemotactic activity and support less phagocytic activity than normal sera. One product of C3 cleavage, C3a, has anaphylotoxic activity. To generate the membrane attack complex, the C4b2a3b complex of the classic pathway and the C3bBbC3b complex of the alternative pathway are required. Thus, the absence of C3 affects adversely all of the activities listed in the question. *(Joklik et al, pp 288–294; Roitt et al, pp 21.8–21.9)*

221. (D) Immediate hypersensitivity (type I reaction) is mediated by IgE. No other classes of immunoglobulin mediate type I reaction. In type I reaction, soluble components responsible for eliciting pharmacologic reactions derive from basophils and mast cells, not from granulocytes. Complement is not directly involved in type I reaction. In the other types of hypersensitivity such as type II reaction, complement-mediated toxicity plays important roles in its pathogenesis. *(Joklik et al, p 319; Roitt et al, pp 22.2–22.4,22.9–22.14)*

222. (C) Heat-shock proteins, also termed stress proteins, are produced in response to stress by virtually all prokaryotic and eukaryotic cells. T cells expressing the gamma, delta T-cell receptor antigen receptors appear to recognize these proteins. The heat-shock proteins represent major antigens of many pathogens and have been identified as targets of host immune responses in numerous autoimmune diseases. Antibodies to specific heat-shock proteins are seen in patients with rheumatoid arthritis, systemic lupus erythematosus, ankylosing spondylitis, and others. *(Joklik et al, p 317; Roitt et al, p 17.11)*

223. (E) All of the examples listed in A through D of the question are well-established examples of antigenic mimicry responsible for autoimmune responses. There is no structural or antigenic similarity between plasma membrane lipids and bacterial endotoxin (lipid A), which is derived from the outer membrane of gram-negative bacteria. *(Joklik et al, p 363; Roitt et al, p 27.9)*

224. (D) Perforin, serine protease, and lymphotoxin (INFα/β and INF-γ) are all implicated in lysis of target cells by cytotoxic T cells. *(Joklik et al, p 327; Roitt et al, pp 9.6–9.8)*

225. (E) All of the events listed in the question (A through D) occur during phagocytosis of bacteria. Phagocytes do not release interleukin-2 (IL-2). IL-2 is a T-cell product. *(Joklik et al, pp 314–315; Roitt et al, pp 1.9,9.1–9.2,13.11)*

226. (D) All of the extracellular matrix proteins listed in the question except keratin are important in cell–cell interaction and cellular adherence. *(Joklik et al, p 292; Roitt et al, p 14.1)*

227. (E) LFA-1 belongs to the beta-2 integrin family and is expressed in all leukocytes except for some peritoneal macrophages. This cell-surface protein is essential for cell–cell and cell–extracellular matrix adhesion. *(Joklik et al, pp 297–301)*

228. (A) A major deficit in children less than 2 years old is their inability to make antibodies against polysaccharide antigens. There is a period of 2 to 3 months after birth when the transferred maternal antibodies are protective, followed by 2 years of relatively high danger from infection as passively transferred antibody declines. When exposed to a polysaccharide antigen, children in this age range can transiently make IgM antibodies, but IgG antibodies do not develop, and no memory B cells are established. *(Joklik et al, p 362)*

229. (C) B cells, rather than T cells, proliferate and differentiate to become antibody-secreting plasma cells; hence, statement C is incorrect. All of the other statements are correct. *(Joklik et al, pp 203–221)*

230. (B) All animals have innate or nonadaptive systems that act as an initial defense system against microbes. In addition to the epithelial surfaces and phagocytic cells, they also consist of nonspecific soluble circulating factors such as complement components, lysozyme, acute-phase proteins (C protein, for example), interferon, etc. Opsonic antibodies are produced specifically against antigens of microbes. When these specific opsonins (antibodies) combine with bacterial surface antigens that normally allow the bacteria to interact with phagocytosis, the bacteria are more readily phagocytosed and killed. Antigens that have bound opsonic antibody, which can then interact with complement and bind C3b complement component, are even more easily phagocytosed than antigen alone. These antigens are more easily phagocytosed because phagocytes have Fc and C3 receptors on their cell surfaces. Complement itself is able to lyse some bacteria nonspecifically. The production of opsonic antibodies is an adaptive response and thus is the correct answer. C-reactive protein binds the bacterial cell surface causing complement to deposit. Such opsonized bacteria are readily engulfed by phagocytes. *(Joklik et al, pp 214,347–351; Roitt et al, pp 1.5,17.6)*

231. (E) Macrophages and neutrophils both are phagocytic and display movement, contain lysosomal granules, and have receptors for the Fc portion of IgG. However, only one subset of macrophages present antigen to T cells; neutrophils cannot present antigens. *(Joklik et al, pp 209,349; Roitt et al, pp 2.1–2.18)*

232. (A) Only IgG is able to cross the human placenta and provide passive immunity to the fetus. This maternally derived antibody is an example of naturally acquired passive immunity. All of the other statements are wrong. If the fetus is infected, it produces IgM. The presence of IgM in the cord blood is a means of identifying that there was a neonatal infection such as congenital syphilis. *(Joklik et al, p 382; Roitt et al, pp 4.2,19.9)*

233. (B) Most infants with agammaglobulinemia remain well during the first 6 to 9 month of life, presumably by virtue of maternally transmitted IgG antibodies. Thereafter, they repeatedly acquire infections with extracellular pyogenic organisms such as pneumococci, streptococci, and *Hemophilus*. To cope with these, the patients should be given gamma globulin therapy and prophylactic antibiotics. *(Joklik et al, p 329)*

234. (C) Patients with chronic granulomatous disease have defective NADPH oxidase. This enzyme normally canalizes the reduction of O_2 to O_2^-. O_2^- is then quickly converted to hydrogen peroxide. As a result, the patients are incapable of forming hydrogen peroxide. Thus, the myeloperoxidase–hydrogen peroxide–halide system (a key microbicidal system in neutrophils) cannot function in the patients. Their neutrophils can phagocytose microorganisms but cannot kill them. As a result, microorganisms remain alive in phagocytes, giving rise to persistent cell-mediated responses to intracellularly growing bacteria. Bacteria and fungi that produce catalase are usually implicated in the infections. *(Roitt et al, 21.9)*

235. (A) HIV-1 is transmitted between humans in three ways: sexually, perinatally, and by exposure to contaminated blood or body fluid. Transmission does not occur through day-to-day nonsexual contact with infected individuals or through insect vectors. This is because of the fragility of the virus and the need for direct mucosal or blood contact. *(Ryan et al, pp 548–549)*

236. (D) Cytochromes are respiratory enzymes located primarily in mitochondria and are not involved in intracellular killing of microorganisms. All of the other statements are correct. Phagocytes kill engulfed bacteria by two distinct mechanisms: oxygen-dependent and oxygen-independent. Effectors involved in the oxygen-dependent mechanism are superoxide, hydrogen peroxide, singlet oxygen, and hydroxyl radical. Molecules responsible for the oxygen-independent mechanism include cationic proteins and hydrolytic enzymes contained in the lysosome. Low intracellular pH of phagocytosing cells also contributes to the killing of phagocytosed bacteria. (*Joklik et al, pp 350–351*)

237. **(A)** In chronic granulomatous disease (CGD) of children, there is a deficit in NADPH oxidase. This oxidase reoxidizes NADPH to NADP, allowing the hexosemonophosphate (pentose–phosphate) pathway to continue operating. As in all oxidase reactions, there is also formation of H_2O_2. Thus, in CGD, there is a deficit in H_2O_2 generation, which is needed for the bactericidal activity of the myeloperoxidase–halide system. As a consequence, the microbes are phagocytosed but are not killed at a normal rate. There are no defects in other components or functions of phagocytes in this disease. (*Joklik et al, pp 340–341; Roitt et al, pp 21.9–21.10*)

238. **(D)** There is a dual role for T cells in antituberculosis immunity: to recruit phagocytic mononuclear cells for the formation of granulomas and to activate the macrophages for enhanced microbicidal activity. Macrophage activation, particularly near the center of granulomas, is the major mechanism of host resistance to tuberculosis. Delayed hypersensitivity does not protect the host against tuberculosis. Humoral antibody, serum calcium, and polymorphonuclear neutrophil (PMN) count play no important role in the host resistance to tuberculosis. (*Joklik et al, pp 351,506; Roitt et al, p 17.8*)

239. **(E)** Secondary immunodeficiencies are those that result from extrinsic or environmental causes. Worldwide, malnutrition is probably the leading cause of immunodeficiency in children; it leads to a profound T-cell deficiency. Malignancy itself also causes immunodeficiency. Most drugs used in cancer chemotherapy are cytotoxic for T cells. The selective destruction of CD4+ T cells and monocyte/macrophage lineages by HIV are known to cause severe immunodeficiency in AIDS patients. (*Roitt et al, pp 21.6–21.10*)

240. **(E)** Bence Jones proteins are monoclonal free light chains appearing in large quantity in serum and/or urine of multiple myeloma patients. Other proteins listed in the question are not at all related to Bence Jones proteins. (*Chapel and Haeney, p 126*)

241. **(E)** A vaccine produced from an extracellular toxic bacterial product, an exotoxin, which is made nontoxic (usually with dilute formaldehyde) but maintains antigenicity, is known as a toxoid. The toxoid induces the formation of specific antitoxin antibodies that serve as the basis for the specific protection from the toxin. Not all toxins can be converted to toxoids by treatment with formaldehyde or heat. (*Joklik et al, p 366; Roitt et al, 19.3*)

242. **(E)** Molecules encoded by MHC class II are proteins, not lipoproteins, and are located on the HLA-D gene locus, not the HLA-B locus, which produces class I molecules (along with regions A and C). The complement proteins are encoded by the class III region. Essentially all human nucleated cells carry the antigens of the A, B, and C class I regions. Class II antigens (HLA-DR, DQ, and DP) have a more restricted distribution; class II antigens are expressed on B cells, macrophages, and dendritic cells. (*Joklik et al, pp 209–210,268–269; Roitt et al, pp 5.3–5.9*)

243. **(C)** European Caucasian patients possessing the HLA-B27 antigens do have an 88% relative risk, compared to patients without the antigen, of having ankylosing spondylitis. Also, the relative risk for patients with the DR3 antigen of having celiac disease is 13%. The maximum relative risk for having rheumatoid arthritis (4%), myasthenia gravis (3%), multiple sclerosis (4%), and psoriasis (9%), depending on which antigen is being compared, is much lower. (*Joklik et al, pp 279–282; Roitt et al, p 11.12*)

244. **(D)** The characteristic marker of cells of B-lymphocyte lineage, which act as the cell-surface antigen receptors, is the possession of

immunoglobulins. Binding of antigens to antigen receptors triggers the process of B-cell activation. All other statements are incorrect. Fc receptors are not antigen-binding receptors. (*Joklik et al, pp 252–253. Roitt et al, pp 2.6–2.7*)

245. (E) Monocytes/macrophages are found primarily in the skin, lymph nodes, spleen, and thymus, not just in lymph nodes. Therefore, statement E is incorrect and is the answer. Monocytes/macrophages are rich in MHC class II antigens and are important for presenting antigens to cells. They are also actively phagocytic. (*Joklik et al, pp 249,348; Roitt et al, pp 1.2–1.4*)

246. (D) An antigen can be defined as a substance that specifically reacts with preformed products of the immune response; it may or may not be an immunogen. A hapten, an incomplete antigen, is a low-molecular-weight substance that is unable to induce an immune response by itself but can become immunogenic by combining with larger molecules (carriers). Homopolymers are usually not good antigens. The minimum size of immunogenicity appears to be about 500 to 1,000 daltons. (*Joklik et al, pp 218–219; Roitt et al, pp 7.7–7.8,8.6*)

247. (B) Freund's adjuvant consists of killed *M. tuberculosis* suspended in oil. This adjuvant is used to elicit stronger T- and B-cell mediated responses when antigens alone do not evoke sufficient immunogenic responses. This adjuvant is emulsified with the aqueous antigen solution before injecting into animals. (*Roitt et al, p 17.4*)

248. (E) The immature B cells, which are derived from pre-B cells, have surface IgM and can develop into the mature B cell without antigen stimulation. Thus, statement E is incorrect. On antigen stimulation, the mature B cell proliferates and develops into the plasma cell. (*Joklik et al, pp 251–252; Roitt et al, 10.8–10.11*)

249. (B) Surface immunoglobulins, which are the characteristic marker of cells of the B-lymphocyte lineage, act as the cell-surface antigen receptors. The surface immunoglobulin

of the immature B cell has surface IgM, and the mature (adult) B cell has other classes of immunoglobulin (IgD in most B cells). The surface immunoglobulins are not dimeric. They also contain, in addition to two heavy chains, a kappa or a lambda light chain, but not both. (*Joklik et al, pp 250–252; Roitt et al, pp 2.6–2.7*)

250. (D) There are a relatively small group of antigens, the T-independent antigens, which can activate B cells to produce antibody without the help of T cells. These T-independent antigens share some common properties: they are large polymers, have repeating antigenic determinants, and show resistance to rapid degradation. In addition, some of them can also, at relatively high concentrations, activate B-cell clones that are not specific for that particular antigen, a process called polyclonal B-cell activation. Serum albumin clearly does not share those properties, ie, it is an animal protein composed of 20 different L-amino acids. Therefore, it is a T-dependent antigen. (*Joklik et al, pp 209,220; Roitt et al, pp 8.5–8.6*)

251. (D) BCG is a bovine strain of tubercle bacilli attenuated in the laboratory, which has been used successfully as a live vaccine in the prevention of tuberculosis, particularly in underdeveloped countries. Although BCG has diminished virulence in normal individuals, it still can cause active infection in individuals (such as AIDS patients) whose immune system is severely compromised. All other vaccines listed in the questions are acellular vaccines posing no danger to immunocompromised patients. (*Roitt et al, pp 19.1–19.7*)

252. (D) Carbohydrates located on the Fc segment provides binding sites for receptors on placental syncytiotrophoblasts, neutrophils, and K cells. The Fc segment may also play a role in Ig secretion by plasma cells. The binding to receptors on placental syncytiotrophoblasts is essential for transplacental transport of IgG molecules. (*Joklik et al, p 382; Roitt et al, p 14.10*)

253. **(C)** The biologic activity of an antibody molecule centers on its ability to specifically bind antigen. The combining site is located on the amino-terminal end of the antibody molecule and is composed of hypervariable segments within the variable regions of both light and heavy chains. Antibody specificity is a function of both the amino acid sequence and its three-dimensional configuration. *(Joklik et al, pp 227–230; Roitt et al, p 4.10)*

254. **(A)** The hypervariable regions are located on the Fab piece, not on the Fc piece. All other statements are correct. *(Joklik et al, pp 226–230; Roitt et al, p 4.10)*

255. **(E)** Conventional antibody responses are polyclonal and include many antibody molecules differing somewhat in their binding affinity. Monoclonal antibody is formed by a single clone of antibody-producing cells. Any given clone may produce any class of immunoglobulin. Characteristically, it has antibody-combining sites that are identical. Monoclonal antibodies are produced by the hybridoma technique (fusion of immune competent B cells to a myeloma cell). They are also produced by neoplastic plasma cells (multiple myeloma). Monoclonal antibodies are widely used for both diagnostic and therapeutic purposes. *(Joklik et al, pp 206,378,941,945; Roitt et al, pp 28.8–28.9)*

256. **(D)** Antigen–antibody reactions are highly specific. The binding of antigen to antibody does not involve covalent bonds but only relatively weak, short-range forces (eg, hydrogen bonding, electrostatic, van der Waals forces). The strength of antigen–antibody bonds depends on the closeness of tie between the configuration of the antigen-determinant site and the combining site of the antibody. Antibodies with the best fit and strongest binding are said to have high affinity for the antigen. *(Joklik et al, pp 336–337; Roitt et al, pp 7.1–7.3)*

257. **(E)** The number of combining sites on an antibody is referred to as antibody valence. This number will be determined by the equilibrium dialysis technique. IgG, IgA, IgD, and IgE have a valence of 2. The valence of IgM is 5 to 10. *(Joklik et al, pp 236–237; Roitt et al, pp 7.2–7.4)*

258. **(D)** Radioimmunoassays are the most sensitive and versatile techniques for the quantitation of antigens or haptene. Radioimmunoassay is particularly applicable to the measurement of serum levels of many hormones, drugs, and other biologic materials. The method is based on competition for a specific antibody between the labeled (known) and unlabeled (unknown) concentration of the antigen or haptens. *(Joklik et al, pp 240–241)*

259. **(C)** Haptens can bind to the host proteins or other carriers to form complete antigens. Many simple chemicals and drugs can function as haptens. *(Joklik et al, pp 207,213,237)*

260. **(E)** Cytotoxic T cells lyse a variety of cells, which include tumor cells, graft cells, cells attacked in autoimmune disease, and virus-infected cells. No bacteriolysis has been demonstrated by cytotoxic T cells. *(Joklik et al, pp 259,297,935–938; Roitt et al, pp 17.1–17.8)*

261. **(D)** Opsonin is a serum component, usually antibody or complement, which coats particulate organisms (bacteria) to promote phagocytosis. Both neutrophils and macrophages have Fc and C3 receptors on the cell surface. Therefore, opsonized bacteria are readily phagocytosed by these phagocytes. Opsonization itself does not lyse bacteria, but when complement is provided, opsonized gram-negative bacteria may undergo lysis. Opsonins neither remove the microbial capsule nor affect lysosomal enzymes. *(Joklik et al, p 350; Roitt et al, pp 1.5–1.7,13.2,13.11)*

262. **(D)** It is known that three mechanisms are involved in the generation of antibody diversity: multiple genes or germ-line diversity (numerous V genes, each encoding one variable-region domain), somatic mutation (primordial V genes mutate during B-cell ontogeny to produce different genes in different B-cell clones), and somatic recombination (heavy-chain gene segments, one of a dozen

D genes and one of four J genes recombine to join the main part of the variable-region gene). The light-chain genes lack D segments; thus, the number of recombinations is smaller. The environment is unlikely to generate antibody diversity. *(Joklik et al, pp 230–234; Roitt et al, pp 6.1–6.14)*

263. **(D)** Somatic mutations tend to involve only the V genes. The mutations affect both the kappa and lambda chains. It is not somatic mutation that scrambles the other genes and gene fragments. See the preceding comments. *(Roitt et al, pp 6.1–6.14)*

264. **(D)** The total or partial absence of C3 (in homozygous deficiency) and the virtual absence of C3 (in C3bINA deficiency) are associated with several bacterial infections, particularly with pneumonococcal septicemia, meningococcal septicemia, and meningitis. The association of C3 deficiency with increased susceptibility to viral or fungal infections is not clinically proven. *(Joklik et al, p 294; Roitt et al, pp 21.8–21.9)*

265. **(C)** The alternative pathway was originally known as the properdin pathway because properdin apparently caused complement activation by this mechanism. It stabilizes the C3 convertase causing massive conversion of C3 to C3b by discharging the feedback loop to exhaustion by forming the alternative pathway C5 convertase. This event causes C5 to C9 consumption. *(Joklik et al, pp 290–291; Roitt et al, p 13.4)*

266. **(E)** No imunosuppressive activity is known for vitamin C. Corticosteroids are antiinflammatory and suppress activated macrophages, decrease antigen-presenting-cell function, and reduce MHC expression. Cyclosporin suppresses lymphokine production by T_H cells by interfering with the activation of lymphokine genes, and directly or indirectly to reduce the expression of the receptors for IL-2 on lymphocytes undergoing activation. Alkylating agents interfere with DNA duplication in the premitotic phase and are most effective in rapidly dividing cells. Lymphoid irradiation produces long-term suppression of T-lymphocyte function. *(Roitt et al, pp 26.10–26.11; Chapel and Haeney, pp 137–139)*

267. **(D)** The C1q component of complement interacts with the C_H-2 domain, which is located on the Fc fragment. *(Joklik et al, pp 288–290; Roitt et al, p 13.3)*

268. **(E)** Anaphylotoxins (C3a and C5a) are split products of C3 and C5 respectively. Both C3a and C5a cause smooth muscle contraction, mast cell degranulation, neutrophil activation, and chemotaxis of neutrophils. C3a and C5a are inactivated by carboxypeptidase B, which removes the arginine group from the C3a and C5a. *(Joklik et al, pp 293; Roitt et al, pp 13.13)*

269. **(D)** C3 convertase of both the classical and alternative pathways may bind C3b to yield the enzymes that activate the next component of the complement system, C5: classical pathway C5 convertase, C4b2b3b, and alternative pathway C5 convertase C3bBb3b. The fixation of C5b and product of C5 convertase to biologic membrane triggers a series of events that results in the assembly of the membrane-attack complex. *(Joklik et al, pp 291–292; Roitt et al, pp 13.9–13.10)*

270. **(E)** Poststreptococcal glomerulonephritis is primarily a disease of childhood, characterized by edema, hypertension, hematuria, and proteinuria. The disease may follow either respiratory or cutaneous group A streptococcal infection. This causes an increase in ASO titers. Immunoglobulins, complements, and antigens that react with antibodies against group A streptococci have been detected in the affected glomerulus. This causes a transient decrease of serum C3 level. The M proteins of some nephritogenic strain have been shown to share antigenic determinants with glomeruli, which suggests an autoimmune mechanism similar to rheumatic fever. *(Ryan et al, pp 273–274)*

271. **(A)** The majority of NK cells are CD16+ (IgG Fc receptor), NKH1+, and CD3−, and do not contain productive rearrangement of the

T-cell receptor genes. NK cells vary in their sensitivity to regulatory actions of interferon, interleukins, and in the spectrum of cells they will lyse. *(Joklik et al, pp 214,375; Roitt et al, pp 1.5,2.7–2.8,9.5)*

272. (D) The pathogenic antibody to nuclei (DNA) is seen in systemic lupus erythematosus. In Hashimoto's thyroiditis, antithyroglobulin is the pathogenic antibody. In Addison's disease, antiadrenal cell antibody is implicated. Antiacetylcholine receptor antibody is the pathogenic antibody in myasthenia gravis. *(Joklik et al, p 321; Roitt et al, pp 27.1–27.12)*

273. (A) Insulin-dependent diabetes mellitus is believed to be initially caused by an environmental agent such as a virus infection of chemical poison. The destruction of insulin-secreting beta cells in the pancreas triggers an autoimmune response which perpetuates the damage. The pathogenic antibody in this disease is antipancreatic inslet cells. Thus, this type of diabetes mellitus is considered to be an organ-specific autoimmune disease. *(Roitt et al, pp 27.1–27.6)*

274. (B) Measurement of total IgE is useful in patients in whom parasites are suspected. The measurement is best performed by a radioimmunoassay since the normal level of IgE in the serum is extremely low (120 to 480 ng/mL). Other assay methods are either nonquantitative or less sensitive. *(Chapel and Haeney, p 427; Roitt et al, pp 28.6–28.)*

275. (C) Antibodies (IgM or IgG) develop after interferon production. Thus, they do not constitute the first line of defense against viruses. *(Joklik et al, pp 352–357; Roitt et al, pp 16.1–16.8)*

276. (D) B cells are characterized by their surface immunoglobulins. These immunoglobulin markers are made by the cells themselves, and are inserted into the surface membrane where they act as specific antigen receptors. Stem cells, monocytes, T cells, and neutrophils have no such surface membrane associated immunoglobulin markers. Pre-B cells express cytoplasmic μ chains only. The

immature B cell has surface IgM, and the mature B cell has other immunoglobulin isotypes (IgM, IgD). *(Roitt et al, pp 2.6,10.10–10.11)*

277. (D) INF-γ is produced by antigen-activated T lymphocytes and NK cells and serves to activate macrophages to enhanced levels of cytotoxicity. Interferons α and β act on virus-infected cells and block viral replication. *(Joklik et al, pp 316,861–862; Roitt et al, pp 16.1–16.8)*

278. (E) Since M proteins are not adherence-promoting cell-surface molecules of *Streptococcus pyogenes*, antibodies against M proteins do not affect the adherence of this bacterium to the epithelial surface. Since *S. pyogenes* is not a gram-negative bacterium, it has no lipid-containing outer membrane. Thus, complement-mediated bacteriolysis does not occur in this bacterium even in the presence of complement. The activity of natural killer cells has not been shown to be influenced by antibody to streptococcal M proteins. Finally, gram-positive bacteria are not killed by exposure to antibodies specific to their cell-surface components. Such antibody-coated bacteria are, however, engulfed by host phagocytes. *(Joklik et al, pp 79,420–422; Roitt et al, pp 1.5–1.7,13.2–13.11)*

279. (C) Resistance of microbes to killing by polymorphs and macrophages can be attributed to the production of phagocyte repellents, such as microbial toxins, by blockage of the attachment of phagocytes via the C3b receptor to microbes, or blockage of microbial engulfment via capsules. Phagocytosed microbes can defy destruction by preventing fusion of the lysosomes with the phagosomes. This engulfment of microbes results in the release of antimicrobial substances into the phagolysomes and the killing of microbes. In patients with the rare congenital disease known as Chediak–Higashi syndrome, there is a diminished capacity of the lysosomes to fuse with phagosomes. This diminished capacity leads to recurring bacterial infections involving bacteria of low pathogenicity. *(Joklik et al, pp 314–315,339-340,350-351; Ryan et al, p 817)*

280. (B) Innocuous antigens such as pollens stimulate B cells to produce specific IgE. Antigen-specific IgE binds to mast cells by the Fc receptors. This binding leads to the degranulation of the mast cells and the secretion of histamine, serotonin, and other pharmacologic mediators of inflammation that cause the symptoms encountered in type I allergy. Type I allergy (hypersensitivity) includes asthma, eczema, hay fever, and urticaria. *(Joklik et al, p 319; Roitt et al, pp 22.1–22.17)*

281. (E) Type II, or antibody-dependent cytotoxic hypersensitivity, is manifested when antibody combines with its antigen on cells leading to phagocytosis, killer-cell involvement, or complement-induced lysis. Examples of this type of reaction include autoimmune hemolytic anemia and Goodpasture syndrome. All other statements are either incorrect or incomplete. *(Joklik et al, pp 319–321; Roitt et al, pp 23.1–23.10)*

282. (A) Antigen-specific IgE is historically assessed by passive cutaneous anaphylaxis (PCA). An experimental animal is injected intracutaneously with serum containing IgE, which attaches to mast cells and sensitizes them. Two days later the specific antigen for IgE and a dye are injected intravenously. The antigen induces degranulation of mast cells and release of pharmacologic mediators (histamine, serotonin, bradykinin, slow-reacting substance, heparin, etc.) at the skin site where IgE was injected. The area of the dye in the skin is a measure of the antigen-specific IgE injected. Type IV hypersensitivity is a delayed-type allergy, and this type of hypersensitivity cannot be transferred by serum. Complement does not mediate PCA. The IgE participating in PCA, in contrast to other immunoglobulins, is destroyed by heating at 50°C for 30 minutes. It is risky to perform PCA in atopic individuals who genetically tend to develop sudden hypersensitivity states such as asthma or hay fever. *(Joklik et al, p 319; Roitt et al, pp 22.10–22.11)*

283. (C) Arthus allergy is a type III hypersensitivity that is usually initiated by complement-fixing IgG and natural killer cells. The reaction occurs within hours after antigen challenge. It produces cell death and extensive local destruction of tissues. *(Joklik et al, p 322; Roitt et al, pp 24.4–24.5)*

284. (D) IgE levels are frequently elevated in type I hypersensitivity (as in hay fever, perennial rhinitis, asthma, and atopic eczema) and are elevated in parasitic diseases. Arthus hypersensitivity is a type III reaction (immune complex) in which IgG is primarily involved. Tuberculosis and leprosy are diseases that can lead to delayed-type hypersensitivity (type IV reaction) in which IgE is not involved. *Brucella* infection elicits both IgM and IgG production, and also cell-mediated immunity. *(Joklik et al, pp 359–362; Roitt et al, pp 22.2–22.6)*

285. (D) T cells account for 65 to 80% of leukocytes in peripheral blood. B cells account for 8 to 15% in peripheral blood. T cells lack IgG receptors, but have CD3 antigen and T-cell receptors. IgG and IgM receptors are found in B cells. Monocytes/macrophages, polymorphonuclear leukocytes, and NK cells have Fc receptors. T cells are not involved in phagocytosis or antibody-dependent cellular cytotoxicity. *(Joklik et al, p 250; Roitt et al, pp 2.6–2.12)*

286. (C) MHC class I molecules are normally expressed on most nucleated cells. In some species, it is expressed on erythrocytes and platelets. In contrast to this, MHC class II molecules are restricted to antigen-presenting cells, and in some species, to activated T cells and vascular endothelial cells. *(Roitt et al, pp 8.3,26.2–26.3)*

287. (E) MHC class II molecules are expressed on antigen-presenting cells, which include macrophages, monocytes, B cells, and vascular endothelial cells. Erythrocytes are unable to present antigens and do not express class II molecules. *(Roitt et al, p 8.3)*

288. (A) Rheumatoid arthritis is an immune complex disease. Rheumatoid factor (RF) is a term used for autoanti-IgG antibodies that are reactive with determinants in the Fc region of IgG. It can combine with antibodies to DNA to form immune complexes. The immune complexes activate complement and release chemical attractants. As a result, neutrophils are attracted and hydrolytic enzymes are released. RF is a polymer of IgG molecules and is produced by B cells (plasma cells). (Joklik et al, pp 319,321)

289. **(B)** Class I restricted T cells (Tc cells) recognize endogenous antigens synthesized within the target cell, whereas class II restricted T cells (T$_H$ cells) recognize exogenous antigen. Antigens to be recognized by T cells may or may not be of microbial origin. Peptide–MHC molecule complexes on the cell surface can be recognized by a specific T-cell receptor and processed immunologically to elicit appropriate immune responses. (Roitt et al, p 7.1)

290. **(C)** Both the C3 component of complement and IgG appear to be necessary for the removal of particulate immune complexes. Size is very important for the removal of immune complexes. Generally large complexes are removed in several minutes. However, small complexes require hours to several days for their removal. In vivo, the main site where immune complexes are eliminated is the liver where the Kupffer cells are actively engaged in phagocytosis of the complexes. (Roitt et al, pp 24.6–24.10)

291. **(E)** It has been indicated that low-affinity antibody can lead to production of small immune complexes in type III hypersensitivity. When an individual forms antibodies to autoantigens, only a limited number of epitomes on the antigen are recognized by the immunologic system, and this situation can cause the production of small immune complexes. None of the others contribute to the formation of small immune complexes. (Roitt et al, pp 24.1–24.10)

292. **(D)** The tuberculin-type hypersensitivity is type IV or delayed-type hypersensitivity, requiring a maximum reaction time of 48 to 72 hours. (Joklik et al, pp 507–508; Roitt et al, p 25.7)

293. **(A)** Delayed-type hypersensitivity (type IV) cannot be transferred by serum, but it can be transferred from one individual to another by T lymphocytes. Although it may be associated with T-cell protective immunity, it does not necessarily run parallel with it. TD cells participate in type IV hypersensitivity. However, they often act in conjunction with other cell types (monocytes) at the reaction site. The damage seen in type IV reactions is largely the result of inflammatory mediators released from activated macrophages, lymphocytes, and sometimes basophils. Histamine is not essential. There are four clinical categories of delayed-type hypersensitivity. (Joklik et al, pp 322–323; Roitt et al, pp 25.1–25.9)

294. **(E)** IL-12 is a new class of lymphokine that is produced by monocytes. The lymphokine favors TH-1 responses, with macrophage and NK cell activation and induces INF-γ production. IL-1 stimulates T cells and B cells, and induces inflammatory responses stimulating the production of prostaglandin and degradative enzymes such as collagenase. IL-2 stimulates the proliferation and activation of T cells and B cells. IL-4 promotes B-cell activation and differentiation. IL-6 stimulates B-cell differentiation and induces acute-phase proteins. (Roitt et al, pp 8.9–8.10)

295. **(C)** From the clinical point of view, granulomatous hypersensitivity is the most significant form of type IV hypersensitivity producing numerous pathologic lesions in diseases in which T-cell-mediated immunity is involved. Granulomatous hypersensitivity is believed to be due to the lengthy presence of microorganisms within macrophages. Individuals suffering from such chronic infections as tuberculosis, leprosy, schistosomiasis, and other diseases are likely to manifest granulomatous hypersensitivity, which can be tested by either the macrophage migration inhibition test, or the lymphocyte transformation test. (Joklik et al, pp 322–323; Roitt et al, pp 25.6–25.7)

296. **(A)** Clonal abortion is a pathway to B-cell tolerance. In clonal abortion, immature B

cells, during their first exposure to low levels of antigen, become tolerant to this antigen so that they are unable to respond subsequently to antigenic challenge. Repeated antigenic challenge with a T-independent antigen may remove all mature functional B-cell clones resulting in clonal exhaustion. *(Joklik et al, pp 260–261; Roitt et al, pp 12.2,12.9)*

297. **(B)** Clonal exhaustion is another mechanism by which B-cell tolerance can be established. Repeated challenges with immunizing concentrations of T-independent antigens can induce clonal exhaustion. When such challenges are made, mature B cells that can respond to the T-independent antigen differentiate into very short-lived antibody-producing cells, so that there are no B cells that can respond to subsequent challenges with the T-independent antigen. *(Joklik et al, pp 260–261; Roitt et al, p 12.8)*

298. **(E)** In the fluorescence-activated cell sorter, cells in the sample are first stained with specific fluorescent reagents to detect surface molecules and are then introduced into the vibrating chamber. The cell stream passing out of the chamber is encased in a sheath of buffer fluid. The stream is illuminated by laser light and each cell is measured for size and granularity, as well as for red and green fluorescence, to detect two different surface markers. The vibration in the cell stream causes it to break into droplets which are charged and may then be steered by deflection plates under computer control to collect different cell populations according to the parameters measured. *(Roitt et al, p 28.5)*

299. **(A)** During the primary response, some of the stimulated T and B cells, which are lymphocytes, differentiate into long-lived memory T and B cells. These memory cells are small lymphocytes and are able to circulate in the body for many years. A second exposure to that antigen allows them to proliferate rapidly in the more intense secondary response. All other cells do not serve as memory cells. *(Joklik et al, p 235; Roitt et al; pp 8.16,10.14)*

300. **(E)** Polymorphonuclear (PMN) leukocytes in the capillaries are the first to arrive in acute inflammation by pyogenic cocci. The PMN in the capillaries sticks to the walls and then crosses the capillaries and proceeds to the site of the inflammation, stimulated by chemotactic attractants in the inflammatory exudate. After phagocytosis of the pyogenic cocci by PMN, the inflamed area becomes more acidic and the proteases induce lysis of the PMN, forming pus. The large mononuclear phagocytes arrive later, to finish killing the cocci and cleaning up the debris. *(Joklik et al, pp 348–349; Roitt et al, p 2.15)*

301. **(C)** The macrophage population, which was once thought to be homogeneous, is now found to be heterogeneous, as are lymphocytes, with various functions. Macrophages/monocytes can be divided into two subsets on the basis of a cell marker. One subset is phagocytic and removes particulate antigens, while the second subset plays an important role in the initiation and regulation of immune responses. The latter subset contains specialized antigen-presenting monocytes, which can be found in skin (Langerhans' cells) and the dendritic macrophages of all lymphoid tissues. Pre-B cells cannot present antigens, but mature B cells can. T-cells, NK cells, and eosinophils cannot present antigen. *(Joklik et al, p 209; Roitt et al, p 8.3)*

302. **(E)** Eosinophils can be triggered to degranulate, by fusion of the intracellular granules with the plasma membrane, releasing the granule contents to the outside of the cell. This mechanism is particularly useful against cells that are too large to be phagocytosed. In helminth (worm) infections, the eosinophil count is greatly increased. Allergies also cause an increased eosinophil count. *(Joklik et al, pp 312,348,361; Roitt et al, pp 2.15–2.16)*

303. **(D)** In the complement-fixation test, red blood cells coated with antibody against the red blood cells (hemolysin) are used as the indicator system. The indicator system undergoes hemolysis when complement is left unfixed in the test system. Antibody-coated red cells are not used in the other methods listed in the question. *(Joklik et al, pp 241–242; Roitt et al, pp 29.3–28.4)*

304. (B) Immunoelectrophoresis is the method of choice for identifying the light- and heavy-chain isotype of a multiple myeloma protein. In this technique, the complex antigen mixture is separated electrophoretically before antiserum is added. Diffusion of separated antigens and the antiserum give rise to the arcs of visible precipitation. This technique is also used for analysis of sera suspected of IgA deficiency, polyclonal proliferation, and hypogammaglobulinemia. *(Joklik et al, pp 240–241; Roitt et al, pp 28.2–28.3)*

305. (C) C4b coatings act similarly to C3b but are less effective. Phagocytes and some other immune cells have receptors for C3b. C3a and C5a are chemotactic for phagocytes. *(Joklik et al, pp 292–293; Roitt et al, pp 13.2,13.11)*

306. (E) The fixation of C5b to biologic membranes is followed by the sequential addition of four more proteins C6 and C7 to form C567, which is relatively stable and can interact with C8 and C9 to exert a destructive effect on the membrane. *(Joklik et al, pp 291–292; Roitt et al, pp 13.9–13.10,13.13–13.14)*

307. (B) Anaphylotoxins (C3a and C5a) are the only components of complement that cause degranulation of mast cells and other cells (neutrophils, macrophages, and platelets). Degranulation of mast cells releases biologically active mediators responsible for anaphylaxis. *(Joklik et al, p 293; Roitt et al, pp 13.12–13.13)*

308. (C) The primary humoral defense mechanism against viruses is antibody-mediated neutralization. Virus-specific immunoglobulins, mostly the IgA class, are present in virtually all body secretions. The process of neutralization can occur with antibodies that (1) bind to the virus and hinder the absorption of the virus to a cell surface; (2) stabilize the virus capsid so that the nucleic acids within the capsid cannot be released; or (3) fix complement on the protein coat causing struc-

tural or toxic damage. A virus that has been properly neutralized by antibodies is no longer infectious. Other items are either incorrect or incomplete. *(Joklik et al, pp 353–354; Roitt et al, p 16.3)*

309. (E) *Mycobacterium tuberculosis* is a facultative intracellular pathogen that causes tuberculosis in humans. This bacterium cannot be killed within neutrophils or resident macrophages. The organism can be killed by activated macrophages, which are the major effector cells for this pathogen. Both oxygen intermediate metabolites, nitric oxide, and possibly hydrolytic enzymes are involved in mycobacterial killing by activated macrophages. *(Joklik et al, pp 350–351,506; Roitt et al, pp 17.8–17.10)*

310. (B) Exotoxin produced by *Clostridium tetani* is responsible for the clinical symptoms of tetanus. Tetanus can be prevented if individuals are vaccinated with tetanus toxoid and maintain sufficient levels of antitetanus antibody, because specific antitetanus antibody neutralizes tetanus toxin elaborated in vivo by *C. tetani.* *(Joklik et al, pp 365–367; Roitt et al, p 19.3)*

311. (D) Heparin sulfate is the major preformed proteoglycan that binds histamine and inhibits complement activation. It has several other functions. By binding histamine, it removes a very important pharmacologic mediator of immediate hypersensitivity. *(Joklik et al, p 320; Roitt et al, pp 22.6–22.14)*

312. (A) Tryptase is a proteolytic enzyme that activates C3. Leukotriene B4 and ECF-A are chemoattractants for neutrophils, eosinophils, monocytes, and basophils. *(Roitt et al, pp 22.6–22.14)*

313. (C) Prostaglandin DX2 is involved with the contraction of bronchial smooth muscle that occurs in type I hypersensitivity. *(Joklik et al, pp 314–315; Roitt et al, pp 22.6–22.14)*

314. (C) Prevention of measles (rubeola) can best be accomplished by vaccination. The vaccine is composed of live attenuated Edmonston strain of measles virus. It provides the most dependable and lasting protection against rubeola. The vaccine is usually administered shortly after 1 year of age. No toxins associated with viruses are known. *(Joklik et al, pp 365–366,1011; Roitt et al, pp 19.1–19.10)*

315. (D) An effective vaccine is available for the prevention of whooping cough. The vaccine is composed of killed phage I *Bordetella pertussis* cells, and it is given in three injections during the first year of life. The vaccine has been associated with encephalopathy, which is thought to occur once in 5 to 10 million injections in America. To reduce the side effect, an acellular vaccine (hemagglutinin and pertussis toxin) is being tested. *(Joklik et al, p 479; Roitt et al, pp 19.1–19.10)*

316. (A) Prevention against tetanus can be effectively achieved by the administration of tetanus toxoid, which constitutes the key protective component of the vaccine. The toxoid is given intramuscularly in combination with diphtheria and pertussis, with diphtheria, or alone to individuals of questionable immunization status after injuries from which clinical tetanus may result. *(Joklik et al, pp 647–648; Roitt et al, pp 19.1–19.10)*

317. (A) Local patterns of cytokine and hormone expression help to select the effector mechanism to be activated. If an organism triggers release of IL-12 and INF-γ from macrophages and NK cells, the T_H subset that develop will be biased toward T_H-1. Release of IL-4 and IL-10 will bias it toward T_H-2. *(Roitt et al, p 9.3)*

318. (B) Release of IL-4, IL-5, IL-6, and IL-10 will be biased toward T_H-2. *(Roitt et al, pp 9.3–9.4)*

319. (E) MHC class I antigens are heterodimers of a heavy chain that is noncovalently bound to a small highly conserved molecule called beta-2 microglobulin. Class I antigens are found on virtually every cell and tissue of the body, including T cells, B cells, macrophages, and dendritic cells. In contrast to this, MHC class II antigens are not expressed on all classes of cells. They are present on B cells,

macrophages, and dendritic cells. *(Joklik et al, pp 209–210; Roitt et al, p 26.2)*

320. (B) Surface immunoglobulin acts as the membrane receptor for antigen on B cells. Unlike B cells, T cells, macrophages, and dendritic cells do not carry surface immunoglobulins. T cells recognize the MHC class I or II molecules plus antigen with receptor, that is, heterodimer of disulfide-linked alpha or beta chains of T-cell receptor. This complex is structurally somewhat similar to rearranged immunoglobulin gene product (immunoglobulin superfamily). *(Joklik et al, pp 206, 252–253,297; Roitt et al, pp 2.6–2.7)*

321. (E) Although there is great homology between the constant (C) regions of all immunoglobulins, certain amino acid sequences in the C region are characteristic of each major class (eg, delta, mu, and alpha). Limited substitutions characterize subclasses or isotypes (eg, gamma-1 and alpha-2) of the heavy (H) chain of IgG and IgA of all members of a species. Other limited substitutions of different amino acid residues of the C region occur only in the kappa chains of the gamma-1 H chains of an individual. These individual specific markings are called allotype: the Km and Gm allotypes. The function of the variable region is to confer antibody specificity. The function of the C region, especially of the H chains, is to confer different biologic properties on the immunoglobulin molecules. No other regions of an immunoglobulin molecule determine allotype. *(Joklik et al, p 205; Roitt et al, pp 4.1–4.11)*

322. (C) See the answer to question 321.

323. (D) See the answer to question 321.

324. (E) IgE is involved in type I hypersensitivity reaction (immediate hypersensitivity). IgE is present in very low concentration in the bloodstream and tends to be bound, through Fc, by IgE receptors on the surface of two related and highly specialized granular cells known as tissue master cells and blood basophils. When IgE bound to a mast cell reacts with its appropriate antigen, the cell releases histamine and other permeases from its granules; thus, IgE is the immunoglobulin responsible for allergic or anaphylactic reactions. *(Joklik et al, pp 206,319–321; Roitt et al, pp 4.2–4.3,4.10–4.12,18.4–18.6)*

325. **(C)** In primary humoral immune response, the predominant immunoglobulin is IgM, which appears first in the serum and is followed by IgG. *(Joklik et al, pp 248–249; Roitt et al, pp 4.2–4.3,6.10)*

326. **(A)** During the secondary humoral immune response (a second exposure to the same antigen), a more rapid and greater response ensues, which is predominantly composed of IgG, not IgM, as the major class of antibody. *(Joklik et al, p 249; Roitt et al, pp 4.2–4.3,6.10)*

327. **(B)** IgA is the predominant immunoglobulin in extracellular secretions. IgA is, in its multimeric form, the immunoglobulin of mucous surface, and in its monomeric form, the immunoglobulin in blood. Like IgG and IgM, IgA has protective functions against microorganisms or their products. *(Joklik et al, pp 206,224; Roitt et al, pp 4.2–4.3,4.6–4.7)*

328. **(D)** No function is yet known for IgD other than as a membrane receptor. Because it is found on the surface of maturing B lymphocytes, IgD is believed to play a role in preventing immunologic tolerance. *(Joklik et al, p 206; Roitt et al, pp 2.6–2.7,4.2–4.3)*

329. **(B)** These two diseases belong to type II hypersensitivity reaction and are mediated by cytotoxic antibody. In Goodpasture syndrome, host immunoglobulin autoantibodies bind in situ to collagen antigens expressed on glomerular and alveolar basement membranes, leading to localized complement activation and inflammation. These reactions result in glomerulonephritis and hemorrhagic alveolitis. *(Joklik et al, pp 319–320; Roitt et al, pp 23.1–23.9)*

330. **(A)** These diseases result from type I hypersensitivity reaction (immediate hypersensitivity). These types of hypersensitivity reactions are mediated by IgE antibodies, which

bind via characteristic Fc domains with very high affinity to the specific Fc receptors on the surface of mast cells and basophils. Such binding is independent of the antigen specificity of the IgE molecules. Crosslinking of such antibodies by multivalent antigens stimulates the effector cell to release preformed and newly formed soluble pharmacologically active mediators including histamine, chemotactic factors, proteolytic enzymes, and heparin. The release of histamine results in almost immediate increased vascular permeability and smooth muscle contraction, whereas heparin inhibits coagulation, and chemotactic factors attract eosinophils. *(Joklik et al, p 319; Roitt et al, pp 22.1–22.17)*

331. **(D)** These diseases are mainly due to delayed-type hypersensitivity (type IV reaction). Unlike other types (I, II, and III) of immunopathologic reactions, type IV responses are initiated by antigen-specific T cells. The histologic picture of this reaction is characterized by the presence of mononuclear cells (lymphocytes and macrophages). The damage seen in type IV reactions is largely the result of inflammatory mediators released from activated macrophages and sometimes basophils. This type of reaction can be transferred in vivo with sensitized T cells alone. *(Roitt et al, pp 24.1–24.11)*

332. **(E)** These diseases are caused by microbial exotoxins. The diseases themselves are not immunologic diseases, although they can be treated by specific antitoxin antibodies. *(Joklik et al, p 365; Ryan et al, pp 155–156)*

333. **(B)** Hashimoto's thyroiditis is an autoimmune disease mediated by antithyroglobulin. The formation of antithyroglobulin is a result of altered host immune regulation. In Graves' disease patients, autoantibody against the receptor for thyroid-stimulating hormone (TSH) is produced. *(Joklik et al, pp 320–321; Roitt et al, 27.1–27.12)*

334. **(A)** Rheumatoid arthritis is characterized by a chronic inflammation of the joints, which is associated with autoantibodies directed against the Fc portion of the patient's IgG.

These autoantibodies (anti-immunoglobulin antibodies) are called rheumatoid factor and are either IgM or IgG. These antibodies form immune complexes with IgG that are the main cause of the disease. More recently, however, delayed-type hypersensitivity reaction involving T cells has been suspected of participating in the disease process. *(Joklik et al, pp 321–322)*

335. **(D)** This disease is an autoimmune disease mediated by antibodies against DNA. *(Joklik et al, p 321; Roitt et al, pp 27.2–27.10)*

336. **(E)** In this disease, the host produces antibodies against acetylcholine receptors. *(Joklik et al, p 321; Roitt et al, p 27.6)*

337. **(D)** The syndromes of severe combined immunodeficiency disorder (SCID) are characterized by the absence of all adaptive immune functions from birth and great cellular, molecular, and genetic diversity. Some infants with SCID have profound lymphopenia, and their lymphocytes do not respond to mitogens, antigens, and allogenic cells. Unless immunologic reconstitution can be achieved through immunocompetent tissue transplants or enzyme replacement therapy, or gnotobiotic isolation can be carried out, death usually occurs before the patient's first birthday and almost invariably before the second. *(Joklik et al, p 333; Roitt et al, p 21.4–21.5)*

338. **(B)** This disease is a result of thymic hypoplasia or aplasia due to dysmorphogenesis of the third and fourth pharyngeal pouches during early embryogenesis. Patients with DiGeorge syndrome have decreased T cells that respond poorly to mitogen stimulation. *(Joklik et al, pp 332–333; Roitt et al, p 21.5)*

339. **(A)** In this disease, granulocytes cannot generate sufficient quantities of hydrogen peroxide due to the defect in the NADPH-oxidase system. Because of the lack of sufficient hydrogen peroxide, the myeloperoxidase-H_2O_2-halide system, the key microbicidal system of human neutrophils, cannot function. Thus, neutrophils of chronic granulomatous disease patients cannot kill phagocytosed "cata-

lase-positive" bacteria such as staphylococci and fungi. *(Joklik et al, p 340; Roitt et al, pp 21.9–21.10)*

340. **(D)** Antibody diversity is generated by gene arrangements that affect a cluster of heavy chains located on the chromosome. The heavy-chain genes include V (variability), D (diversity), J (joining), and C (constant) genes. In the germ-line state, these genes are quite far apart. During B-cell development, one of several hundred V genes is translocated to lie close to one of about a dozen D genes and one of four J genes to form a V-D-J complex. The process involved in this complex formation is DNA rearrangement. *(Joklik et al, p 206; Roitt et al, pp 6.4–6.12)*

341. **(A)** The V-D-J complex formed as a result of DNA rearrangement constitutes the immunologic profile of the heavy chain of that B cell. The V-D-J complex lies close to the mu constant region gene. By the excision of portions of the C-region and intervening genes, the V-D-J complex may be translocated to lie next to a delta, gamma, epsilon, or alpha C-region gene. To achieve this, the transcribed RNA (V-D-J- and C-region genes including intervening genes) is processed to splice out the intervening sequences. *(Joklik et al, pp 206,230–233; Roitt et al, pp 6.4–5.12)*

342. **(A)** Interferons are proteins with antiviral activity elaborated by infected cells and stimulated lymphocytes in response to certain intracellular stimuli. Interferon-β belongs to type I interferons, which can protect cells that have not yet been infected and additionally can stimulate NK cells into lytic and replicative states. Interferon-β is predominantly produced by fibroblasts in response to viral infection or other inducing agents. In many systems, interferon-induced inhibition of virus multiplication involves interference with the ability of parental or early viral messenger RNA molecules to be translated. As a result, no viral-specific proteins are synthesized, no progeny viral genomes are formed, and infection is aborted. The effect of interferon is remarkably specific: cellular protein synthesis is unaffected and viral protein syn-

thesis is inhibited. Other cytokines are either ineffective or not as active as interferon-β. *(Joklik et al, pp 355,863–864; Roitt et al, p 16.2)*

343. **(E)** There are two types of tumor necrosis factor (TNF): TNF-α and TNF-β. TNF-α is cachectin produced by macrophages and lymphocytes. TNF-β is lymphotoxin produced by T cells. The ability to cause fever (pyrogenicity) is one of the important biologic activities associated with TNF-α. IL-1 and IL-6 also function as pyrogen. *(Joklik et al, pp 87,314–317; Roitt et al, p 9.8)*

344. **(C)** Only IgG can bind to rheumatoid factor, which is an antibody against the Fc portion of IgG. *(Joklik et al, p 224; Roitt et al, pp 4.2–4.3)*

345. **(A)** IgA, secretory immunoglobulin, contains a secretory component, which is synthesized by epithelial cells, not plasma cells. *(Joklik et al, p 227; Roitt et al, pp 4.2–4.3,4.6)*

346. **(A)** Only IgA (secretory immunoglobulin) is secreted in the milk of lactating women. *(Joklik et al, pp 224–227; Roitt et al, pp 4.6,6.2–6.3)*

347. **(J)** Only plasma cells can produce and secrete immunoglobulins extracellularly. Although B cells produce certain classes of immunoglobulin (IgM and IgD), which are inserted into the cell membrane (surface immunoglobulin), they do not secrete IgA, IgG, and IgE. No other cells listed in the question produce and secrete immunoglobulin. *(Joklik et al, pp 205–206,233–234; Roitt et al, pp 1.4,2.9,4.1)*

348. **(A)** Although neutrophils and eosinophils can phagocytose foreign particles, they do not present antigens. B cells can present antigens, but they are not phagocytic. All other cells are neither phagocytic nor antigen-presenting cells. *(Joklik et al, pp 209,254; Roitt et al, 2.11–2.14)*

349. **(G)** Eosinophilia and the production of high levels of IgE are the common consequences of infection by parasitic worms and the eosinophil appears to be a major effector cell against helminths. The increase in the number of eosinophils in worm infections such as schistosomiasis and ascariasis is T-cell-dependent. *(Roitt et al, pp 2.15–2.16)*

350. **(J)** Natural killer cells, macrophages, and cytotoxic T cells can kill tumor cells. Killing of tumor cells by cytotoxic cells is major histocompatibility complex-restricted. Macrophages that can kill antibody-coated tumor cells are phagocytes. *(Joklik et al, pp 276–278; Roitt et al, pp 2.7–2.8)*

351. **(J)** All of the data shown in this question are in the normal ranges except for the number of neutrophils. The normal range of neutrophils in healthy individuals is 6,000 to 9,000/mm^3 of peripheral blood. *(Joklik et al, pp 338–339)*

352. **(H)** Severe combined immunodeficiency disorder (SCID) is characterized by the absence of all adaptive immune function from birth. Infants with SCID have profound lymphopenia; an absence of lymphocytes' proliferative response to mitogens, antigens, and allogenic cells in vitro; and delayed cutaneous anergy. Serum immunoglobulin concentrations are diminished to absent, and no antibody formation occurs after immunization. Unless immunologic reconstitution can be achieved through immunocompetent tissue transplants or enzyme replacement therapy or germ-free isolation can be carried out, the patient will not survive beyond his or her first birthday. *(Joklik et al, pp 333–334)*

353. **(A)** Chronic granulomatous disease of children is characterized by chronic suppurative infections, draining adenopathy, pneumonia, hepatomegaly with liver abscesses, osteomyelitis, splenomegaly, hypergammaglobulinemia, and dermatitis, with onset of symptoms usually before 1 year of age. The cause of these problems is the genetic defect in NADPH-oxidase. Neutrophils contain myeloperoxidase, which utilizes hydrogen peroxide and halide ions to produce hypohalite ions such as hypochlorite, which is highly microbicidal. Because of the defective NADPH-oxidase, the patient's phagocytes cannot generate sufficient hydrogen peroxide, thus, the myeloperoxidase–hydrogen peroxide and halide system cannot function normally. Neutrophils from these patients can phagocytose bacteria and fungi normally, but phagocytosed agents cannot be killed efficiently because of the defective myeloperoxidase–H_2O_2–halide system. Streptococcal infections in chronic granulomatous disease patients are rare because the defective myeloperoxide–H_2O_2–halide system can utilize hydrogen peroxide accumulated by phagocytosed streptococci (streptococci are catalase-negative). *(Joklik et al, pp 340–341, 350–351; Roitt et al, pp 21.9–21.10)*

354. **(F)** Systemic lupus erythematosus (SLE) is an autoimmune disease (type III hypersensitivity or immune-complex disease). All other diseases listed in the question are not autoimmune diseases. SLE patients produce antinuclear, anti-DNA antibodies. Immune complexes are detected by immunofluorescent staining of kidney sections, and antinuclear antibodies have been detected in serum by indirect immunofluorescence. *(Joklik et al, pp 221–222; Roitt et al, p 27.2)*

355. **(I)** Macrophage-activating activity is primarily constituted by interferon-gamma (INF-γ) and is important in enhancing macrophage activity, promoting the killing of intracellular organisms. INF-γ is known as immune interferon and produced by NK cells and stimulated T cells. Endotoxin often triggers activation of INF-γ–primed macrophages. Tissue necrosis factor beta (TNF-β) is produced by some T cells and activates macrophages, but it is not produced by NK cells. When combined with INF-γ or endotoxin, some lymphokines (IL-2 and IL-4) and cytokines can activate macrophages. The functions of lymphokines and cytokines are complex. New functions associated with various lymphokines and cytokines are being discovered constantly. *(Joklik et al, p 316; Roitt et al, pp 8.8,9.10)*

356. **(K)** Prostaglandin E2 (PGE_2) modulates a number of inflammatory events. It enhances vascular permeability, is pyrogenic, and increases sensitivity to pain. PGE_2 also stimulates the formation of cyclic adenosine monophosphate in many types of inflammatory cells and thereby suppresses a number of immunologic responses, including lymphocyte blastogenesis, lymphocyte-mediated cytotoxicity, and the release of mediators from mast cells. *(Joklik et al, p 315; Roitt et al, p 25.4)*

357. **(C)** Interleukin-3 is a product of T cells, and its primary target is stem cells. It is known as multilineage colony-stimulating factor. *(Joklik et al, p 255; Roitt et al, p 8.9)*

REFERENCES

Chapel N, Haeney M. *Essentials of Clinical Immunology*, 2nd ed. Oxford: Blackwell Scientific Publications; 1984

Joklik WK, Willett HP, Amos DB, Wilfert CM. *Zinsser Microbiology*, 20th ed. Norwalk, CT: Appleton & Lange; 1992

Roitt I, Brostoff J, Male DK. *Immunology*, 4th ed. London and New York: Mosby; 1996

Ryan KJ, Champoux JJ, Falkow S, Plorde JJ, Drew WL, Neidhardt FC, Ray CG. *Sherris Medical Microbiology*, 3rd ed. Norwalk, CT: Appleton & Lange; 1994

Morbidity and Mortality Weekly Report 1991;40:27–31

CHAPTER 4

Antibiotics
Questions

DIRECTIONS (Questions 358 through 390): Each of the numbered items or incomplete statements in this section is followed by answers or by completions of the statement. Select the ONE lettered answer or completion that is BEST in each case.

358. Antibiotics A and B are added alone, or combined, to cultures of *Streptococcus pyogenes*. The results presented in the figure below illustrate

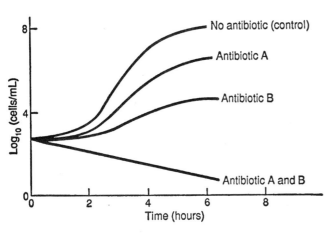

Figure 4–1

(A) antagonism
(B) indifference
(C) addition
(D) synergism

359. The structure shown in the figure below is the antibiotic

(A) ofloxacin
(B) penicillin
(C) polymyxin
(D) streptomycin
(E) chloramphenicol

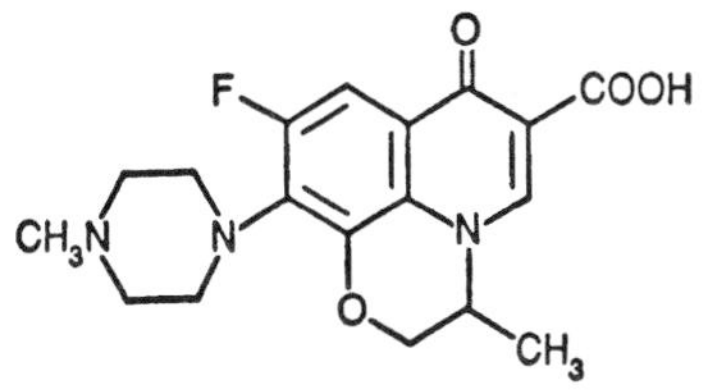

Figure 4–2

360. A burn patient developed a wound infection, and a bacteriological culture of the site indicates a gram-negative rod that was oxidase-positive and produced a bluish-green pigment. The organism was relatively resistant to antibiotics but susceptible to ticarcillin, gentamicin, and tobramycin. The organism is likely to be identified as

(A) *Escherichia coli*
(B) *Klebsiella pneumoniae*
(C) *Proteus mirabilis*
(D) *Serratia marcescens*
(E) *Pseudomonas aeruginosa*

361. A spinal fluid specimen from a 28-year-old man shows *Neisseria meningitidis*. This patient should be treated with

    (A) penicillin G
    (B) amikacin
    (C) kanamycin
    (D) ethambutol
    (E) gentamicin

362. Incorporation of uracil into macromolecules would be inhibited in a culture of sensitive bacteria by the addition of

    (A) streptomycin
    (B) rifampin
    (C) kanamycin
    (D) amikacin
    (E) tobramycin

363. A tetracycline may be the drug of first choice for treatment of all of the following diseases EXCEPT

    (A) lymphogranuloma venereum
    (B) inclusion conjunctivitis
    (C) trachoma
    (D) hospital-acquired pneumonia due to *Klebsiella*
    (E) psittacosis

364. Penicillin is the drug of first choice for infections caused by all of the following EXCEPT

    (A) *Treponema pallidum*
    (B) *Actinomyces israelii*
    (C) *Bacteroides fragilis*
    (D) *Streptococcus pyogenes*
    (E) *Clostridium perfringens*

365. The antibiotic selected for a patient with hepatic insufficiency is

    (A) amikacin
    (B) amphotericin B
    (C) kanamycin
    (D) sulfamethoxypyrimidazine
    (E) ampicillin

366. Which of the following is responsible for a rapid bactericidal action of penicillin G against *Streptococcus pneumoniae*?

    (A) polysaccharide capsule
    (B) M-protein
    (C) autolytic enzyme
    (D) the 50S ribosomal subunit
    (E) β-lactamase

367. All of the following agents affect primarily the cytoplasmic membrane EXCEPT

    (A) sodium deoxycholate
    (B) colistin
    (C) cycloheximide
    (D) nystatin
    (E) polymyxin

368. An adult patient with a history of severe penicillin allergy has a sore throat and low-grade fever. Results of a throat culture show a large number of β-hemolytic streptococcal colonies. Of the following, the most likely antibiotic selected would be

    (A) ampicillin
    (B) oxacillin
    (C) cephalothin
    (D) tetracycline
    (E) phenoxymethylpenicillin

369. Organisms that are inhibited but not killed by penicillin because they have defective autolytic enzymes are called

    (A) tolerant
    (B) sensitive
    (C) insensitive
    (D) resistant
    (E) indifferent

370. Which of the following statements about chemotherapy is true?

    (A) peak attainable serum levels can determine whether or not a particular antibiotic will be useful in treating a given disease

(B) administration of two different antibiotics at the same time never leads to treatment failure

(C) none of the antibiotics require host activation to produce the active agent

(D) the location of the infection cannot determine the degree to which it will respond to chemotherapy

(E) if an organism is sensitive to the antibiotic in vitro, it must also be sensitive to that antibiotic in vivo

371. In order for an organism from a soft-tissue infection to be considered susceptible to an antibiotic, the

(A) minimal inhibitory concentration (MIC) must be equal to the achievable blood level.

(B) MIC must be two to four times greater than the achievable blood level

(C) achievable blood level must be less than the MIC

(D) achievable blood level must be two to four times greater than the MIC

(E) Kirby–Bauer zone diameter must be two to four times greater than the MIC

372. Which of the following statements about β-lactam antibiotics is true?

(A) benzylpenicillin (penicillin G) is not resistant to penicillinase

(B) all penicillins do not contain the four-member β-lactam ring and a fused five-member ring containing a sulfur atom

(C) penicillinase destroys the activity of penicillin by hydrolyzing the β-lactam ring, producing penicilloic acid

(D) charged R groups are added to produce semisynthetic penicillins showing smaller activity against gram-negative organisms

373. All of the following statements about metabolic inhibitors are true EXCEPT

(A) sulfonamides block the synthesis of dihydropteroic acid, a crucial intermediate in the synthesis of tetrahydrofolic acid

(B) isonicotinic acid resembles nicotinamide and blocks synthesis of pyridine-containing cofactors such as NAD

(C) puromycin causes early termination of translation and the release of incomplete peptides

(D) methotrexate is more active against mammalian dihydrofolate reductase than it is against the same enzyme present in bacteria

(E) trimethoprim blocks the activity of dihydrofolate reductase and therefore acts synergistically with sulfonamides

374. The antibiotic that interferes with the function of the cell membrane is

(A) penicillin

(B) neomycin

(C) rifampin

(D) amphotericin

(E) streptomycin

375. The antibiotic that is MOST toxic to humans is

(A) polymyxin B

(B) sulfamethoxazole

(C) sulfadiazine

(D) trimethoprine

376. All of the following statements are false EXCEPT

(A) mitomycin C will cross-link DNA in vitro

(B) cross-linked DNA can be partially denatured but will not reanneal with fidelity when rapidly cooled

(C) the target-binding site of an antibiotic is not necessarily the site at which it exerts its antibiotic action

(D) metronidazole is not clinically useful against both prokaryotic and eukaryotic pathogens

(E) amantadine is therapeutic for influenza A_2 viral infections

377. All of the following statements about antibiotics are true EXCEPT

  (A) chloramphenicol interacts with the 50S ribosomal subunit and blocks the peptidyl transferase reaction

  (B) sulfonamides and trimethoprim act synergistically because they inhibit two different steps of tetrahydrofolate synthesis

  (C) rifampin inhibits translation by interacting with the sigma subunit of DNA polymerase

  (D) some mutants of *Escherichia coli* actually require streptomycin for growth

  (E) puromycin mimics a charged rRNA molecule and causes premature termination and release of incomplete peptides

378. All of the following statements about antibiotic resistance in bacteria are true EXCEPT

  (A) low to moderate levels of resistance to penicillin are usually associated with altered (mutated) penicillin-binding proteins

  (B) resistance due to an altered target site or enzyme is often expressed at high antibiotic concentrations

  (C) bacteria harboring R plasmids are usually resistant to more than one antibiotic

  (D) antibiotic resistance can be transferred from one bacterium to another by transformation, transduction, or conjugation

  (E) most antibiotics are mutagenic, both inducing and selecting resistant mutants

379. All of the following statements about resistance to β-lactam antibiotics by β-lactamases are true EXCEPT

  (A) β-lactamases are generally inducible in gram-positive bacteria and constitutive in gram-negative bacteria

  (B) cleavage of the β-lactam ring reduces, but does not destroy, antibiotic activity

  (C) β-lactamases usually are the mechanism for high-level resistance

  (D) β-lactamases usually are inactivated by clavulinic acid

  (E) β-lactamases are generally plasmid coded

380. R plasmid-mediated resistance is usually due to

  (A) mutational events in an existing cellular structure

  (B) a mutational event that makes cells impermeable to one antibiotic

  (C) a mutational event that makes cells impermeable to a class of antibiotics

  (D) a mutational event that renders specific target sites within microorganisms indifferent to the presence of antibiotics

  (E) the synthesis of new distinct proteins that make the microbe resistant, ie, enzymatically destroy or modify the antibiotics

381. Possible target sites of activity of antibacterial drugs include all of the following EXCEPT

  (A) the cell walls

  (B) the cytoplasmic membranes

  (C) the nucleic acids

  (D) ribosomes

  (E) the bacterial nuclear membrane

382. β-lactam antibiotics are correctly described as all of the following EXCEPT

  (A) semisynthetic or produced naturally by microbes

  (B) generally low-molecular-weight compounds (less than 10,000 daltons)

  (C) those having some deleterious side effects on the host

  (D) more bactericidal against growing bacteria than against nongrowing bacteria

  (E) potent antimycotic agents

383. L forms of bacteria should be sensitive to all of the following EXCEPT

  (A) streptomycin

  (B) amikacin

  (C) tetracycline

  (D) erythromycin

  (E) amantadine hydrochloride

384. All of the following contribute to the killing action of β-lactam antibiotics EXCEPT

(A) binding of the antibiotic to certain proteins associated with the bacterial cytoplasmic membrane

(B) the inability of the bacterial cytoplasmic membrane to resist increased osmotic pressure

(C) inhibition of the transpeptidation reaction

(D) activity of autolytic hydrolases

(E) binding of the antibiotic to bacterial nuclear membrane

385. All of the following statements concerning protein synthesis inhibitors are false EXCEPT

(A) chloramphenicol is bactericidal and inhibits the translocation reaction on the 30S ribosomal subunit

(B) tetracycline is active only against the 70S ribosomes from mammalian mitochondria

(C) erythromycin is a bactericidal aminoglycoside

(D) resistance to one form of tetracycline gives cross-resistance to all others

386. Nalidixic acid is correctly described by all of the following statements EXCEPT

(A) it inhibits the "swivelase" activity of *E. coli* DNA gyrase

(B) it inhibits the A subunit of *E. coli* DNA gyrase

(C) it is used in the treatment of uncomplicated urinary tract infections

(D) high-level resistance mutations are fairly common

(E) it inhibits dihydropteroate synthetase

387. Protoplasts can be produced by treatment of certain gram-positive bacteria with

(A) capsular antibody and complement

(A) streptomycin

(C) lysozyme

(D) chloramphenicol

(E) rifampin

388. A poorly controlled diabetic patient has osteomyelitis. A bone marrow specimen taken aseptically from this patient contains gram-positive cocci in clusters. The bacterium you might expect to isolate from this patient

(A) probably has a thick peptidoglycan layer in its cell wall

(B) has endotoxin in its cell wall

(C) would no doubt respond to amphotericin B

(D) cannot be cultured on blood agar

(E) requires hemin (factor X) and nicotinamide adenine nucleotide (factor V)

389. Penicillins and cephalosporins were initially derived from

(A) molds

(B) yeasts

(C) *E. coli*

(D) viruses

390. The antibiotic which may incorporate into human teeth and bone is

(A) polymyxin

(B) streptomycin

(C) chloramphenicol

(D) tetracycline

DIRECTIONS (Questions 391 through 419): Each group of items in this section consists of a list lettered headings followed by several numbered words or phrases. For each numbered word or phrase, select the ONE lettered heading that is most closely associated with it. Each lettered heading may be selected once, more than once, or not at all.

Questions 391 and 392

(A) streptomycin

(B) iododeoxyuridine (IUDR)

(C) rifampin

(D) chloramphenicol

(E) nalidixic acid

391. Misreading of messenger RNA

392. Treatment of herpetic conjunctivitis

Questions 393 and 394

    (A) benzylpenicillin (penicillin G)

    (B) streptomycin

    (C) erythromycin

    (D) chloramphenicol

    (E) tetracycline

393. A bactericidal antibiotic that inhibits protein synthesis

394. Chromosomal mutation to resistance that alters protein L4 of the 50S ribosomal subunit

Questions 395 and 396

    (A) metronidazole

    (B) griseofulvin

    (C) nystatin

    (D) polymyxin

    (E) isoniazid

395. Effective given orally in *Microsporum*-induced disease of hair

396. Indicated in the chemoprophylaxis of tuberculosis

Questions 397 and 398

    (A) brown discoloration of the teeth

    (B) bone marrow depression and pancytopenia

    (C) cardiac damage

    (D) vestibular damage

    (E) erythema nodosum leprosum

397. Dapsone

398. Streptomycin

Questions 399 and 400

    (A) benzylpenicillin

    (B) penicillin G plus streptomycin

    (C) erythromycin

    (D) primaquine

    (E) thiabendazole

399. Atypical pneumonia due to *Mycoplasma pneumoniae*

400. Subacute bacterial endocarditis due to *Enterococcus faecalis*

Questions 401 and 402

    (A) amphotericin B

    (B) colistin

    (C) methicillin

    (D) carbenicillin

    (E) cycloserine

401. Polypeptide antibiotic inhibiting *Pseudomonas*

402. Inhibits mucopeptide synthesis by affecting alanine racemase

Questions 403 through 405

    (A) inducible oxicillinase production

    (B) TEM-1 β-lactamase

    (C) overproduction of target enzyme

    (D) lack of oxidative metabolism and active transport

    (E) alteration of intracellular target site (ribosomes)

    (F) active pumping out of substrate (efflux)

    (G) mutation of nuclear membrane

    (H) mutation in anionic transporter

    (I) hydrophobicity of antibiotic

    (J) production of high levels of acetylating and phosphorylating enzymes

    (K) alteration in penicillin-binding proteins (PBPs)

    (L) porin mutation in OmpF

    (M) mutation that alters binding of dihydropteroate synthetase

403. The predominant mechanism of resistance of bacteria to erythromycin

404. Predominant mechanism of resistance of *Staphylococcus aureus* to methicillin

405. The predominant mechanism of plasmid-dependent resistance of bacteria to aminoglycosides

Questions 406 through 408

(A) metronidazole

(B) flucytosine

(C) ketoconazole

(D) epinephrine

(E) phenoxymethylpenicillin

(F) acyclovir

(G) chloramphenicol

(H) enviroxime

(I) chloroquine

(J) 3-azidothymidine

406. A healthy medical student clearing trees in Lyme, Connecticut was bitten by ticks. One week later she complained of a fever, stiff neck, stiff joints, and arrhythmias. An expanding skin lesion known as erythema chronicum migrans with sharply formed borders was found on her leg. The antibiotic of first choice for the acute phase of this disease is:

407. A 22-year-old nurse who had been in excellent health complained of fatigue and diarrhea. Then he developed pneumonia that was caused by *Pneumocystis carinii*. Repeated blood tests showed depletion of the CD4$^+$ T lymphocytes. Treatment of this illness is difficult but may depend on use of:

408. A 33-year-old man spent the summer in the jungles of Brazil. Suddenly, he developed shaking chills and was hospitalized with anemia, pigmentation, hypertrophy of the spleen, and intermittent fever. Giemsa stain blood smears showed kidney-bean–shaped gametocytes with round pointed ends. Treatment of this disease rests on the use of:

Questions 409 and 410

(A) doxycycline

(B) mitomycin

(C) erythromycin

(D) ciprofloxacin

(E) cefazolin

(F) clindamycin

(G) sulfadiazine

409. Blocks the completion of murein layer in growing bacteria

410. Inhibits DNA gyrase

Antibiotics
Answers and Explanations

358. (D) An examination of the bacterial cell population per mL indicates that the combination of antibiotic A plus B yields a cell count per mL that is smaller than that achieved by either antibiotic A or B used alone. Thus, a synergistic action between antibiotics A and B, or synergism, has been obtained. Antagonism between antibiotics A and B would have been indicated if the combination of antibiotics A and B yielded a cell population per mL that was higher than that achieved by A alone. Indifference refers to the inability of antibiotic A to alter the antibacterial properties of B and vice versa, while addition refers to an additive antibacterial action between antibiotics A and B. (*Brooks et al, pp 158–159*)

359. (E) The structure shown in this question represents ofloxacin, a fluoroquinolone which is a synthetic analogue of nalixidic acid. Fluoroquinolones are active against many gram-negative and gram-positive bacteria. Fluoroquinolones block the action of DNA gyrase and thus inhibit bacterial DNA synthesis. The structures of penicillin, polymyxin, streptomycin, and chloramphenicol, which act on the cell wall, the cell membrane, the 30S subunit, and the 50S subunit of the bacterial chromosome respectively, are shown in the following figure. (*Brooks et al, pp 163–177, Joklik et al, pp 161,165,170,174*)

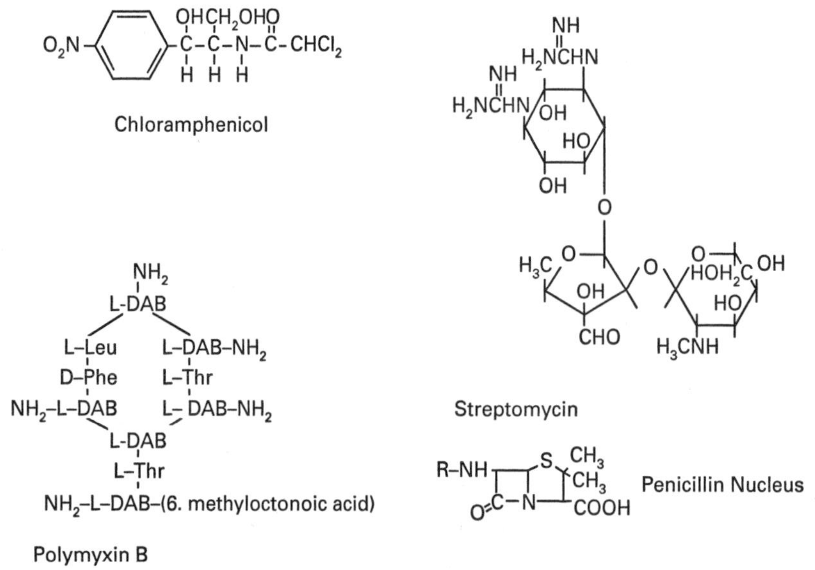

Chloramphenicol

Streptomycin

Polymyxin B

Penicillin Nucleus

Figure 4–3

360. (E) *Pseudomonas aeruginosa* is a gram-negative, oxidase-positive rod that produces a bluish-green pigment. It can cause the disease in immunocompromised individuals, ie, patients with severe burns, leukemia, or lymphoma who have been treated with radiation and antineoplastic drugs. *P. aeruginosa* becomes resistant to many antibiotics. However, it tends to be susceptible to ticarcillin, mezlocillin, and peperacillin especially, when used in combination with the aminoglycosides gentamicin, tobramycin, or amikacin. *E. coli, K. pneumoniae, P. mirabilis,* and *S. marcescens* are gram-negative, oxidase-negative rods, that do not produce a bluish-green pigment. *(Brooks et al, pp 212–217,224–225)*

361. (A) Penicillin G is the most suitable antibiotic for the treatment of meningitis of adults caused by *N. meningitidis.* Adults who are allergic to penicillin should be given cefotaxime, ceftriaxone, or chloramphenicol. The aminoglycosides amikacin, kanamycin, or gentamicin are not the drugs of choice for treating meningococcal disease. Ethambutol is employed for the treatment of tuberculosis, because many strains of *Mycobacterium tuberculosis* or other atypical mycobacteria such as *Mycobacterium kansasii* which causes tuberculosis are susceptible (1–5 µg/mL) to ethambutol. *(Brooks et al, pp 174,255)*

362. (B) Rifampin binds tightly to DNA-dependent RNA polymerase and thus inhibits RNA synthesis in bacteria. A key component of RNA is uracil. Thus, its incorporation will be blocked by rifampin. Streptomycin, kanamycin, amikacin, and tobramycin are aminoglycosides which bind to the 30 subunit of the bacterial ribosome and inhibit polypeptide synthesis. Therefore, all these antibiotics will interfere with the incorporation of amino acids and not uracil in sensitive bacteria. *(Joklik et al, pp 168–173)*

363. (D) *Klebsiella pneumoniae,* causing about 3% of bacterial pneumonias, can present a treatment problem because no single specific antibiotic therapy is available. This is particularly true for hospital-acquired pneumonia due to various *K. pneumoniae* strains which show multiple antibiotic resistances due to the possession of transmissible plasmids. Thus, variation in susceptibility to tetracycline is encountered and antibiotic susceptibility tests are required to determine the antibiotic of first choice for the treatment of hospital-acquired pneumonia due to *Klebsiella.* Lymphogranuloma venereum, inclusion conjunctivitis, trachoma, and psittacosis are caused by chlamydiae for which the drug of first choice is tetracycline. *(Brooks et al, pp 217,300–306)*

364. (C) *Bacteroides fragilis* is part of the normal flora of the lower gastrointestinal tract and present to health at its normal habitat. However, in the event of spillage of colonic contents into the peritoneal cavity due to diverticulitis, colon cancer, following surgery or trauma, a poorly understood chain of events leads frequently to abscess formation. The abscesses contain a mixed bacterial population, in which *B. fragilis* tends to be the predominant species. In contrast to many other species of the genus *Bacteroides, B. fragilis* produces β-lactose that inactivates penicillin. In general, *T. pallidum, A. israelii, S. pyogenes,* and *C. perfringens* are susceptible to penicillin, which is the drug of first choice for treatment of infections caused by these microorganisms. *(Brooks et al, pp 186,207,261,282,329)*

365. (E) Ampicillin shows relatively good activity against both gram-positive and gram-negative bacteria. It inhibits the action of transpeptidases involved in the synthesis of the bacterial cell wall peptidoglycan. Mammalian cells lack peptidoglycan and are not affected by ampicillin. Like any other antibiotic belonging to the penicillin group, ampicillin does not possess any renal toxicity. Most sulfonamides are excreted quickly in urine. However, sulfamethoxypyrimidazine is excreted slowly and thus it tends to be toxic. Amphotericin B is the drug of choice for the treatment of blastomycosis, candidiasis, coccidioidomycosis, cryptococcosis, and histoplasmosis. It binds to the sterols of the fungal membrane and disturbs their function. However, amphotericin B frequently produces renal failure and other toxic effects. The aminoglycosides amikacin and kanamycin, which are active against many gram-negative bacteria, like the majority of aminoglycosides, are nephrotoxic. *(Brooks et al, pp 162–166,172,176–178)*

366.   **(C)** Penicillin G is bactericidal for *S. pneumoniae* and other bacteria because it inhibits cell-wall synthesis. The sequence of events terminating in the death of the bacterial cell is as follows: Penicillin G and other β-lactam antibiotics bind to 3–6 chromosomally controlled proteins known as PBP. Some of the PBPs are transpeptidation enzymes involved with the synthesis of the peptidoglycan of the cell wall. Following binding of penicillin G to removal of PBPs or inactivation of an inhibitor of autolytic enzymes present in the cell wall occurs. This leads to the activation of autolytic enzymes and the lysis of the *S. pneumoniae*, or other penicillin G-susceptible cells. *(Brooks et al, p 150)*

367.   **(C)** Cycloheximide, a by-product of the metabolism of genus *Streptomyces* inhibits protein synthesis in the 80S ribosomes of eukaryotes, but does not inhibit the 70S ribosomes of prokaryotes. Cycloheximide blocks peptide bond formation. Colistin (polymyxin E) and polymyxin B are simple polypeptides produced by *Bacillus polymyxa*. They bind to the outer membrane of the gram-negative bacteria, altering their structure and osmotic properties. This leads to leakage of cellular metabolites following secondary damage of the cytoplasmic membrane. Mystatin, an antifungal polyene antibiotic, binds to the sterols of the fungal cytoplasmic membrane and causes leakage of the cytoplasmic contents. Finally, sodium deoxycholate is an anionic detergent that causes gross disruption of the lipoproteins of the cell membranes and lysis of the bacterial cell. *(Joklik et al, pp 164–165,191,528)*

368.   **(D)** Individuals that are allergic to penicillin usually tend to show allergy to other β-lac-

tam antibiotics, such as ampicillin, oxacillin, cephalosporin, or phenoxymethylpenicillin. The responsible antigens appear to be degradation moieties of the penicillin molecule. Skin test with undegraded and degraded penicillin-containing solutions identify individuals allergic to penicillin. Persons hypersensitive to penicillin usually are treated with tetracycline. *(Brooks et al, pp 161–169)*

369.   **(A)** Antibiotic tolerance is manifested by the requirement of high levels of antibiotic for killing, with only normal antibiotic levels required for inhibition of the bacteria. In other words, the minimal bactericidal concentration (MBC) is 30 or more times the MIC. Although a number of bacteria have been demonstrated to have this antibiotic tolerance in vitro, it only appears to be of clinical significance in staphylococcal heart valve infections among drug addicts. The reason for this antibiotic tolerance is related to defective autolytic enzymes in the staphylococci. *(Brooks et al, pp 150)*

370.   **(A)** If a microbe is sensitive to the antibiotic in vitro, it may or may not be sensitive to the antibiotic in vivo. Many problems must be overcome, such as the protein binding of the antibiotic (only the free antibiotic is effective); intracellular location of the microbe; inability of the antibiotic to reach acceptable levels in serum, urine, or serous fluids because of permeability problems or rapid excretion or destruction of the agent; and so on. *(Brooks et al, pp 155–156)*

371.   **(D)** The achievable blood level of the antibiotic must be greater than the MIC; ie, it takes higher levels to kill than to inhibit the microbe. Minimal bacterial concentrations are generally used at levels two to four times greater than the MIC. *(Brooks et al, pp 154–165)*

372.   **(A)** The benzylpenicillin β-lactam ring is hydrolyzed by penicillinase to the inactive penicilloic acid. *(Brooks et al, pp 161–166)*

373. (D) Methotrexate, like trimethoprim, blocks the activity of dihydrofolate reductase. Since the same enzyme is present in mammalian cells and in those bacteria that synthesize folic acid, methotrexate would have to be less, rather than more, active against the mammalian enzyme. *(Joklik et al, p 179)*

374. (D) Amphotericin B is an antifungal antibiotic that interacts with the membrane component ergosterol that leads to the formation of pores in the fungal membrane. This results in loss of vital metabolites from the cell. Rifampin binds strongly to DNA-dependent RNA polymerase and inhibits RNA synthesis. Neomycin and streptomycin inhibit polypeptide synthesis while penicillin blocks cell-wall synthesis. *(Joklik et al, pp 158–183)*

375. (A) Polymyxin B is a basic polypeptide that is bactericidal to many gram-negative bacteria including *Pseudomonas* and *Serratia*, but it is nephrotoxic and neurotoxic. Because of its toxicity and poor distribution to tissues, it is now used only topically. It binds to the phosphatidylethanolamine of the bacterial membranes and interferes with membrane functions of active transport. Sulfadiazine trimethoprim and sulfamethoxazole are sulfonamides and are well-tolerated by humans. *(Joklik et al, pp 165,178–180)*

376. (C) Mitomycin C will not cross-link DNA in vitro. It first requires metabolic processing to an active quinine methide. Cross-linked DNA, when partially denatured, will reanneal upon cooling. Metronidazole is useful for prokaryotic and eukaryotic pathogens. Amantadine is prophylactic for the influenza A_2 virus. *(Ryan et al, p 211)*

377. (C) Rifampin, whose antimicrobial action is through inhibition of nucleic acid synthesis, binds strongly to DNA-dependent RNA polymerase in bacteria but not in mammalian cells, blocking initiation of mRNA synthesis. It binds covalently to the β subunit of RNA polymerase but it does not involve the sigma subunit, a promoter-specific protein. *(Joklik et al, p 168)*

378. (E) Antibiotics are *not* mutagenic. Rather, they select the few spontaneous mutants (one out of a million or billion), allowing them to multiply in the presence of the antibiotic. *(Joklik et al, p 128)*

379. (B) Cleavage of the β-lactam ring by β-lactamase completely destroys the activity of the β-lactam drug. *(Brooks et al, p 161)*

380. (E) Plasmid-mediated resistance is usually due to the synthesis of a new, distinct protein. *(Brooks et al, pp 152–153; Joklik, pp 147–149)*

381. (E) Bacteria lack nuclear membranes. The cell wall, the nucleic acids, the cytoplasmic membranes, and ribosomes are all target sites for the activity of antibacterial drugs. *(Brooks et al, p 149)*

382. (E) β-lactam drugs are ineffective antimycotic agents, because fungi lack bacterial cell walls. β-lactam antibiotics generally have low to intermediate molecular weights rather than high molecular weights. For example, the β-lactams have molecular weights in the 300 to 400 dalton range, certainly less than 10,000 daltons. Also, β-lactams are bactericidal only against growing rather than nongrowing bacteria. *(Brooks et al, pp 163–169)*

383. (E) Amantadine hydrochloride is an anti-influenza drug. It blocks uncoating of influenza A virus. L forms, lacking cell walls, would not be sensitive to antibiotics that block peptidoglycan synthesis, such as bacitracin and penicillin. Streptomycin, tetracycline, amikacin, erythromycin, and L forms should be sensitive to them, because they block protein synthesis rather than peptidoglycan synthesis. *(Brooks et al, pp 22,270–271)*

384. (E) Bacteria lack nuclear membranes. The penicillin-binding proteins, which are found in the cytoplasmic membranes of all bacteria with peptidoglycans, bind covalently to the β-lactam antibiotics. *(Joklik et al, pp 154–157)*

385. (D) Chloramphenicol is not bactericidal and it binds exclusively to the 50S ribosomal subunit, not to the 30S subunit, blocking the peptidyl transferase reaction. Tetracycline binds mainly to the 30S ribosomal subunit of rapidly growing bacteria, as well as to the 70S ribosomes of mammalian mitochondria. Erythromycin is bacteriostatic rather than bactericidal, and it is not an aminoglycoside. *(Joklik et al, pp 173–175)*

386. **(E)** Sulfonamides, not nalixidic acid, inhibit dihydropteroate synthetase. Nalidixic acid blocks DNA replication in *E. coli* by inhibiting the A subunit of DNA gyrase. It inhibits the nicking and closing activity of the swivelase portion of DNA gyrase, which relieves the stress on supercoiled DNA. Mutation on the *nalA* gene locus confers high-level resistance to nalidixic acid, a fairly common problem in nalidixic acid treatment of uncomplicated urinary tract infections. *(Joklik et al, pp 166–167)*

387. **(C)** A protoplast is a bacterial cell from which its cell wall has been completely removed. This can be achieved by treating certain gram-positive bacteria with appropriate concentrations of lysozyme or by blocking peptidoglycan synthesis with penicillin. In media that are absolutely protective, such treatments liberate protoplasts from certain gram-positive bacteria. Streptomycin induces misreading of mRNA, with resultant synthesis of protein with a number of "wrong" amino acids. Chloramphenicol blocks the peptidyl transferase reaction. Nalidixic acid inhibits DNA gyrase. Rifampin inactivates the DNA-dependent polymerase. *(Joklik et al, pp 170–172)*

388. **(A)** The presence of gram-positive cocci in clusters in a bone marrow specimen obtained aseptically from a poorly controlled diabetic patient with osteomyelitis suggests *Staphylococcus aureus* as the most likely cause of osteomyelitis in this patient. In general, gram-positive bacteria contain thick cell walls composed of peptidoglycan and teichoic or teichuronic acids. The peptidoglycan layer of gram-negative bacteria is thin, consisting of a single molecule of murein (peptidoglycan). Gram-negative bacteria contain endotoxin in the outer membrane of their cell wall. *S. aureus* and other gram-positive bacteria can be cultured on blood, agar, and since they do not have ergosterol in their cytoplasmic membrane are resistant to the antifungal agent amphotericin B. *Hemophilus influenzae* requires hemin and nicotinamide adenine nucleotide for growth (factors X and V), which are produced by *S. aureus*. *(Joklik et al, pp 76–87,165,401–412)*

389. **(A)** The first member of the β-lactam antibiotics, such as penicillin, was derived from molds of the genus *Penicillium*. Penicillin and other natural, semisynthetic, and synthetic β-lactams have a β-lactam ring which is necessary for their antibacterial activity. The first cephalosporin antibiotic was also derived from cultures of molds of the genus *Cephalosporium*. Yeasts have been used to obtain various water-soluble vitamins. *E. coli* produces vitamin K in the human intestinal tract. Viruses have not been shown to produce penicillins or cephalosporins. *(Ryan et al, pp 192–195)*

390. **(D)** The tetracyclines display a strong affinity for developing teeth and bone, which they stain yellow, and thus should not be administered to children up to 8 years old. Other undesirable side effects of tetracyclines include gastrointestinal disturbances due to modification of the normal flora, superinfection by tetracycline-resistant bacteria, and oral or vaginal infections caused by *Candida albicans*. Divalent catious chelate tetracyclines and reduce their absorption as well as their activity. Therefore, they should not be taken with dairy products or antiacid compounds. *(Ryan et al, p 201)*

391. **(A)** Streptomycin induces misreading of messenger RNA, with resultant synthesis of protein with a number of "wrong" amino acids. Chloramphenicol blocks the peptidyl transferase reaction. Nalidixic acid inhibits DNA gyrase. Rifampin inactivates the DNA-

dependent RNA polymerase. *(Joklik et al, pp 170–172)*

392. **(B)** IUDR, an analogue of thymidine, inhibits the replication of herpesviruses. It is used clinically for the topical treatment of herpetic conjunctivitis. Although the IUDR is probably incorporated into both host and viral DNA, it is accessible to relatively few host cells in the limited access of the eye. Because of mismatching, since IUDR does not pair with adenine as faithfully as thymine, defective DNA and then defective messenger RNA result. *(Joklik et al, pp 856–857)*

393. **(B)** Although all of the antibiotics listed in the question, other than benzylpenicillin, inhibit protein biosynthesis, only streptomycin is considered bactericidal. *(Brooks et al, pp 150–151)*

394. **(C)** Erythromycin, a macrolide antibiotic, blocks the translocation step in protein synthesis. Resistance to erythromycin due to a chromosomal mutation is a genetically controlled property of the 50S ribosomes so that the ribosomes have a reduced ability to bind the antibiotic. This resistance appears to be the result of an altered 50S ribosomal subunit protein component, either protein L4 or L12. *(Joklik et al, p 175)*

395. **(B)** Dermatomycosis is a disease of hair, skin, or nails caused by over 42 species of the genera *Microsporum, Trichophyton,* and *Epidermophyton.* It is transmitted by direct and indirect contact from one individual to another, or from infected animals to humans. The infection begins in the hair follicles from which extension occurs into the surrounding hair, skin, and nails. The most effective antibiotic is griseofulvin, which must be given orally for a long time. Griseofulvin is concentrated in the stratum corneum and it inhibits the growth of the etiological agent. Nystatin, another antifungal agent, is used for the treatment of cutaneous candidiasis. Metronidazole, polymyxin, and isoniazid are therapeutic drugs that lack antifungal activity. *(Joklik et al, pp 1125–1144)*

396. **(E)** It has been demonstrated that isoniazid chemoprophylaxis is a good way of preventing tuberculosis. To be effective, isoniazid must be administered in suitable daily doses to individuals at risk of infection. Isoniazid chemoprophylaxis is usually administered in any child who develops a positive tuberculin test before 4 years of age, in tuberculin-positive persons who live in close contact with active tuberculosis, and in healthy physicians, nurses, or hospital attendants whose tuberculin tests have recently become positive. Chemoprophylaxis is often employed for patients known to have a positive tuberculin test and to be either suffering from leukemia or lymphoma, or receiving immunosuppressive drugs which alter host resistance and predispose to activation of subclinical, or inactive, tuberculosis. Griseofulvin, nystatin, metroidazole, or polymyxin are unsuitable for chemoprophylaxis against tuberculosis. *(Joklik et al, pp 180–181,509)*

397. **(E)** Leprosy is rare in the United States and Europe. However, there are approximately 12 million cases of leprosy in Africa, Asia, and parts of Central and South America. This disease is caused by the acid-fast bacillus *Mycobacterium leprae,* which tends to be susceptible to 4,4'-diaminodiphenylsulfone (dapsone). Dapsone has been the mainstay for the treatment of leprosy. The range of resistance of *M. leprae* to dapsone is 2 to 19%. Now the World Health Organization recommends combined therapy for lepromatous leprosy consisting of dapsone, rifampin, and clofazimine. There are two forms of leprosy: the tuberculoid form, which is mild leprosy characterized by the appearance of a hypopigmenter macule, and the severe form of leprosy known as lepromatous leprosy. The severe form of the disease is characterized by severe, multiple, deforming, nodular, erythematous lesions called erythema nodosum leprosum. Brown discoloration of the teeth, bone marrow depression, and cardiac or vestibular damage are not the key features of leprosy. *(Joklik et al, pp 516–521)*

398. (D) Streptomycin is an aminoglycoside, which may be bactericidal for many gram-positive, gram-negative bacteria, and *Mycobacterium tuberculosis*. The bacterial action of streptomycin has not been adequately explained. Apparently, binding of streptomycin to 30S ribosome moiety and the subsequent misreading of the genetic message is contributing to the lethal action of streptomycin, but it does provide a clear explanation of its bactericidal activity. Some of the undesirable side effects of streptomycin include its marked toxicity for the vestibular portion of the eighth cranial nerve, leading to vertigo and ataxia. Streptomycin has also been shown to be nephrotoxic and allergenic. Teeth discoloration may be a side effect of tetracycline administration. Chloramphenicol may induce bone marrow depression, and erythema nodosum leprosum presents the lesions of lepromatous leprosy. *(Brooks et al, pp 170–173; Joklik et al, pp 173–174)*

399. (C) *Mycoplasma pneumoniae* is one of the agents that causes primary atypical pneumonia. Other microorganisms such as adenovirus, parainfluenza or influenza virus, respiratory syncytial virus, and *Chlamydia psittaci* can also cause primary atypical pneumonia. This disease is an acute bronchopneumonia with a slight fever, nonproductive cough, pulmonary infiltrate, and headache. Eryth-romycin or tetracycline for 2–3 weeks is used for treatment. The organisms may persist for up to 2 months after treatment but the symptoms disappear. Primaquine is an antiprotozoan drug used for the treatment of malaria. Thiabendazole is employed for the treatment of trichinosis. Mycoplasmas lack cell walls, and therefore cannot be expected to respond to penicillin. *(Joklik et al, pp 733–736)*

400. (B) *Enterococcus faecalis (Streptococcus faecalis)* has been implicated in the development of subacute bacterial endocarditis, particularly in old persons or individuals with valvular heart disease. *E. faecalis* tends to be resistant to penicillin G, ampicillin, or the penicillinase-resistant penicillins. Plasmid-mediated resistance to high levels of streptomycin has also been a critical factor in reducing the administration of streptomycin for the treatment of subacute bacterial endocarditis caused by *E. faecalis* or other microorganisms. However, combined use of streptomycin and penicillin reduces the emergence of plasmid-mediated resistance to streptomycin. Therefore, streptomycin in combination with penicillin or vancomycin is useful in the therapy of subacute bacterial endocarditis due to *E. faecalis*. See the previous answer for reasons why the other therapeutic drugs are not suitable. *(Joklik et al, pp 427–428)*

401. (B) Colistin (polymyxin E) is a polypeptide antibiotic produced by *Bacillus polymyxa* which inhibits the growth of many species of the genus *Pseudomonas*. Colistin binds to the outer membrane of the cell wall and alters its structure so that there is leakage of cytoplasmic contents. *Pseudomonas* are resistant to most β-lactam antibiotics, including penicillin G and methicillin, because these antibiotics cannot penetrate the outer membrane of the cell wall of *Pseudomonas* and the small amount that enters the outer membrane is hydrolized by periplasmic lactamases. Carboxy derivatives of ampicillin such as carbenicillin and ticarcillin can be active against *Pseudomonas*. However, these drugs are not polypeptide antibiotics. Cyclosine resembles D-alanine which, due to its neurotoxicity, had found limited use in the treatment of tuberculosis. Amphotericin B is an antifungal antibiotic. *(Joklik et al, pp 163–165)*

402. (E) Cycloserine is a bactericidal antibiotic that resembles D-alanine, a component of the bacterial cell wall peptidoglycan. The enzyme alanine racemase converts the L-alanine, which is supplied to the bacterial culture medium, to its isomer D-alanine. Cycloserine, due to its similarity to D-alanine, inhibits mucopeptide synthesis by interfering with the activity of alanine racemase. See the previous answer for reasons why the other drugs are inappropriate. *(Joklik et al, pp 163–164)*

403. (E) Erythromycin is obtained from *Streptomyces erythreus*, and in concentrations of

0.1 to 2 μ/mL is active against many gram-positive and gram-negative bacteria such as streptococci, pneumococci, corynebacteria, *Mycoplasma*, *Chlamydia trachomatis*, spirochetes, *Legionella*, etc. The 50S ribosomal subunit is the site of action of erythromycin. Bacteria that become resistant to erythromycin under chromosomal or plasmid-mediated control synthesize ribosomes that have a diminished affinity for erythromycin. This is correlated with a reduced affinity of the L4 and L12 50S ribosomal proteins to bind erythromycin. *(Joklik et al, p 175)*

404. **(K)** Methicillin is a semisynthetic penicillin which is resistant to penicillinase (β-lactamase). The production of penicillinase in gram-positive bacteria tends to be under chromosomal and plasmid control. However, in *Staphylococcus aureus* the plasmid penicillinase gene is obtained from that on the staphylococcal chromosome via a transposon (jumping gene). Since methicillin is resistant to hydrolysis by β-lactamases, another mechanism must be the basis for the observed resistance of staphylococci to methicillin. The current belief is that methicillin resistance of *S. aureus*, *S. pneumoniae*, and *Neisseria gonorrhoeae* to methicillin is due to an alteration in the penicillin-binding proteins. *(Joklik et al, p 157)*

405. **(J)** Chromosomal-dependent resistance to aminoglycosides depends primarily on absence of specific aminoglycoside receptors on the 30S ribosomal subunit. However, the predominant mechanism of plasmid-dependent resistance of bacteria to aminoglycosides is the synthesis of high or adequate levels of acetylating, phosphorylating, or adenylating enzymes by the bacteria. These enzymes add an acetyl, phosphate, or adenyl group to aminoglycosides and thus render them inactive bacteria. *(Brooks et al, p 151)*

406. **(E)** The lesion known as erythema chronicum migrans (ECM) is a diagnostic hallmark of Lyme disease. This disease is transmitted to humans by bites of infected ticks carrying the causative agent of Lyme disease, *Borrelia burgdorferi*. The clinical manifestations of Lyme disease include fever, a stiff neck and joints, an expanding skin lesion called erythema chronicum migrans, and cardiovascular or neurological symptoms. The antibiotic of first choice for the acute phase of the disease is phenoxymethylpenicillin. Metronidazole is an antiprotozoal drug used to treat *Trichomonas*, *Giardia*, and amebic infections. It is also effective against anaerobic bacteria such as *Bacteroides* species or *Clostridium difficile*. Flucytosine is an antifungal agent used for the treatment of infections caused by *Candida*, *Cryptococcus*, and *Torulopsis*. Ketoconazole is another antifungal drug. Epinephrine is used for the treatment of immediate-type hypersensitivity. Chloramphenicol is the drug of choice for typhoid fever and meningitis caused by *Hemophilus influenzae*. Chloroquine is employed to treat malaria. The antiviral drugs acyclovir, enviroxime, and 3′-azidothymidine are used for the treatment of infections caused by the herpesviruses, rhinoviruses, and the human immunodeficiency virus, respectively. *(Brooks et al, pp 176,178,284,398–401)*

407. **(J)** The major characteristic of acquired immunodeficiency syndrome (AIDS) is depletion of the CD4+ lymphocytes within which multiplication of the human immunodeficiency virus (HIV) occurs. Constitutional symptoms include unexplained fatigue, diarrhea, and infections caused by such protozoa as *Pneumocystis carinii* and *Toxoplasma gondii*. Several antiviral drugs are currently being investigated for the treatment of HIV infections. However, at the present moment, 3′-azidothymidine, also known as zidovudine or AZT, is the only antiviral drug approved for the treatment of AIDS. Another antiviral drug called dideoxyinoside (ddI) is also being used for treatment. *(Brooks, pp 574–580)*

408. **(I)** Malaria is caused by various species of protozoa of the genus *Plasmodium*. The main species are *P. falciparum*, *P. vivax*, and *P. malariae*. Chloroquine is the drug of choice for the treatment of malaria. For chloroquine-resistant plasmodia, primaquine or quinine sulfate plus pyrimethamine-sulfadoxine (Fansidar) may be used. Plasmodia are

strictly parasitic and have two hosts—the anopheline mosquito and humans. In humans they live inside the erythrocytes, and the morphology of the plasmodia, or their gametocytes, is used to determine the specific plasmodium that caused malaria. For example, the presence of a kidney-bean–shaped gametocyte in Giemsa stain blood smears indicates malaria caused by *P. falciparum*. Malaria due to *P. falciparum* is common in tropical jungles where anopheline mosquitoes are abundant. Individuals infected with *P. falciparum* develop shaking chills, intermittent fever, anemia, hypertrophy of spleen, and tissue pigmentation due to deposition of red blood cell pigment. *(Brooks et al, pp 349–351)*

409. **(E)** Cefazolin is a cephalosporin that interferes with the transpeptidation reactions which are required for the formation of peptide cross-links between peptidoglycan chains. The antibacterial action of cefazolin is thought to be due to the chemical similarity of the D-alanyl–D-alanine end of the pentapeptide. Thus, cefazolin blocks the completion of the murein layer in growing susceptible bacterial cells. Doxycycline, erythromycin, and clindamycin inhibit protein synthesis. Mitomycin interferes with the synthesis of nucleic acids, while sulfadiazine inhibits dihydropteroate synthetase. *(Ryan et al, pp 192–196,200–206)*

410. **(D)** Ciprofloxacin is a fluoroquinolone that inhibits DNA gyrase and is an enzyme involved in the supercoiling, nicking, and joining of bacterial DNA. Ciprofloxacin is active against aerobic and facultative anaerobic bacteria; it binds slightly to protein, is widely distributed in body tissues, has a prolonged half-life in serum, and it is able to penetrate phagocytes. At the recommended dosages, ciprofloxacin and other fluoroquinolones do not usually cause adverse reactions. However, they may concentrate in the cartilage and thus are not recommended for children and pregnant women. *(Ryan et al, pp 203–204)*

REFERENCES

Joklik WK, Willett HP, Amos BD, Wilfert CM. *Zinsser Microbiology*, 20th ed. Norwalk, CT: Appleton & Lange; 1992.

Brooks GF, Butel JS, Ornston LN, Jawetz E, Melnick JL, Adelberg EA. *Medical Microbiology*, 19th ed. Norwalk, CT: Appleton & Lange; 1991.

Ryan KJ, Champoux JJ, Drew WL, et al. *Sherris Medical Microbiology*, 3rd ed. Norwalk, CT: Appleton & Lange; 1994.

CHAPTER 5

Medical Bacteriology
Questions

DIRECTIONS (Questions 411 through 654): Each of the numbered items or incomplete statements in this section is followed by answers or by completions of the statement. Select the ONE lettered answer or completion that is BEST in each case.

411. All of the following statements about plasmids that contribute directly to microbial pathogenicity are true EXCEPT

    (A) the capacity of *Corynebacterium diphtheriae* strains to produce diphtheria toxin is due to the presence of plasmids

    (B) plasmids responsible for production of a toxin may be cured and toxin production ability lost without deleterious effect on the microbes

    (C) plasmids for two classes of *Escherichia coli* enterotoxins are involved in travelers' diarrhea

    (D) one class of ent plasmid encodes for a heat-labile enterotoxin, which is functionally and structurally similar to cholera toxin

    (E) to be enteropathogenic, *E. coli* ent strains also require plasmids that encode for pili that bring about specific adherence to mammalian epithelial cells

412. Which of the following is NOT a facultative intracellular pathogen?

    (A) *Listeria monocytogenes*
    (B) *Histoplasma capsulatum*
    (C) *Mycobacterium tuberculosis*
    (D) *Staphylococcus aureus*
    (E) *Brucella abortus*

413. All of the following statements about *Staphylococcus aureus* are true EXCEPT

    (A) it clots mammalian plasma
    (B) it causes erysipelas
    (C) cell walls contain ribitol phosphate teichoic acid
    (D) it causes furuncles
    (E) it causes carbuncles

414. All of the following statements about staphylococcal infections are true EXCEPT

    (A) the very young and the elderly are particularly susceptible to staphylococcal infections

    (B) exfoliative toxin is responsible for the scalded skin syndrome

    (C) *S. epidermidis* is responsible for increasing numbers of infections in immunosuppressed patients

    (D) *S. saprophyticus* is responsible for urinary tract infections in young, sexually active nonhospitalized women

    (E) coagulase is the sole staphylococcal virulence factor

415. All of the following are true statements about staphylococci EXCEPT

(A) toxic shock syndrome may affect both males and females

(B) many individuals are nasal carriers of *S. aureus*

(C) impetigo is caused only by *S. aureus*

(D) *S. epidermidis* is often responsible for infective endocarditis in intravenous drug abusers

(E) the phage type is a list of the strain numbers of those standard bacteriophages that can lyse a given *S. aureus* strain

416. When neonatal meningitis is caused by streptococci, they usually are

(A) *Streptococcus pyogenes* (group A)

(B) *Streptococcus agalactiae* (group B)

(C) *Streptococcus sanguis* (viridans streptococci)

(D) *Streptococcus pneumoniae* (serotype B)

(E) *Streptococcus mitis* (viridans streptococci)

417. Following a skin infection with *S. pyogenes* group A, type 12, one can expect

(A) common sequelae to include rheumatic fever

(B) common sequelae to include acute glomerulonephritis

(C) a rise in antistreptolysin O titer

(D) deep suppurative ulcers

(E) to be unable to culture the bacteria from the skin during the infection

418. The normal flora of the throat does NOT include moderate numbers of which of the following bacteria?

(A) alpha-hemolytic streptococci

(B) beta-hemolytic staphylococci

(C) alpha-hemolytic pneumococci

(D) beta-hemolytic group A streptococci

(E) gram-negative diplococci

419. There is a mechanism for antibiotic resistance to penicillin and the penicillin-derivative methicillin, NOT due to a beta-lactamase, by all of the clinically important bacteria EXCEPT

(A) *Staphylococcus aureus*

(B) *Escherichia coli*

(C) *Streptococcus pneumoniae*

(D) *Neisseria gonorrhoeae*

(E) *Neisseria meningitidis*

420. The pneumococcal antigen that reacts with a nonantibody serum globulin present in inflammatory states is

(A) capsular polysaccharide

(B) penicillin-binding protein 2

(C) C substance (phosphocholine-containing teichoic acid)

(D) pneumolysin

(E) purpura-producing principle

421. A gram-positive coccus that grows in pairs or short chains and that is alpha-hemolytic and optochin-sensitive is

(A) *Streptococcus pyogenes*

(B) *Streptococcus agalactiae*

(C) *Streptococcus faecalis*

(D) *Staphylococcus aureus*

(E) *Streptococcus pneumoniae*

422. The antibody that develops after an episode of pneumococcal pneumonia may not protect against subsequent pneumococcal disease because

(A) the antibody is only against the pneumococcal C substance (phosphocholine-containing teichoic acid)

(B) antibody levels are present for only a few weeks

(C) the polysaccharide is not immunogenic

(D) the 84 different pneumococcal polysaccharides and their antibodies do not cross-protect

(E) anticapsular antibody is not protective

423. All of the following statements about meningococcal disease are true EXCEPT

(A) serogroups A and C are associated with epidemic disease and B with endemic disease

(B) there is no human carrier state (without disease) for the meningococcus

(C) acquisition of meningococci in the nasopharynx by nonimmune individuals may result in bacteremia

(D) bacteremia results in disease

(E) meningococcemia results in a syndrome of sudden overwhelming fever and shock with a hemorrhagic (petechial) rash

424. The most likely component responsible for the production of overwhelming septic shock complicating bacteremia with *Neisseria meningitidis* is the

(A) capsular polysaccharide

(B) pili

(C) lipopolysaccharide in the outer membrane

(D) low-molecular-weight outer membrane proteins

(E) peptidoglycan

425. All of the following statements about the major microbes that may cause meningitis are true EXCEPT

(A) in neonates, they include *E. coli*, group B streptococci, and *Listeria monocytogenes*

(B) in children from 1 month to 6 years of age, they include *Hemophilus influenzae* type b, Neisseria meningitidis, and *Streptococcus pneumoniae*

(C) in young adults, they include *N. meningitidis* and *S. pneumoniae*

(D) among the elderly, they are due only to *N. meningitidis*

(E) in closed populations of adults (military recruits, college dormitories), they are due only to *N. meningitidis*

426. The major mechanism of host resistance to tuberculosis is

(A) humoral antibodies

(B) delayed hypersensitivity

(C) high level of calcium in serum

(D) increased microbicidal activity of activated macrophages

(E) massive proliferation of polymorphonuclear leukocytes

427. The characteristics of *Mycobacterium tuberculosis* include which of the following?

(A) obligate requirement for oxygen

(B) niacin production

(C) acid-fastness

(D) slow growth

(E) all of the above

428. A positive tuberculin skin test indicates

(A) no immunity to *M. tuberculosis* infections

(B) a parasitic infection

(C) prior exposure to *M. tuberculosis*

(D) active pulmonary tuberculosis

(E) active nontubercular mycobacterial infections

429. The purified protein derivative

(A) fails to induce delayed hypersensitivity upon repeated injection

(B) contains only tuberculoproteins

(C) contains tuberculoproteins and trehalose 6,6-dimycolate (Cord factor)

(D) is usually administered at 1 tuberculin unit

(E) is usually extracted with phenol from the tubercle bacilli

430. *Mycobacterium kansasii*

(A) causes cervical adenitis

(B) grows best at 30 to 33°C

(C) is a scotochromogen

(D) is considered a "rapid grower"

(E) causes chronic pulmonary tuberculosis

431. *Mycobacterium intracellulare*

(A) contain lipids, polysaccharides, and peptidoglycan in its cell wall

(B) causes pulmonary infections that can be easily spread by person-to-person transmission

(C) cannot be grown on the Jensen–Lowenstein medium

(D) produces severe infections in guinea pigs

(E) is an obligate intracellular parasite

432. *Mycobacterium leprae*

(A) forms non-acid–fast serpentine cords

(B) contains 80S ribosomes

(C) does not respond to sulfones and rifampin

(D) does not induce delayed-type hypersensitivity

(E) cannot be cultured on artificial media

433. Human mycobacterial pathogens other than *M. tuberculosis*

(A) include the photochromogens that cause scrofula in young children

(B) include such rapid growers as *M. kansasii*

(C) respond readily to antituberculosis drugs

(D) produce purified protein derivatives (PPDs) that are used in skin tests

(E) are usually pathogenic for the guinea pig

434. The causative organisms of which of the following diseases are not introduced into hosts in the form of spores?

(A) tetanus

(B) gas gangrene

(C) anthrax

(D) diphtheria

(E) pseudomembranous colitis (antibiotic associated)

435. All of the following statements concerning *Pseudomonas aeruginosa* and *Pseudomonas* infections are true EXCEPT

(A) *P. aeruginosa* produces an exotoxin similar in its mode of action to diphtheria toxin

(B) *P. aeruginosa* is one of the most common organisms that cause infections in burn patients

(C) pus associated with *Pseudomonas* infections usually appears greenish

(D) *P. aeruginosa* is quite susceptible to penicillin G

(E) *P. aeruginosa* is a gram-negative, motile rod found commonly in our environment

436. Antibiotic-associated pseudomembranous colitis is caused by an exotoxin elaborated by

(A) *Bacteriodes fragilis*

(B) a toxigenic strain of *E. coli*

(C) *Vibrio cholerae*

(D) *Clostridium difficile*

(E) *Listeria monocytogenes*

437. The effectiveness of immunization with diphtheria toxoid is based on the fact that the

(A) toxoid stimulates a state of hypersensitivity to corynebacteria

(B) toxoid stimulates production of antibodies that opsonize invading corynebacteria for rapid phagocytosis

(C) toxoid is converted into immune globulins that are bactericidal

(D) toxoid stimulates the production of specific antitoxin that neutralizes diphtheria toxin

(E) antitoxin prevents invasion of the bloodstream by corynebacteria

438. The simplest way to determine the susceptibility of an individual to diphtheria is to perform

(A) an agglutination test with *Corynebacterium diphtheriae*

(B) a flocculation test with toxin

(C) a flocculation test with toxoid

(D) a skin test

(E) a complement fixation test

439. Toxin of *E. coli* that is very similar to the shiga toxin of *Shigella dysenteriae* is

(A) heat-labile enterotoxin

(B) heat-stable enterotoxin

(C) adherence-promoting toxin

(D) verotoxin

(E) exfoliative toxin

440. Which of the following statements correctly describes *Neisseria gonorrhoeae?*

(A) types 2 and 4 are pathogenic

(B) it lacks indophenol oxidase

(C) it grows best anaerobically (80% CO_2 tension)

(D) it may cause blindness in the newborn

(E) it produces a protease that cannot degrade IgA

441. *Chlamydia trachomatis* is a widely prevalent human pathogen that

(A) is the most common cause of nongono-coccal urethritis

(B) does not respond to chemotherapy

(C) produces a protease that degrades IgA

(D) is a flagellated protozoan

(E) is not usually transmitted sexually

442. All of the following statements concerning *N. gonorrhoeae* are correct EXCEPT

(A) it can be cultured on the Thayer–Martin medium

(B) it grows best in the presence of 2 to 10% carbon dioxide

(C) it confers solid immunity to subsequent reinfections

(D) it can cause pelvic inflammatory disease (PID)

(E) virulent organisms possess pili

443. Congenital syphilis can best be detected by the use of

(A) dark-field examination

(B) silver nitrate staining of the spirochetes

(C) the Wassermann complement fixation test

(D) IgM-FTA-ABS test

(E) x-rays

444. The most recently discovered sexually transmitted disease is

(A) trichomoniasis

(B) condyloma acuminata (venereal warts)

(C) hepatitis

(D) acquired immunodeficiency syndrome (human immunodeficiency virus)

(E) candidiasis

445. Which of the following statements correctly describes enterotoxins?

(A) they are not produced by *Salmonella* species

(B) they are not produced by *E. coli*

(C) they stimulate adenyl cyclase

(D) they are not antigenic

(E) they contain lipid A

446. Which of the following statements correctly describes *Pseudomonas* infections?

(A) they are often encountered in cystic fibrosis patients

(B) they do not occur in patients suffering from burns

(C) they can be easily treated with antibiotics

(D) they are caused by *P. aeruginosa*, which produces a red pigment

(E) they do not respond to a combined gentamicin and carbenicillin treatment

447. *P. aeruginosa* is accurately described as

(A) nonmotile

(B) a fastidious microorganism

(C) utilizing lactose

(D) producing large amounts of urease

(E) producing an exotoxin

448. 2-Keto-3-deoxyoctonate is correctly described as

(A) the toxic moiety of the somatic O antigen

(B) a constituent of the inner core of *Salmonella* lipopolysaccharide

(C) usually not found in endotoxin

(D) responsible for the variation in phase type within Enterobacteriaceae

(E) a dideoxyhexose

449. The H antigens of *Salmonella* are known to be

(A) located on the cell wall

(B) composed of polysaccharides

(C) found mostly in virulent strains

(D) used to characterize these species

(E) encountered primarily in the lactose-fermenting strains

450. Humans acquire *Salmonella typhimurium* by

(A) aerosols

(B) tick bites

(C) mosquito bites

(D) penetration of the broken skin

(E) the ingestion of contaminated food and water

451. The reservoir of *S. typhi* is

(A) dogs

(B) cats

(C) turtles

(D) pigs

(E) humans

452. The Vi antigen of *S. typhi* is

(A) part of the O antigen

(B) its main virulence factor

(C) stable to heating at 60°C for 1 hour

(D) now considered a major adhesin

(E) often hindering agglutination by anti-O antibodies

453. The best specimen for the diagnosis of typhoid fever in the first week of illness is

(A) sputum

(B) blood

(C) stool

(D) urine

(E) bone marrow

454. In the diagnosis of urinary tract infections, all of the following results indicate infection EXCEPT

(A) culture resulting in more than 105 bacteria per mL of urine

(B) one or two bacteria per oil immersion field seen on a Gram stain of uncentrifuged urine

(C) greater than 10 white blood cells per high power field of centrifuged urine

(D) white blood cell casts in the urine sediment

(E) urine pH of 6.0

455. Most organisms that cause urinary tract infection come from

(A) toilet seats

(B) the environment

(C) sexual partners

(D) normal bowel flora

(E) normal skin flora

456. All of the following statements about urinary tract infections (UTIs) are true EXCEPT

(A) ascending UTIs are more common than descending UTIs

(B) nontreatment of UTIs in young girls is not considered an acceptable practice even though the UTIs are asymptomatic

(C) it is important to determine if the UTI is localized in the lower or upper urinary tract

(D) community-acquired and hospital-acquired UTIs are equally susceptible to the same antibiotics

(E) the finding of any viable bacteria in urine samples removed by suprapubic aspiration denotes a UTI

457. The most likely candidate responsible for the production of overwhelming septicemic shock complicating bacteremia with *Neisseria meningitidis* is

(A) capsular polysaccharide

(B) pili

(C) lipopolysaccharide in outer membrane

(D) low-molecular-weight outer membrane proteins

(E) glucose fermentation

458. A curved gram-negative rod that is a common cause of diarrhea and is associated with animal exposure and sometimes food- or water-borne outbreaks is

(A) *Campylobacter jejuni*

(B) *Escherichia coli*

(C) *Shigella sonnei*

(D) *Yersinia enterocolitica*

(E) *Klebsiella pneumoniae*

459. In cholera, oral rehydration can be accomplished because sodium absorption is linked to

(A) potassium

(B) chloride

(C) bicarbonate

(D) glucose

(E) none of the above

460. Enterotoxins have been shown to be the principal mechanism for diarrhea in all of the following EXCEPT

(A) *Escherichia coli*

(B) *Bacillus cereus*

(C) *Staphylococcus aureus*

(D) *Shigella sonnei*

(E) *Clostridium difficile*

461. The main virulence factor of *Yersinia pestis* is/are the

(A) K antigen

(B) endotoxin

(C) V and W antigens

(D) lecithinase

(E) erythrogenic toxin

462. The germane diagnostic feature of *Y. pestis* is the

(A) bipolar staining

(B) large capsule

(C) flagella

(D) short and thick pili

(E) siderophores

463. A suitable antibody response to F-1 and V and W antigens will usually be sufficient for protection against

(A) relapsing fever

(B) leptospirosis

(C) brucellosis

(D) plague

(E) Lyme disease

464. *Yersinia enterocolitica* is correctly described as

(A) antigenically similar to other *Yersinia* species

(B) not cross-reacting with *Brucella abortus*

(C) causing gastroenteritis in humans

(D) resistant to aminoglycosides

(E) transmitted to humans by deer flies

465. All of the following statements concerning the treatment of gram-negative anaerobes are true EXCEPT

(A) therapy follows surgical drainage

(B) therapy follows the identification of all organisms involved

(C) infections can be treated with penicillin, though *Bacteroides fragilis* is often resistant

(D) use of clindamycin can lead to enteric colitis

(E) therapeutic decisions are made in the absence of susceptibility data

466. The single most important factor for pathogenicity in *Bacteroides* is

(A) a reduced environment
(B) collagenase production
(C) possession of superoxide dismutase
(D) slime secretion
(E) presence of indophenol oxidase

467. All of the following statements concerning *Bacteroides fragilis* are true EXCEPT

(A) its endotoxin is less toxic than that of *E. coli*
(B) it tends to be resistant to aminoglycosides
(C) it is frequently isolated from postoperative intra-abdominal abscesses
(D) it is the least predominant member of the normal flora in the human intestine
(E) it produces low levels of superoxide dismutase

468. Mycoplasmas are pleomorphic gram-negative bacteria that

(A) are sensitive to penicillin
(B) lack cell walls in all stages of growth
(C) cannot divide by binary fission
(D) require high salt concentration to maintain cellular integrity
(E) do not produce "fried egg" colonies

469. *Mycoplasma pneumoniae* (the Eaton agent) is an infectious agent that

(A) lacks sterols in its cytoplasmic membrane
(B) contains muramic acid in its cell wall
(C) contains only DNA
(D) causes primary atypical pneumonia
(E) is susceptible to penicillin

470. L forms are correctly characterized as

(A) generally susceptible to amphotericin B
(B) containing sterols in their membrane
(C) not induced by penicillin or ultraviolet light

(D) unable to revert to their bacterial parental types
(E) unable to produce the characteristic toxins of their parental strains

471. L forms are correctly described as

(A) generally susceptible to amphotericin B
(B) not producing hemolysins or toxins
(C) possessing defective cell walls
(D) needing low osmotic environments for survival
(E) forming spider-like colonies on blood sugar

472. The spirochete that is tightly coiled, thin, and has a hook at its end is

(A) *Leptospira icterohaemorrhagiae* (interrogans serogroup)
(B) *Borrelia recurrentis*
(C) *Treponema pallidum*
(D) *Vibrio cholerae*
(E) *Spirillum minus*

473. *Campylobacter fetus* subspecies *jejuni* is correctly described as

(A) transmitted by rat bites
(B) a nonmotile gram-negative rod
(C) detected in clinical specimens by agglutination of Proteus OX-K
(D) one of the most common causes of diarrhea
(E) resistant to erythromycin

474. The body louse is the vector for

(A) leptospirosis
(B) pinta
(C) epidemic relapsing fever
(D) bejel
(E) meningitis

475. An organism that can be grown on artificial media is

(A) *Rickettsia rickettsii*
(B) *Chlamydia trachomatis*

(C) *Mycobacterium leprae*

(D) *Treponema pallidum*

(E) *Campylobacter fetus* subspecies *jejuni*

476. The primary virulence determinant of invasive *Hemophilus influenzae* is

(A) an extremely potent endotoxin

(B) pili

(C) a ribose- and ribitol-containing capsule

(D) a heat-stable exotoxin

(E) its ability to be transformed by *Hemophilus influenzae* or *Streptococcus pneumoniae* DNA

477. *Hemophilus ducreyi* is correctly described as

(A) causing soft chancre (chancroid)

(B) complicating the diagnosis of gonorrhea

(C) producing large amounts of mucopolysaccharidase

(D) possessing axial filaments

(E) possessing periplasts

478. The *H. influenzae* strains found in cases of acute bacterial meningitis are usually

(A) serotype c

(B) serotype d

(C) encapsulated

(D) exotoxin producers

(E) isolated from young adults

479. In the diagnosis of pertussis, *Bordetella pertussis* is most likely isolated from

(A) blood culture during the bacteremic phase of the disease

(B) a throat swab during the convalescent phase of the disease

(C) a nasopharyngeal swab cultured on Bordet–Gengou medium

(D) abscess sites on the skin

(E) a spinal fluid

480. *Bordetella pertussis* is correctly described by which of the following statements?

(A) it is commonly transferred to humans from infected animals

(B) it commonly colonizes the gastrointestinal tract

(C) it commonly causes disease in children older than 5 years

(D) it produces several determinants of pathogenicity

(E) transition from phase I to phase IV is associated with virulence

481. All of the following statements correctly describe bacterial properties of *Chlamydia* EXCEPT

(A) they possess both RNA and DNA

(B) they possess a peptidoglycan cell wall

(C) they have ribosomes

(D) they multiply by binary division

(E) their growth is inhibited by antibacterial agents

482. All of the following statements about chlamydiae are true EXCEPT

(A) there are three species

(B) infected host cells develop inclusion bodies

(C) they are transmitted by insect vectors

(D) the infectious developmental form is the element body

(E) they are obligately intracellular bacteria

483. *Chlamydia trachomatis* infection may result in

(A) Brill's disease

(B) ornithosis

(C) undulant fever

(D) Pontiac fever

(E) nongonococcal urethritis

484. All of the following statements about *Listeria monocytogenes* are true EXCEPT

(A) it primarily causes a disease among animals that is occasionally passed to humans

(B) meningoencephalitis (meningitis) in the adult is the most commonly recognized form of listeriosis

(C) the microbe can only be cultured in human trophoblastic cells

(D) neonatal listeriosis occurs as a result of genital tract infection in the gravid female

(E) human infections characteristically yield a striking monocytic blood reaction

485. All of the following statements about brucellae are true EXCEPT

(A) dairy cattle in the United States may be infected with *Brucella abortus*

(B) *Brucella suis* infects goats

(C) brucellae do not produce exotoxin but do elaborate endotoxin

(D) brucellae tend to localize in the pregnant uterus of animals

(E) human placentas, which lack erythritol, are not especially susceptible to brucellae

486. All of the following statements about *Legionella* are true EXCEPT

(A) *Legionella pneumophila* is a small, facultatively intracellular gram-negative bacillus

(B) with paired sera, a four-fold rise in titer relative to acute-phase serum, is considered diagnostic

(C) antibodies to *Legionella* infections normally appear in humans within 7 to 10 days

(D) the nonpneumonic form of legionellosis is called Pontiac fever

(E) upper respiratory symptoms are rare in Legionnaires' disease

487. All of the following statements about *Legionella pneumophila* are true EXCEPT

(A) intravenous erythromycin is the antibiotic treatment of choice for legionellosis

(B) hospitalized patients with legionellosis should be kept in single rooms to prevent transmission to other patients

(C) people over 50 who are heavy cigarette smokers are more susceptible to legionellosis than are young adults who are not cigarette smokers

(D) *Legionella* is primarily a water-borne organism, spread via aerosols

(E) *Legionella* prevents phagosome–lysosome fusion when phagocytosed by phagocytic cells

488. A 55-year-old Caucasian male was hospitalized with pneumonitis after 5 days of unremitting fever (104°C) and recurrent rigors. He is suspected of having legionellosis. Which of the following statement about such cases is FALSE?

(A) for fastest diagnosis, a monoclonal antibody test for *Legionella* species should be requested on a serum sample

(B) there is no good antibiotic treatment for legionellosis

(C) a request should be made for culture of the suspected *Legionella*

(D) misdiagnosis is common unless *Legionella* is suspected

(E) there is no secondary transmission of *Legionella*

489. The rickettsial microorganism that can be cultured on blood agar is

(A) *Rickettsia prowazeki*

(B) *Coxiella burnetii*

(C) *Rickettsia typhi*

(D) *Rochalimaea quintana*

(E) *Rickettsia akari*

490. Members of the genus *Rickettsia* are gram-negative bacteria that

(A) are facultative intracellular parasites

(B) can be classified as energy parasites

(C) derive most of their energy from oxidation of glutamate

(D) retain excessive levels of coenzyme A, nicotinamide–adenine dinucleotide, and adenosine triphosphate in their cytoplasm

(E) do not multiply in endothelial cells of small blood vessels

491. All of the following can serve as vectors of rickettsiae EXCEPT

(A) lice
(B) mosquitoes
(C) fleas
(D) ticks
(E) mites

492. *Coxiella burnetii* is readily transmitted by

(A) mites
(B) lice
(C) fleas
(D) ticks
(E) aerosols

493. All of the following characterize *C. burnetii* EXCEPT that it

(A) can resist pasteurization
(B) produces infections that are not associated with a rash
(C) causes pneumonia
(D) shows strong cross-serologic reactivity with other rickettsiae
(E) can cause fetal infection

494. Trench fever is correctly described as

(A) transmitted by the body louse
(B) caused by *Rickettsia typhi*
(C) diagnosed by the Weil–Felix reaction
(D) treated with penicillin
(E) prevented by vaccination

495. Brill–Zinsser disease is correctly described as

(A) not responding to tetracycline or chloramphenicol treatment
(B) transmitted by ticks
(C) representing a relapse of prior epidemic typhus

(D) leading to the production of high levels of Weil–Felix agglutinins
(E) caused by *Borrelia recurrentis*

496. Scrub typhus is accurately described by which of the following statements?

(A) it has not been associated with skin rashes
(B) it is caused by *Rickettsia akari*
(C) second attacks are rare
(D) it can lead to the production of *Proteus* OX-K agglutinins
(E) it is transmitted by rat fleas

497. Which of the following statements concerning *Nocardia* is true?

(A) *Nocardia asteroides* is not acid-fast
(B) *N. asteroides* causes infections that cannot be treated with sulfonamides
(C) *N. asteroides* is not distributed widely in soil
(D) it causes infections in patients who receive corticosteroids
(E) it enters the human body via the genitourinary tract

498. In humans, *Actinomyces israelii* causes disease that is characterized by

(A) rapidly advancing abscesses
(B) confinement to the cervicofacial region
(C) presence of sulfur granules in the lesion
(D) involvement of the thyroid gland
(E) absence of lesions at the lower jaw region

499. *A. israelii* is a nonmotile gram-positive bacterium that

(A) gives rise to an effective human response
(B) is aerobic
(C) causes abscesses with draining sinuses
(D) produces a neurotoxin
(E) cannot be found in scrapings of the oral mucosa

500. A Gram stain of appropriate collected clinical specimens may be useful in the diagnosis of all the following infectious diseases EXCEPT

(A) acute bacterial meningitis

(B) streptococcal pharyngitis

(C) bacterial pneumonia

(D) gas gangrene

(E) *Neisseria gonorrhoeae* urethritis in males

501. It can usually be determined in the laboratory whether a proper sputum specimen has been collected for the diagnosis of bacterial pneumonia by determining the

(A) viscosity of the material

(B) ratio of white blood cells to epithelial cells in a gram stain

(C) ratio of gram-positive to gram-negative cocci

(D) ratio of aerobic to anaerobic bacteria

(E) presence of *Streptococcus pneumoniae* on culture

502. In the laboratory diagnosis of the enteric pathogens *Salmonella* and *Shigella,* the screening procedure includes testing their inability to

(A) ferment glucose

(B) ferment lactose

(C) ferment sucrose

(D) produce oxidase

(E) reduce nitrates

503. In the diagnosis of acute bacterial meningitis, the specific identity of the organism can often be determined rapidly by the use of

(A) culture of cerebrospinal fluid (CSF) on solid media

(B) culture of CSF in liquid media

(C) antibody detection in CSF counterimmunoelectrophoresis

(D) bacterial antigen detection in CSF by agglutination

(E) acute and convalescent serum antibody titers

504. When using acute and convalescent antibody titers in the diagnosis of a microbial infection, in the absence of isolation of the pathogen, confirmation of the disease is made by observing

(A) an acute titer of greater than 16

(B) a convalescent titer of greater than 16

(C) a change of any magnitude in the antibody titer

(D) a two-fold rise in titer

(E) a four-fold rise in titer

505. All of the following bacteria CANNOT be successfully Gram stained EXCEPT

(A) *Borrelia burgdorferi*

(B) *Chlamydia trachomatis*

(C) *Mycobacterium tuberculosis*

(D) *Vibrio vulnificus*

(E) *Yersinia pestis*

506. All of the following are aerobic gram-positive rods EXCEPT

(A) diptheroids

(B) *Nocardia* spp.

(C) *Actinomyces* spp.

(D) *Listeria monocytogenes*

(E) *Lactobacillus* spp.

507. All of the following statements about the normal intestinal flora of human newborns are true EXCEPT

(A) their intestines are sterile at birth

(B) microbes are soon introduced with food after birth

(C) *Bifidobacterium,* gram-positive nonmotile microbes, aerobic and anaerobic, are found in large numbers in breast-fed children

(D) bottle-fed children and breast-fed children have a similar flora

(E) bowels of newborns in intensive-care nurseries tend to be heavily colonized by Enterobacteriaceae

508. All of the following statements concerning the normal adult colon are true EXCEPT

(A) the stomach's acidity keeps the total stomach microbial content practically germ-free

(B) 96 to 99% of resident bacterial flora consists of anaerobes

(C) *Bacteroides fragilis* is the most common gut anaerobe

(D) only 1 to 4% of gut contents are facultative aerobes

(E) vitamin K is supplied to humans mainly by intestinal bacteria

509. Which of the following bacteria are aerobic?

(A) *Bacteroides fragilis*

(B) *Actinomyces* spp.

(C) *Moraxella catarrhalis*

(D) *Fusobacterium nucleatum*

(E) *Clostridium tetani*

510. Which of the following is NOT a fastidious microorganism?

(A) *Bordetella pertussis*

(B) *Actinomyces israelii*

(C) *Legionella pneumophila*

(D) *Campylobacter jejuni*

(E) *Hemophilus influenzae*

511. Humans acquire *Salmonella* gastroenteritis by means of

(A) mosquito bites

(B) tick bites

(C) penetration of the broken skin by animal bites

(D) aerosols

(E) the ingestion of contaminated food or water

512. All of the following statements about Lyme borreliosis are true EXCEPT

(A) it is caused by the bite of a tick from a deer infected with *Borrelia burgdorferi*

(B) infections are found only in Connecticut, New England, and the mid-Atlantic states

(C) there is an effective antibiotic treatment for acute infections

(D) it is often associated with an infective arthritis of one joint

(E) production of antibodies is often late (more than 4 to 6 weeks), making serologic diagnosis difficult

513. Which of the following cannot serve as a vector of rickettsiae?

(A) lice

(B) mosquitoes

(C) fleas

(D) ticks

(E) mites

514. All of the following statements about staphylococci are true EXCEPT

(A) toxic shock syndrome, which may be caused by either *Staphylococcus aureus* or beta-hemolytic group A *Streptococcus pyogenes*, may affect both males and females

(B) many individuals are nasal carriers of *S. aureus*

(C) impetigo is caused only by *S. aureus*

(D) *Staphylococcus epidermidis* is often responsible for infectious endocarditis in intravenous drug abusers

(E) the phage type is a list composed of the strain numbers of those standard bacteriophages that can lyse a given *S. aureus* strain

515. Latent syphilis is NOT associated with

(A) the presence of clinical lesions

(B) a negative dark-field examination

(C) normal cerebrospinal fluid

(D) positive nontreponemal serologic tests

(E) positive treponemal serologic tests

516. *Chlamydia trachomatis*

(A) is the most common cause of nongonococcal urethritis

(B) does not respond to chemotherapy

(C) produces a protease that degrades IgA

(D) is a flagellated protozoan

(E) is not usually transmitted sexually

517. All of the following statements about anaerobic infections are true EXCEPT

(A) the pus often has a sweet smell

(B) they are often contiguous with a mucosal surface

(C) they tend to form discrete closed-space infections, eg, lung

(D) they can form infections by burrowing through tissue layers

(E) they are favored by reduced blood supply

518. Pigmented *Serratia* were at one time thought to be harmless saprophytes; which of the following statements about them is FALSE?

(A) they are not associated with underlying disease

(B) they have emerged as major entities in nosocomial infections

(C) *Serratia marcescens* is the major *Serratia*

(D) they provide extracellular deoxyribonuclease

(E) 75 to 90% of *Serratia* infections are hospital acquired

519. All of the following statements about Lyme borreliosis (disease) are true EXCEPT

(A) *Borrelia burgdorferi* is the causative organism

(B) there is no vaccine currently available

(C) initial symptoms are flu-like chills, fever, headache, dizziness, fatigue, and stiff neck

(D) a good way to prevent Lyme disease is to carefully inspect one's arms and legs for any ticks and then crush any tick between one's fingers

(E) the size of a deer tick is about the size of a poppy seed

520. All of the following statements about *Erysipelothrix rhusiopathiae* are true EXCEPT

(A) it is nonsporogenous, nonmotile, and nonencapsulated in humans

(B) it causes erysipeloid, a disease most prevalent in abattoir employees

(C) it is a gram-positive rod

(D) its colonies are similar to those of *Streptococcus viridans*

(E) animals are never infected with *E. rhusiopathiae*

521. All of the following statements about mycobacteria are true EXCEPT

(A) *Mycobacterium avium* and *Mycobacterium intracellulare* overlap in their properties as two major slowly growing nonphotochromogenic pathogens

(B) *M. avium* and *M. intracellulare* produce symptoms similar to tuberculosis but the symptoms are quite mild

(C) *M. avium* and *M. intracellulare* infections are common infections of individuals with acquired immune deficiency syndrome (AIDS)

(D) *Mycobacterium kansasii* is a rapidly growing photochromogen

(E) *Mycobacterium fortuitum* is a rapidly growing mycobacterium that is only very occasionally pathogenic to humans

522. All of the following statements about tularemia are true EXCEPT

(A) tularemia is a major zoonotic disease caused by *Francisella tularensis*

(B) one bacterium of *F. tularensis* can infect highly susceptible animals such as mice and guinea pigs

(C) most tularemia infections in the United States are acquired by direct inoculation from the bite of contaminated arthropods

(D) there are no clinical manifestations of tularemia

(E) tularemia antibodies are found in the serum by the end of the second to third week

523. All of the statements about the G protein that plays the role of "middle man" in the communications system responsible for coordinating cellular activities are true EXCEPT

(A) it is activated by guanosine triphosphate

(B) it rests on the inner surface of the bilayered membrane

(C) when a cell receives a signal, perhaps by a neurotransmitter, protein does not enter directly

(D) protein G binds with a receptor that extends through the cell membrane

(E) when the receptor-signal unit attaches to a G protein in a membrane, the G protein switches off

524. All of the following statements about the members of the genus *Pasteurella* are true EXCEPT

(A) they are primarily parasites of animals

(B) they can produce a variety of diseases in humans

(C) *Pasteurella multocida* is the species most frequently associated with human infections

(D) they are very small, gram-positive bacteria

(E) they are facultatively anaerobic and show bipolar staining

525. Which of the following bacteria are often isolated from humans?

(A) *Gardnerella vaginalis*, which appears to act in concert with certain aerobes to cause nonspecific vaginitis

(B) *Cardiobacterium hominis*, a gram-negative rod that is most frequently associated with endocarditis in individuals with damaged or prosthetic heart valves

(C) *Enterobacter cloacae*, a gram-positive rod isolated entirely from the cloacal infections

(D) *Actinobacillus* spp., found both as commensals and as pathogens in domestic animals and birds

(E) *Streptobacillus moniliformis*, which causes the systemic febrile disease by direct contact with rats

526. All of the following statements about verotoxins are true EXCEPT

(A) they are cytotoxins

(B) they are produced by *Escherichia coli* and called verotoxin *E. coli* (VTEC)

(C) they are shiga-like toxins

(D) the majority of VTEC isolates have been isolated in Africa

(E) vero tissue culture cells are a cell line developed from monkey kidney cells

527. All of the following statements concerning syphilis are true EXCEPT

(A) the *Treponema pallidum* immobilization (TPI) test is a confirmative test for syphilis

(B) the fluorescent *Treponema* antibody absorption test (FTA-ABS) is not a confirmative test for syphilis

(C) live *T. pallidum* cells are required in the TPI test

(D) the TPI test is very expensive and technically difficult

(E) the FTA-ABS test does not require live *T. pallidum* cells

528. All of the following statements are true EXCEPT

(A) both the Mantoux test and the multiple puncture test require purified protein derivative

(B) injection of *Neisseria meningitidis* serogroup A yields human protective antibodies in adults

(C) there is no evidence that *Mycobacterium kansasii* is transmitted directly from patients to healthy contacts

(D) *Mycobacterium intracellulare* is sensitive to the routine levels of streptomycin, isoniazid, and para-aminosalicylic acid that are effective against *Mycobacterium tuberculosis*

(E) individuals with human immunodeficiency virus are more susceptible to tuberculosis than are normal individuals

529. All of the following statements about Legionnaire's disease are true EXCEPT

(A) Pontiac fever has relatively mild flu-like symptoms, although it is caused by *Legionella pneumophila*

(B) *L. pneumophila* in air conditioning equipment transmits legionellosis

(C) the microbe is motile and is easy to gram stain

(D) seroconversion after *L. pneumophila* infections may take 6 to 8 weeks

(E) *L. pneumophila* can be grown clinically since the development of charcoal yeast extract agar

530. All of the following statements about mycoplasmas are true EXCEPT

(A) mycoplasmas are the smallest procaryote capable of self-replication

(B) mycoplasmas were first isolated from cattle as the pleuropneumonia organism

(C) cold agglutinins (nonspecific antibodies that agglutinate red blood cells in the cold) appear in the convalescent serum of infected humans

(D) *Ureaplasma urealyticum* are mycoplasmas frequently isolated from the urogenital tract

(E) vaccines for *Mycoplasma pneumoniae* can completely prevent infections in outbreaks

531. All of the following statements are true EXCEPT

(A) *Proteus vulgaris* can be typed with specific antiserum in a quellung reaction

(B) *Klebsiella pneumoniae* and *Streptococcus pneumoniae* can be typed with specific antiserum in a quellung reaction

(C) *Proteus vulgaris* is a possessor of urease

(D) *Proteus mirabilis* and *Proteus vulgaris* are two *Proteus* strains isolated from urine

(E) all urinary tract infections caused by urease-producing *Proteus* strains are characterized by an alkaline urine

532. All of the following statements about *Salmonella* and *Shigella* are true EXCEPT

(A) typhoid fever is treated with chloramphenicol or ampicillin as the drug of choice

(B) uncomplicated *Salmonella* gastroenteritis is treated with ampicillin as the drug of choice

(C) in shigellosis the natural habitat of *Shigella sonnei* (and other shigellae) is limited to the intestinal tracts of humans and some primates

(D) salmonellae are motile gram-negative rods that do not ferment lactose and do not produce H_2S

(E) shigellae are nonmotile and usually do not ferment lactose but ferment other carbohydrates and do not produce H_2S

533. All of the following statements are true EXCEPT

(A) endemic relapsing fever is caused by mosquito bites from infected animals

(B) Lyme disease is caused by tick bites from infected deer

(C) *Borrelia burgdorferi* is the causative microbe for Lyme disease

(D) *B. burgdorferi* can be grown in pure culture in special media

(E) epidemic relapsing fever occurs in all parts of the world and is transmitted from one individual to another by the body louse

534. Which of the following current instructions regarding prevention of brucellosis is FALSE?

(A) drink pasteurized milk only

(B) eat cheeses made from pasteurized milk only

(C) goat cheese can never cause brucellosis, even overseas

(D) be wary of eating pork unless you are sure it is well cooked

(E) have animals inspected by veterinarians

535. All of the following statements about *Actinomyces* and *Nocardia* are true EXCEPT

   (A) *Actinomyces* do not contain peptidoglycan in their cell walls

   (B) *Nocardia* do contain peptidoglycan in their cell walls

   (C) *Actinomyces* are anaerobic

   (D) *Nocardia* are aerobic

   (E) *Actinomyces* and *Nocardia* are prokaryotic

536. Which of the following statements about common themes in transport proteins in bacteria is FALSE?

   (A) in gram-positive bacteria, depending on their reaction to the Gram stain, the plasma membrane is surrounded only by a rigid and porous cell wall made of peptidoglycan

   (B) gram-negative bacteria produce a second membrane (the outer membrane) that is located outside the plasma (cytoplasmic) membrane

   (C) a fundamental role of the membrane is to serve as a selective permeability barrier

   (D) the outer envelope of gram-positive bacteria do not contain transport proteins

   (E) the outer membrane serves as a permeability barrier that protects gram-negative bacteria from a number of harmful compounds, such as antibiotics

537. Which of the following statements about *Listeria* and listeriosis is FALSE?

   (A) *Listeria* are easily grown on ordinary media when it is the only organism present, eg, in bacteremia

   (B) *Listeria* are difficult to grow in the presence of many other bacteria, eg, from feces

   (C) meningitis is the most commonly recognized form of listeriosis in the adult

   (D) genital tract infection with resulting infection of the offspring is the most distinctive infection caused by *Listeria monocytogenes*

   (E) most of the *L. monocytogenes* clinical syndromes are mild and resolve spontaneously

538. Which of the following statements about *Bacillus cereus*, which is an infrequently recognized cause of food-borne illness in the United States, is FALSE?

   (A) it causes a clinical syndrome that has a short period of incubation, about 4 hours

   (B) the short incubation syndrome is characterized by severe nausea and vomiting and is frequently mistaken for staphylococcal food poisoning

   (C) the second syndrome it causes is characterized by abdominal cramping and diarrhea and takes about 17 hours to appear

   (D) *B. cereus* food poisoning is initiated when the spore forms survive cooking and the contaminated food, eg, rice, is allowed to reach spore germination temperatures

   (E) chloramphenicol is the antibiotic of choice for the short-term incubation syndrome

539. Which of the following staphylococci are coagulase-positive?

   (A) *Staphylococcus xylosus*

   (B) *Staphylococcus hominis*

   (C) *Staphylococcus aureus*

   (D) *Staphylococcus saprophyticus*

   (E) *Staphylococcus epidermidis*

540. Which of the following are not genera of opportunistic Enterobacteriaceae?

   (A) *Klebsiella*

   (B) *Citrobacter*

   (C) *Enterobacter*

   (D) *Eubacterium*

   (E) *Escherichia*

541. All of the following statements about scarlet fever toxin are true EXCEPT

(A) *Streptococcus pyogenes* elaborate group A pyrogenic factor type A

(B) *S. pyogenes* elaborate group A pyrogenic factor type B

(C) *S. pyogenes* elaborate group A pyrogenic factor type X

(D) *S. pyogenes* elaborate group A pyrogenic factor type C

(E) it is possible that a child might have more than one infection with scarlet fever at different times

542. *Staphylococcus epidermidis* is a gram-positive bacterium that

(A) is coagulase-positive

(B) contains protein A

(C) contains endotoxin

(D) ordinarily forms golden colonies

(E) humans ordinarily have on their skin

543. All of the following statements concerning viridans streptococci are true EXCEPT

(A) they often colonize the mouth or upper respiratory tract

(B) they are bile soluble

(C) they are a leading cause of infective (subacute bacterial) endocarditis

(D) they are not sensitive to penicillin

(E) they are alpha-hemolytic

544. Group B streptococci (*Streptococcus agalactiae*) are of clinical significance because of their association with

(A) rheumatic fever

(B) scarlet fever

(C) impetigo

(D) neonatal meningitis

(E) sore throats

545. *Streptococcus pyogenes* (group A) is NOT correctly described by which of the following statements?

(A) M proteins do produce protective antibodies

(B) not all strains can cause rheumatic fever

(C) capsular polysaccharides exist in over 60 antigenic types

(D) strains are typed based in part on their M proteins

(E) M proteins do prevent phagocytosis

546. Characteristics of virulent *Streptococcus pneumoniae* cultures do not include

(A) alpha-hemolysis

(B) sensitivity to optochin

(C) lancet-shaped diplococci

(D) hyaluronic acid capsules

(E) polysaccharide capsules

547. Predisposing factors for pneumococcal disease do not include

(A) sickle cell anemia

(B) hypogammaglobulinemia

(C) splenectomy

(D) heart failure

(E) young adulthood

548. Characteristics of the genus *Neisseria* do NOT include

(A) cocci

(B) gram-negative

(C) oxidase-positive

(D) acid-fast

(E) found only in humans

549. Which of the following statements about colonization by meningococci is FALSE?

(A) it is in part mediated by pili

(B) it is increased in household contacts of individuals with meningococcal disease

(C) it is accompanied by development of immunity

(D) it does not invariably lead to serious infections

(E) it does not have to be taken into consideration by the physician

550. Studies with *Neisseria meningitidis* show that virulence may NOT be associated with

(A) capsular polysaccharide serotype

(B) the polysaccharide capsule composition

(C) pili

(D) IgA protease

(E) the lipopolysaccharide (endotoxin)

551. Bacillus Calmette–Guérin (BCG) vaccination makes it impossible to use the tuberculin test for

(A) evidence of recent mycobacterial infection in an individual

(B) human immunodeficiency virus screening

(C) the location of sources of infection

(D) differential diagnosis in diseases with some similarity to tuberculosis

(E) a screening device prior to x-ray examination in the diagnosis of tuberculosis

552. In addition to *Mycobacterium tuberculosis* and *Mycobacterium bovis* as mycobacterial species that cause human tuberculosis, the third species to cause the disease is

(A) *M. leprae*

(B) *M. simiae*

(C) *M. africanum*

(D) *M. ulcerans*

553. Which of the following statements concerning diphtheria toxin is FALSE?

(A) it is not the major pathogenic determinant

(B) its production by *Corynebacterium diphtheriae* is influenced by the concentration of iron in the growth medium

(C) its production is dependent on the presence of phage genome in *C. diphtheriae*

(D) its toxin consists of two fragments, A and B

(E) it loses its toxicity when converted to a toxoid

554. Malignant pustules associated with cutaneous anthrax are lesions that

(A) are characterized by central necrotic lesions surrounded by reddish swelling of adjacent skin

(B) contain abundant *Bacillus anthracis* spores

(C) tend to develop on the body surface usually exposed to outside environments

(D) are the terminal sign of fatal anthrax

(E) can never be prevented by immunization

555. All of the following statements about bacteria are true EXCEPT

(A) *Bordetella pertussis* requires added growth factors X and V

(B) *Hemophilus influenzae* requires added growth factors X and V

(C) *Chlamydia trachomatis* can be transmitted sexually

(D) *Legionella* is a water-borne bacterium

(E) brucellosis is not associated with unremitting high fever and shaking chills (rigors)

556. Which of the following statements about *Staphylococcus aureus* is FALSE?

(A) it is ubiquitous in the environment and can withstand drying well

(B) it can grow aerobically, but not anaerobically

(C) infections are usually by hand contamination from a person colonized in the nose or in the axillary or perineal region

(D) carriage is higher in individuals with diffuse dermatologic disease and those using needles (eg, insulin-requiring diabetics, heroin addicts, hemodialysis patients) than in the normal population

(E) phage typing of strains may be useful in targeting the strain source in an epidemiologic investigation of a hospital outbreak

557. Which of the following statements about diphtheria toxin is FALSE?

(A) it is not produced by *Corynebacterium diphtheriae* in vitro

(B) it is immunogenic

(C) it is the active agent in the Schick test

(D) it is used as a toxoid to vaccinate infants

(E) individuals exhibit local general hypersensitivity

558. All of the following are true statements about species of *Clostridium* EXCEPT

(A) they are generally sporogenic and gram-positive

(B) they obtain energy by oxidizing one molecule and reducing another

(C) they produce exotoxins

(D) they are sensitive to growth in oxygen

(E) they do not cause disease in humans breathing air

559. The pathogenicity of *Clostridium perfringens* is NOT associated with

(A) saccharolytic properties

(B) proteolytic properties

(C) production of lecithinase C (lipase)

(D) production of endotoxin

(E) ability to cause food poisoning

560. All of the following statements about gonorrhea are true EXCEPT

(A) it is caused by a gram-negative, oxidase-positive diplococcus

(B) it can be caused by penicillinase-producing gonococci

(C) it is very readily diagnosed in females using the Gram stain

(D) it may be provisionally diagnosed in males with a Gram stain in acute cases

(E) it is not prevented by vaccination

561. All of the following are components of *Neisseria gonorrhoeae* that contribute to its virulence EXCEPT

(A) pili

(B) axial filaments (fibrils)

(C) lipopolysaccharide (endotoxin)

(D) IgA protease

(E) outer membrane components

562. All of the following statements concerning sexually transmitted diseases are true EXCEPT

(A) herpes simplex virus type II causes most of the genital lesions in women

(B) most cases of nongonococcal urethritis are caused by *Chlamydia*

(C) *Hemophilus ducreyi* is the causative agent of soft chancre

(D) they are now controlled by vaccination

(E) *Neisseria gonorrhoeae* is a nonmotile gram-negative coccus

563. All of the following statements about gonorrhea are true EXCEPT that it

(A) is an infection of the columnar epithelial cells

(B) is caused by a gram-negative, oxidase-positive diplococcus

(C) can cause blindness in infants

(D) can be associated with β-lactamase–producing strains of *Neisseria gonorrhoeae*

(E) is not contagious

564. Appropriate specimens for the diagnosis of gonorrhea include pus from all of the following EXCEPT the

(A) urethra

(B) cervix

(C) appendix

(D) conjunctiva

(E) anus

565. Positive Venereal Disease Research Laboratories, rapid plasma reagin, and fluorescent treponemal antibody-absorption tests may NOT be obtained in patients with

(A) candidiasis

(B) pinta

(C) bejel

(D) syphilis

(E) yaws

566. All of the following statements about distinctive properties of *Treponema pallidum* are true EXCEPT

(A) possession of fibrils (axial filaments)

(B) inability to grow on artificial media

(C) ability to survive 1 to 4 days in blood stored at 4°C

(D) lack of cross-reactivity with *Treponema pertenue*

(E) spirochete detection in lesions of primary and secondary syphilis

567. The Venereal Disease Research Laboratories test is NOT correctly described as

(A) a widely used nontreponemal test

(B) requiring diphosphatidylglycerol (cardiolipin)

(C) useful in screening large numbers of persons

(D) used to follow the efficiency of penicillin treatment

(E) a rapid plasma reagin test

568. All of the following statements about latent syphilis are true EXCEPT that it is associated with

(A) the absence of clinical lesions

(B) a negative dark-field examination

(C) the period between primary and secondary disease

(D) positive nontreponemal and treponemal serologic tests

(E) infection of the fetuses of pregnant women

569. Prevention of salmonellosis includes

(A) water sanitation

(B) proper food cooking

(C) refrigeration of food

(D) treatment of carriers

(E) all of the above

570. Virulence factors of microorganisms associated with urinary tract infections include all of the following EXCEPT

(A) pili

(B) beta-lactamase production

(C) urease production

(D) high pH

(E) obstruction produced by calculi

571. All of the following bacteria are important pathogens in urinary tract infections EXCEPT

(A) *Escherichia coli*

(B) *Streptococcus pneumoniae*

(C) *Streptococcus faecalis*, group D

(D) *Proteus* spp.

(E) *Staphylococcus saprophyticus*

572. Urinary tract infection is suggested by all of the following EXCEPT

(A) culture disclosing greater than 10^5 bacteria per milliliter of urine

(B) two bacteria per oil immersion field seen on a smear of unspun urine

(C) greater than 10 white blood cells per high-power field in a specimen of spun urinary sediment

(D) urine pH less than 5.5

(E) presence of red blood cells in the urine

573. All of the following statements are true EXCEPT

(A) liquid cultures with less than 10^5 bacteria per mm^3 do not appear turbid to the eye

(B) contamination by skin bacteria is suggested when only one of several blood cultures shows growth by *Staphylococcus epidermidis* or diptheroids

(C) "sore throats" in children are most often due to viral infection

(D) pus from an anaerobic infection often has a foul smell

(E) pus from a pseudomonae infection is always yellow

574. All of the following statements concerning endotoxins of gram-negative bacteria are true EXCEPT

(A) they differ markedly in their toxicity according to their specific bacterial origins

(B) they are found in the blood of patients suffering from endotoxic shock

(C) they consist mainly of lipopolysaccharide complexes

(D) they induce the release of endogenous pyrogens from leukocytes

(E) they are found only in gram-negative bacteria

575. All of the following statements concerning endotoxin are true EXCEPT

(A) it is a cell-wall–associated toxin found in gram-negative bacteria

(B) it is responsible for fatal shock often experienced in the terminal stage of bacteremia due to gram-negative bacteria

(C) it may activate complement via the alternative pathway

(D) it is, like many exotoxins, proteinaceous in nature

(E) there is no immunization against it

576. All of the following results obtained with urine from a patient with suspected urinary tract infection (UTI) indicate a likely positive UTI EXCEPT

(A) a positive spot indole test

(B) the finding that the organism is beta-hemolytic

(C) the finding that the organism is lactose-fermenting

(D) the finding that the organism is anaerobic

(E) the finding of a single species of microbe at $10^6/mm^3$

577. Which of the following statements about staphylococci is FALSE?

(A) toxic shock syndrome, which may be caused by either *Staphylococcus aureus* or beta-hemolytic group A *Streptococcus*

pyogenes, may affect both males and females

(B) many individuals are nasal carriers of *Staphylococcus aureus*

(C) impetigo is caused only by *S. aureus*

(D) *Staphylococcus epidermidis* is often responsible for infectious endocarditis in intravenous drug abusers

(E) the phage type is a list composed of the strain numbers of those standard bacteriophages that can lyse a given *S. aureus* strain

578. Endotoxin is a heat-stable toxin that is

(A) "cleared" from plasma by C1q

(B) a potent activator of C1q

(C) an inhibitor of C1 esterase

(D) a potent activator of the alternative complement pathway

(E) bound to the cell nucleus

579. Anaerobic gram-negative wound infections are NOT correctly described by which of the following statements?

(A) they are usually of endogenous origin

(B) they may not be easily amenable to antibiotic therapy

(C) they are favored if the tissue Eh is reduced by growth of aerobic bacteria

(D) they may produce various toxins

(E) they are usually due to a single microbe infection

580. All of the following factors are involved in the transmission of *Campylobacter jejuni* EXCEPT

(A) person-to-person spread

(B) association with farm animals

(C) ingestion of municipal or stream water

(D) ingestion of raw seafood

(E) contact with domestic animals

581. Which of the following statements regarding activity of cholera toxin is FALSE?

(A) inhibited cation (Na^+ for H^+) and anion (Cl^- for HCO_3^-) exchange

(B) increased adenylate cyclase activity

(C) enhanced chloride secretion

(D) inhibited glucose-linked sodium absorption

(E) increased intracellular cyclic adenosine monophosphate

582. Which of the following statements concerning characteristics of verotoxin-positive *Escherichia coli* is FALSE?

(A) its toxin is cytotoxic to vero cells

(B) it is associated with outbreaks of hemorrhagic colitis

(C) its toxin is similar to the shiga toxin of *Shigella dysenteriae* type I

(D) its toxin activates adenylate cyclase, causing net loss of water and electrolytes in the stool

(E) it occurs in some fast-food chains in the United States and Canada

583. Which of the following pathogenic mechanisms has NOT been described in diarrhea-producing *Escherichia coli*?

(A) invasiveness

(B) heat-stable enterotoxicity

(C) cytotoxicity (vero toxin)

(D) lack of tight adhesiveness

(E) heat-labile enterotoxicity

584. The normal flora of the throat may NOT include moderate numbers of which of the following?

(A) alpha-hemolytic streptococci

(B) gamma-hemolytic streptococci

(C) alpha-hemolytic pneumococci

(D) beta-hemolytic group A streptococci

(E) gram-negative diplococci

585. Fecal leukocytes are seen in stools of persons infected with

(A) *Campylobacter jejuni*

(B) *Vibrio cholerae*

(C) *Staphylococcus aureus*

(D) enterotoxigenic *Escherichia coli*

(E) human immunodeficiency virus

586. Activation of adenylate cyclase is the biochemical event leading to diarrhea mediated by

(A) pseudomonal toxin

(B) *Clostridium difficile* toxin A

(C) heat-labile toxin of *Escherichia coli*

(D) heat-stable toxin of *E. coli*

(E) *Clostridium botulinum* toxin

587. Invasion of the intestinal mucosa occurs with

(A) enterotoxigenic *Escherichia coli*

(B) *Vibrio cholerae*

(C) *Giardia lamblia*

(D) *Shigella dysenteriae*

(E) *Enterobacter cloacae*

588. Members of the genus *Rickettsia* are bacteria that

(A) are facultative intracellular parasites

(B) are gram-positive

(C) derive most of their energy from oxidation of glutamate

(D) retain excessive levels of coenzyme A, nicotinamide–adenine dinucleotide, and adenosine triphosphate in their cytoplasm

(E) do not multiply in endothelial cells of small blood vessels

589. Which of the following is NOT a portal of entry for *Francisella tularensis*?

(A) broken skin

(B) a tick bite (*Dermacentor*)

(C) a deer fly bite (*Chrysops*)

(D) the respiratory tract

(E) sexual contact

590. A reservoir of infection for plague is

(A) squirrels

(B) cats

(C) dogs

(D) armadillos

(E) cows

591. Tularemia is an infectious zoonotic disease that

(A) cannot be confirmed by an appropriate skin test

(B) is usually acquired by drinking unpasteurized milk

(C) cannot be treated with streptomycin or tetracycline

(D) is associated with univalent or blocking antibodies

(E) can be obtained by skinning infected rabbits

592. All of the following statements concerning anaerobic infections are true EXCEPT

(A) they are caused by gram-positive spore-forming anaerobic bacteria and by non–spore-forming anaerobes

(B) they are usually characterized by pus or exudate that emits a foul odor

(C) anaerobic clinical samples may be stored in a refrigerator for up to 2 hours

(D) they are usually of polymicrobial origin

(E) clinical samples should be taken to the clinical laboratory immediately

593. The organism NOT responsible for anaerobic pulmonary infection is

(A) *Fusobacterium* spp.

(B) *Peptostreptococcus* spp.

(C) *Bacteroides* spp.

(D) *Moraxella* spp.

(E) *Clostridium perfringens*

594. Anaerobic gram-negative wound infections are correctly described by all of the following statements EXCEPT

(A) they are usually of endogenous origin

(B) they are polymicrobial

(C) they are favored if the tissue Eh is reduced by trauma or by growth of aerobic bacteria

(D) they are not amenable to antibiotic treatment

(E) they are sometimes most virulent in a reduced environment

595. Proper laboratory diagnosis of gram-negative anaerobes requires all of the following EXCEPT

(A) bladder aspiration for urinary tract infections

(B) unrefrigerated specimens

(C) transtracheal needle aspiration for pulmonary infections

(D) disregarding foul-smelling exudates

(E) immediate transfer of the specimen to the clinical laboratory

596. Beneficial actions of gram-negative anaerobes include all of the following EXCEPT

(A) dehydroxylation of bile acids

(B) synthesis of vitamin K by *Bacteroides fragilis*

(C) conjugation of bile acids

(D) protection against pathogenic bacteria

(E) involvement in the synthesis of vitamin E

597. When neonatal meningitis is caused by streptococci, they usually are

(A) *Streptococcus pyogenes* (group A)

(B) *Streptococcus agalactiae* (group B)

(C) *Streptococcus sanguis* (viridans streptococci)

(D) *Streptococcus pneumoniae* (serotype 8)

(E) *Streptococcus mitis* (viridans streptococci)

598. All of the following statements concerning *Mycoplasma pneumoniae* are true EXCEPT

(A) it is the causative agent of primary atypical pneumonia

(B) it is also known as the Eaton agent

(C) it causes disease that leads to the appearance of cold agglutinins

(D) it is sensitive to tetracycline

(E) it is detected by a hot coagulation test

599. All of the following statements regarding the pertussis vaccine are true EXCEPT

(A) it is effective in preventing pertussis in those under 4 years of age

(B) it has adjuvant properties

(C) it can induce serious neurologic side effects

(D) in the United States it is a killed, whole-cell preparation

(E) it has no available vaccine

600. All of the following are obligately intracellular bacteria EXCEPT

(A) *Chlamydia trachomatis*

(B) *Rickettsia prowazeki*

(C) *Chlamydia psittaci*

(D) *Legionella micdadei*

(E) *Mycobacterium leprae*

601. *Chlamydia trachomatis* may be responsible for all of the various clinical conditions EXCEPT

(A) inclusion conjunctivitis

(B) lymphogranuloma venereum

(C) pneumonitis in the newborn

(D) trachoma and inclusion conjunctivitis

(E) leptospirosis

602. Disease may be transmitted to humans drinking unpasteurized milk or eating cheeses made from such milk that contains any of the following microbes EXCEPT

(A) *Lactobacillus* spp.

(B) *Mycobacterium tuberculosis*

(C) *Brucella abortus*

(D) *Streptococcus pyogenes*

(E) *Listeria monocytogenes*

603. All of the following statements about *Listeria monocytogenes* are correct EXCEPT

(A) it is a facultative intracellular pathogen that can survive within macrophages

(B) it is able to grow at temperatures as low as 2.5°C

(C) it is a gram-positive coccobacillus

(D) it is resistant to all β-lactam antibiotics

(E) it is the cause of disease in adult humans and neonates

604. Which of the following is a true statement about legionellosis?

(A) the *Legionella* species readily stain gram-negative under the usual gram-staining procedures

(B) the causative organisms are intracellular, small gram-negative bacilli

(C) the legionellae are fast-growing bacteria, usually yielding colonies on appropriate solid media after 1 day

(D) Pontiac fever is a nonpneumonic form of legionellosis, causing a self-limited flu-like illness of a few days' duration

(E) legionellae cannot be grown in pure culture

605. All of the following statements about *Legionella* are true EXCEPT

(A) intracellular *Legionella pneumophila* resist destruction by preventing phagosome–lysosome fusion

(B) *Legionella* is often found in lakes, streams, or water supply systems

(C) the ability of *Legionella* to multiply in potable water distribution systems is stimulated by other microflora, such as fresh water protozoa and *Pseudomonas*

(D) aerosols produced by contaminated air conditioning towers may be a source of *Legionella* infections

(E) smokers are not more susceptible to *Legionella* infections

606. Which of the following diseases is caused by an extracellular microbe?

(A) legionellosis

(B) brucellosis

(C) staphylococcal septicemia

(D) tuberculosis

(E) acquired immunodeficiency syndrome (human immunodeficiency virus)

607. All of the following statements correctly describe rickettsiae EXCEPT

   (A) they contain both RNA and DNA
   (B) they divide by binary fission
   (C) they may be maintained by transovarial passage in arthropods
   (D) they are virulent due to the production of exotoxins
   (E) they derive most of their energy from the oxidation of glutamate

608. Which of the following statements concerning rickettsial diseases is FALSE?

   (A) Rocky Mountain spotted fever (RMSF) is now reported in all 48 contiguous United States
   (B) Q fever is essentially a pneumonitis acquired by inhalation
   (C) the skin rash from RMSF is most pronounced on the arms and legs, involving the palms and soles
   (D) Brill–Zinsser disease is a recrudescence of RMSF
   (E) the Weil–Felix test is no longer recommended for RMSF diagnosis

609. Laboratory diagnosis of Rocky Mountain spotted fever by the Weil–Felix reaction (which was previously used for diagnosis of rickettsial diseases) involves all of the following EXCEPT

   (A) tests for the presence of agglutinins for *Proteus* OX-2 and/or OX-19
   (B) complement fixation tests
   (C) indirect fluorescent antibody tests
   (D) isolation of rickettsiae from stools of infected patients
   (E) it has been replaced by an immunofluorescence test

610. The Weil–Felix reaction is only occasionally used in the diagnosis of

   (A) leptospirosis
   (B) toxoplasmosis
   (C) lymphogranuloma venereum
   (D) Rocky Mountain spotted fever
   (E) tularemia

611. All of the following statements concerning rickettsial diseases are true EXCEPT

   (A) Rocky Mountain spotted fever is now reported in all 48 contiguous United States
   (B) Q fever is essentially a pneumonitis
   (C) trench fever is caused by *Rochalimaea quintana*
   (D) Brill–Zinsser disease is the reappearance of epidemic typhus
   (E) rickettsia have no RNA

612. All of the following statements about *Actinomyces*, which are considered bacteria and not fungi, are true EXCEPT

   (A) actinomycosis is characterized by pyogenic lesions with interconnecting sinus tracts
   (B) they are normal inhabitants of the mouth
   (C) they lack chitin in their cell walls
   (D) they are normal inhabitants of the gut
   (E) they contain sterols in their cell membrane

613. "Sulfur granules" are correctly described as

   (A) colonies of *Actinomyces israelii*
   (B) antigen–antibody complexes encountered in actinomycosis
   (C) usually present in nocardiosis
   (D) only formed when *Nocardia* are grown in thioglycollate
   (E) gram-negative filaments

614. *Actinomyces israelii* can be differentiated from *Mycobacterium tuberculosis* by all of the following EXCEPT

   (A) differences in their acid-fast staining properties
   (B) growth characteristics on laboratory media

(C) production of niacin by *M. tuberculosis*

(D) production of niacin by *A. israelii*

(E) *A. israelii* is a member of the normal mouth and gut flora

615. CO₂ is required for primary isolation of

(A) *Treponema pallidum*

(B) *Neisseria gonorrhoeae*

(C) *Mycobacterium tuberculosis*

(D) *Staphylococcus aureus*

(E) *Actinomyces israelii*

616. None of the following bacteria readily stains gram-negative using the standard staining procedure EXCEPT

(A) *Hemophilus influenzae*

(B) *Listeria monocytogenes*

(C) *Bacillus cereus*

(D) *Legionella pneumophila*

(E) *Staphylococcus saprophyticus*

617. All the following bacteria may cause meningitis in neonates or children EXCEPT

(A) *Escherichia coli* type K-1

(B) *Hemophilus influenzae* type b

(C) *Neisseria gonorrhoeae*

(D) *Streptococcus agalactiae* group B

(E) *Neisseria meningitidis* group C

618. Which of the following enzyme(s) is/are used in recombinant DNA technology to manipulate pieces of DNA?

(A) proteases

(B) reverse protein transcriptase

(C) restriction enzymes

(D) reverse protein ligase

(E) hyaluronidase

619. In clusters of clinical infections caused by *Salmonella* species, all of the following methods may be used to define the epidemic EXCEPT

(A) phage typing

(B) serotyping

(C) antibiotic susceptibility

(D) plasmid profile

(E) pyocin typing

620. Which of the following statements about antimicrobial prophylaxis for individuals exposed to persons infected with *Neisseria meningitidis* is FALSE?

(A) penicillin is effective

(B) rifampin is effective

(C) minocycline is effective

(D) ciprofloxin is effective

(E) it is not usually necessary for hospital personnel

621. The microbe responsible for significant numbers of urinary tract infections by gram-positive bacteria in sexually active young women is

(A) *Bacillus subtilis*

(B) *Escherichia coli*

(C) *Staphylococcus saprophyticus*

(D) *Streptococcus pyogenes*

(E) *Listeria monocytogenes*

622. The availability and effectiveness of *Neisseria meningitidis* meningococcal vaccine are true for which of the following meningococcal groups?

(A) group A meningococci

(B) group C meningococci

(C) group D meningococci

(D) group W-135 meningococci

(E) all of the above

623. Virulent *Shigella* and *Salmonella* both share which of the following characteristics?

(A) both genera belong to the family Enterobacteriaceae

(B) they both cause bacterial diarrhea

(C) they both cannot ferment lactose

(D) they both ferment glucose

(E) all of the above

624. The one gram-positive aerobic bacterium in the following list of medically important gram-negative bacteria is

(A) *Neisseria gonorrheae*

(B) *Bordetella purtussis*

(C) *Campylobacter jejuni*

(D) *Listeria monocytogenes*

(E) *Brucella melitensis*

625. The one gram-positive anaerobe in the following list of gram-negative aerobic rods is

(A) *Actinobacillus actinomycetemocomitans*

(B) *Fusobacterium* spp.

(C) *Francisella tularensis*

(D) *Legionella pneumophila*

(E) *Brucella canis*

626. The one anaerobic bacterial gram-positive rod in the following list of fastidious gram-negative rods is

(A) *Campylobacter fetus*

(B) *Hemophilus ducreyi*

(C) *Clostridium histoliticum*

(D) *Pasteurella multocida*

(E) *Brucella suis*

627. The medically important aerobic, gram-positive coccus in the following list of aerobic gram-negative cocci and rods is

(A) *Streptococcus agalactiae* (group B)

(B) *Moraxella catarrhalis*

(C) *Neisseria gonorrheae*

(D) *Helicobacter pylori*

(E) *Haemophilus aphrophilus*

628. The one medically important aerobic gram-positive rod in the following list of gram-negative fastidious rods is

(A) *Bacillus cereus*

(B) *Pasteurella multocida*

(C) *Helicobacter pylori*

(D) *Actinomyces* spp.

(E) *Cardiobacterium hominis*

629. The only bacteria which cannot be gram-stained in the following list of Enterobacteriaceae is

(A) *Citrobacter* spp.

(B) *Treponema pallidum*

(C) *Escherichia coli*

(D) *Enterobacter* spp.

(E) *Shigella sonnei*

630. The only oxidase-positive, glucose-fermenting gram-negative rod in the following list of medically important bacteria which cannot be Gram stained is

(A) *Aeromonas* spp.

(B) *Chlamydia trachomatis*

(C) *Mycobacterium avium* complex

(D) *Rickettsia ricketsii*

(E) *Treponema pallidum*

631. The only medically important glucose-non-fermenting gram-negative rod in the following list of oxidase-positive glucose-fermenting gram-negative rods is

(A) *Plesiomonas shigelloides*

(B) *Vibrio cholerae*

(C) *Vibrio parahemolyticus*

(D) *Pseudomonas aeruginosa*

(E) *Vibrio vulnificus*

632. It is true that urinary tract infections (UTIs) in women

(A) occur when uropathogens from the fecal flora colonize the vaginal introitus, gain access to the urethra, and then ascend to the bladder giving signs and symptoms of infection

(B) the risk of UTIs in women is increased by sexual intercourse or instrumentation of the urinary tract, which act to propel bacteria into the bladder

(C) factors such as type of clothing or regular hygiene practices do not appear to increase the incidence of UTIs in otherwise healthy women

(D) for many years, it was considered that recurrent UTIs might lead to renal (kidney) damage in women; this is *not* the case

(E) all of the above

633. The normal flora of the throat may include moderate numbers of which of the following bacteria?

(A) gamma-hemolytic streptococci

(B) alpha-hemolytic streptococci

(C) alpha-hemolytic pneumococci

(D) gram-negative diplococci

(E) all of the above

634. A 3-year old boy complained of a headache and developed lethargy and emesis. He had a two-day history of a mild upper respiratory illness and a fever of 39.7°C and was extremely lethargic. A lumbar puncture revealed 2529,000 WBC/mm³ polymorphonuclear, and CSF glucose level of 9 mg/dL (normal 15 to 45 mg/dL). The Gram stain was positive for numerous white cells, and gram-negative coccobacilli of CSF was positive. What was the clinical diagnosis of this patient, and what organism was causing this infection?

(A) bacterial pneumonia

(B) bacterial meningitis

(C) staphylococcus pneumonia

(D) *E. coli* septicemia

(E) all of the above

635. A young man had been good health until he came to an emergency room following 2 days of continual, diffuse, dull abdominal pain. Although he had a loss of appetite, he had no nausea, vomiting, or diarrhea. The patient was afebrile (39.2°C) and his blood pressure was 108/60 mm Hg. On examination, the patient had midgastric and right lower quadrant tenderness. Although his white blood cell count was normal, the blood culture taken on admission was subsequently positive for an anaerobic gram-negative rod. The most likely genus of this microbe is

(A) *Bacteriodes*

(B) *Escherichia*

(C) *Staphylococcus*

(D) *Clostridium*

(E) *Blastomyces*

636. In which site are anaerobes ordinarily NOT found?

(A) mouth

(B) gut

(C) vagina

(D) blood

(E) skin

637. A 6-year old girl contracted Rocky Mountain spotted fever (RMSF) when camping with her family. Which of the following statements is FALSE?

(A) she was first treated with tetracycline because the microbe was sensitive to it

(B) no vaccine exists for RMSF

(C) typical rickettsial symptoms (except for Q fever) are fever, rashes, and vasculitis

(D) mammalian reservoirs of RMSF are rodents and dogs

(E) if you have a patient with unexplained fever, you should consider RMSF

638. A 29-year-old man who went fishing in Wisconsin apparently contacted Lyme borreliosis disease. Which of the following statements is FALSE?

(A) the major symptoms of Lyme disease are flu-like chills, fever, headache, dizziness, and fatigue

(B) Lyme borreliosis is caused by the bite of the borrelium *Chronicum nigrans*

(C) Lyme borreliosis was first reported in Lyme, Connecticut, in 1975

(D) if the disease is not treated promptly, it may move into the progressive stage with less common symptoms such as weakness in the legs and facial paralysis

(E) early antibiotic treatment for adults is usually tetracycline or doxycycline

639. All of the following statements are true EXCEPT

(A) brucellosis can be contracted from the slaughter of a pig infected with *Brucella suis*

(B) listeriosis can be contracted by eating Mexican-type cheese infected with *Listeria monocytogenes*

(C) *Listeria monocytogenes* can be easily cultured on laboratory media

(D) brucellosis is associated with spontaneous abortion in pregnant women

(E) fleas, lice, ticks, and mites can all serve as vectors of rickettsiae

640. All of the following statements concerning gonorrhea are true EXCEPT

(A) it is caused by a gram-negative, oxidase-positive diplococcus

(B) it cannot be caused by a penicillinase-producing gonococci

(C) it is not very readily diagnosed with a Gram stain in females

(D) in acute cases in males, it may be provisionally diagnosed with a Gram stain

(E) it is caused by *Neisseria gonorrhoeae*

641. Which of the following statements concerning pneumonia and pneumococcal vaccines is true?

(A) there is no vaccine available that protects individuals against strains of pneumococcal pneumonia

(B) this organism is not responsible for most of the cases of pneumococcal pneumonia in the United States

(C) fewer than 10% of those who should get the shot do so

(D) those individuals over the age of 40 should take the pneumococcal vaccine

(E) people at risk of serious life-threatening complications such as chronic kidney disease, diabetes, lung and heart disease, and HIV should get the vaccine

642. It is true that

(A) tuberculosis (TB) was one of the most intensely researched infectious diseases by physicians and scientists in the first half of this century

(B) with the introduction of streptomycin in 1945 and isoniazid in 1952, TB research had decreased

(C) infection with HIV is associated with increased susceptibility to TB and with accelerated progression of the disease and mortality in the last few years

(D) the situation is more encouraging with respect to leprosy; there is real hope that leprosy can be eliminated as a public health problem

(E) all of the above

643. It is true that

(A) enterotoxin production alone is not the sole factor in the pathogenesis of cholera

(B) *Vibrio cholerae* must also establish themselves in the intestinal tract

(C) the microbe attaches itself to the intestinal lining

(D) virulent microbes can penetrate the intestinal mucosa and attach to the cells

(E) all of the above

644. Which of the following statements is FALSE?

(A) necrotizing fasciitis is a rare outcome of group A streptococcus (GAS) infection

(B) it is the result of a fulminating infection of GAS in which the microbe produces proteases responsible in part for the tissue destruction

(C) the proteases digest the muscle sheath and can rapidly destroy an individual in a matter of hours

(D) there are at least five exotoxins produced by GAS

(E) exotoxin B, a constant feature of all GAS, is an enzyme that degrades fibronectin

645. Given the resurgence of pertussis in a highly immunized population of children, it is true that

(A) throughout the world, pertussis remains a major cause of morbidity and mortality among infants

(B) whole-cell pertussis vaccines have been effective in controlling the disease but have not eliminated circulation of *B. pertussis*

(C) a pertussis epidemic occurred in Cincinnati in 1993 primarily among children who had been appropriately immunized; this is interpreted to mean that the whole-cell vaccine failed to give full protection against the disease

(D) adults and adolescents remain susceptible to pertussis and may be candidates for booster doses of a cellular pertussis vaccine

(E) all of the above

646. It is true that

(A) most of the deaths from pathogens occur in underdeveloped countries as a result of the high incidence of diarrhea

(B) the inflammatory diarrheas tend to be caused by bacterial pathogens such as *Shigella, Salmonella, Campylobacter,* and *Clostridium difficile*

(C) inflammatory diarrheas are much more dangerous than noninflammatory diarrheas

(D) stool specimens from patients with inflammatory diarrhea contain high levels of lactoferrin that can be speedily and accurately detected

(E) all of the above

647. Which of the following statements is FALSE?

(A) most epidemiologic investigations of illness associated with *E. coli* 0157:H7 infections have been directed at restaurants associated with outbreaks

(B) the sources of infection for sporadic cases rarely have been identified

(C) *E. coli* 0157:H7 causes diarrhea (often bloody) and abdominal cramps, although fever is infrequent and hemolytic uremic syndrome (HUS) develops as a complication in 5 to 19% of the cases

(D) there are no subtypings used to distinguish the *E. coli* 0157:H7 strains because there is only a phage type of this strain

(E) children and the elderly are at the highest risk for clinical manifestations and complications of these infections

648. Q fever is an acute infectious disease of worldwide occurrence that

(A) is caused by *Rickettsia akari*

(B) stimulates the production of *Proteus* agglutinins

(C) involves a rash that spreads from the trunk to the extremities

(D) is acquired by inhaling dust containing infected animal excreta

(E) is usually acquired by tick bites

649. Duodenal stomach ulcers have been shown to be linked with which of the following bacteria?

(A) *Streptococcus pyogenes*

(B) *Streptococcus pneumoniae*

(C) *Helicobacter pylori*

(D) *Listeria monocytogenes*

(E) *Vibrio vulnificans*

DIRECTIONS (Questions 650 through 674): Each group of items in this section consists of lettered headings followed by a set of numbered words or phrases. For each numbered word or phrase, select the ONE lettered heading that is most closely associated with it. Each lettered heading may be selected once, more than once, or not at all.

Questions 650 and 651

For each diagnostic procedure listed below, select the most appropriate laboratory finding.

   (A) fermentation of lactose

   (B) inhibition of growth by bacitracin

   (C) inhibition of growth by optochin hydrochloride

   (D) positive coagulase test

650. Differentiation of *Staphylococcus aureus*, from *Staphylococcus saprophyticus*

651. Differentiation of *Streptococcus agalactiae* from other hemolytic streptococci

Questions 652 and 653

   (A) *Helicobacter pylori*

   (B) *Pseudomonas aeruginosa*

   (C) *Mycobacterium smegmatis*

   (D) *Vibrio vulnificus*

   (E) *Campylobacter jejuni*

652. Sensitive to bismuth

653. Alginate glycocalyx

Questions 654 through 659

For each patient discussed below, select the microorganism most likely to have caused the illness described.

   (A) *Hemophilus influenzae*

   (B) *Bordetella pertussis*

   (C) *Listeria monocytogenes*

   (D) *Erysipelothrix rhusiopathiae*

   (E) *Corynebacterium diphtheriae*

   (F) *Mycobacterium tuberculosis*

   (G) *Mycobacterium avium intracellulare*

   (H) *Mycobacterium leprae*

   (I) *Actinomyces israelii*

   (J) *Nocardia asteroides*

   (K) *Campylobacter* spp.

   (L) *Serratia marcescens*

   (M) *Proteus mirabilis*

   (N) *Shigella sonnei*

   (O) *Salmonella typhimurium*

   (P) *Vibrio vulnificus*

   (Q) *Pseudomonas aeruginosa*

   (R) *Yersinia pestis*

   (S) *Francisella tularensis*

   (T) *Pasteurella multocida*

   (U) *Brucella melitensis*

   (V) *Bacillus cereus*

   (W) *Bacteroides fragilis*

   (X) *Escherichia coli*

654. A 28-year-old dairy farmer who was in good health until the preceding day was admitted to the hospital from the emergency room. He felt chilled, feverish, developed nausea, vomiting, diarrhea, and lower abdominal discomfort. His rectal examination revealed occult blood in the stool. A stool examination for fecal leukocytes was positive, and the stool culture was diagnostic. The microbe was a lactose nonfermenter on MacConkey's agar, H_2S-negative (urea-negative), and nonmotile at both 25°C and 37°C.

655. A 6-week-old boy with a 10-day history of choking spells was transferred from another hospital. The spells began with repetitive coughing, progressing until he turned red and was gasping for breath. The child's chest radiograph was clear, and there were no tracheal abnormalities. His white cell count was 15,500 mm^3, with 70% lymphocytes. A nasopharyngeal swab was diagnostic on Bordet–Gengou medium.

656. A 55-year-old man had a 2-month history of fevers, night sweats, increased cough with sputum production, and a 25-lb. weight loss. He denied intravenous drug use or homosexual activity. He drinks about a pint of gin a day. An acid-fast organism grew from the sputum; he had a positive human immunodeficiency virus serology and a low absolute CD4$^+$ lymphocyte count.

657. A 42-year-old man had a renal biopsy in August because of a 20-lb. weight gain with peripheral edema. The biopsy showed minimal changes, so he was admitted to the hospital. Two blood cultures taken at admission grew an oxidase-positive, gram-negative rod on MacConkey agar and were presumptively identified as a *Pseudomonas species*. After this, the organism was shown to ferment glucose, so it was not a pseudomonad. On questioning, the patient stated that he had eaten raw oysters two days before admission.

658. A 2-year-old boy, having had an upper respiratory infection for 2 weeks, was admitted to the hospital after becoming lethargic and anorexic. He had been in the emergency room three days prior to admission, when he had a 39.9°C fever. His chest was clear, and he had exudative pharyngitis. A throat culture was taken, and a course of penicillin was begun. The disease worsened. No group A streptococci developed from the throat culture taken 3 days earlier. On examination of his posterior pharynx, a yellowish, thick membrane was observed, which bled when scraped and removed. The patient's history revealed that he had received no immunizations.

659. A 40-year-old woman had an ulcer on the distal part of her right third finger. She developed chills and fever. Oral antibiotics were not successful, and she was admitted to a hospital 12 days after first noting the finger ulcer. This obese patient had a 40°C temperature and enlarged lymph nodes. Her cultures were negative. Questioning revealed that she had butchered a rabbit two weeks prior to the onset of her illness.

Questions 660 through 665

For each patient discussed below, select the microorganism most likely to have caused the illness described.

   (A) *Staphylococcus aureus*
   (B) *Staphylococcus epidermidis*

   (C) *Streptococcus pneumoniae*
   (D) *Streptococcus pyogenes*
   (E) *Streptococcus agalactiae*
   (F) *Streptococcus viridans*
   (G) *Neisseria meningitidis*
   (H) *Neisseria gonorrhoeae*
   (I) *Borrelia burgdorferi*
   (J) *Hemophilus influenzae*
   (K) *Mycobacterium kansasii*
   (L) *Brucella suis*
   (M) *Listeria monocytogenes*
   (N) *Chlamydia trachomatis*
   (O) *Mycoplasma pneumoniae*
   (P) *Ureaplasma urealyticum*

660. A 15-year-old boy with a history of sickle cell disease had a progressive 4-day productive cough and 2 days of spiking fever. He was admitted to the hospital, and his chest examination was notable for decreased sounds by auscultation and dullness to percussion. Among his initial laboratory results was a leukocyte count of 52,400/mm^3, with 86% neutrophils. A sputum Gram stain was nondiagnostic, but his blood culture was subsequently positive for gram-positive cocci in pairs. The chest radiograph demonstrated a right lower lobe infiltrate.

661. A 19-year-old woman came to a medical clinic with a complaint of right knee and right shoulder pain, nausea, and vomiting. On physical examination, she had a swollen right knee and decreased range of motion of her right shoulder. She also had a thick vaginal discharge. She gave a history of having two recent sexual partners. Cultures were performed on blood, vagina, and joint fluid samples. A Gram stain of joint fluid showed many polymorphonuclear leukocytes, containing gram-negative diplococci. Both the vaginal and joint fluid cultures were positive for the infectious agent.

662. A 47-year-old man had a history of sickle cell disease, which was the cause of many previous hospitalizations to manage his painful crises. He was admitted 9 days earlier to the present hospital. The management of the crisis was successful, and he was discharged after 4 days. On readmission from the emergency room, he noted the presence of right arm discomfort and swelling, a slight fever, and chills. He had no fever in the emergency room, but physical examination showed right arm swelling. A Doppler sonogram of the venous system of his right upper arm showed a right axillary and right subclavian venous thrombosis. Blood cultures were obtained from two separate sites (one from the line and one peripheral), and both sets grew identical gram-positive cocci

663. A 36-year-old woman had an infection on the internal corner of the right eye, and it spread rapidly in a centrifugal pattern to the forehead and cheeks in about 2 days to cause a "butterfly" pattern. The edge of the lesion was sharply defined, particularly on the cheeks. The onset of this infection was very rapid and produced toxicity, chills, and a high fever in a few hours.

664. A 29-year-old man had complained of fatigue, stiff neck, flu-like chills, and headache. Although he lives in a suburb of Chicago, he is an avid fisherman and frequently goes fishing in Wisconsin. Upon questioning, he said he did not remember being bitten by ticks, although about 3 to 4 weeks ago he recalled seeing an expanding red circle surrounding a lighter area with a small welt in the center like a "bull's-eye" on his arm that eventually disappeared. He thought it was an insect bite of some kind.

665. A man in his early 20s came to the emergency room after 3 days of painful urethral discharge. He had been sexually active with his girlfriend for the past few months. The man had noted a similar discharge 1 year prior to this visit, when he was having sexual relations with the same girl. He had a white urethral discharge, and Gram stain and culture for *Neisseria gonorrheae* were negative. A urethral culture was subsequently positive for the causative agent.

Question 666

    (A) antibiotic tolerance
    (B) phage type
    (C) toxic shock syndrome
    (D) enterotoxin
    (E) leukocidin

666. Marked hypotension and scarlatiniform rash followed by desquamation

Questions 667 through 669

    (A) botulinum toxin
    (B) cholera toxin
    (C) diphtheria toxin
    (D) staphylococcal exfoliation
    (E) tetanus toxin

667. Blocks the functioning of the inhibitory transmitter at the inhibitory synapses in the spinal cord, thus causing hyperreflexia and spasms of the skeletal muscles

668. Inhibits the release of acetylcholine at the myoneural junction, thus causing flaccid paralysis

669. Increases the level of cyclic adenosine monophosphate in mucosal epithelial cells by activating adenylate cyclase

Questions 670 and 671

    (A) *Brucella abortus*

    (B) *Listeria monocytogenes*

    (C) *Legionella pneumophila*

    (D) *Chlamydia trachomatis*

    (E) *Hemophilus influenzae*

670. Gram-positive

671 Undulant fever

Questions 672 through 674

    (A) *Rickettsia prowazekii*

    (B) *Rickettsia rickettsii*

    (C) *Rickettsia akari*

    (D) *Coxiella burnetii*

    (E) *Rochalimeaea quintana*

672. Transmitted to humans by lice and is the cause of typhus

673. Enters the human body by inhalation

674. Transmitted to humans by ticks

Medical Bacteriology
Answers and Explanations

411. **(A)** The diphtheria toxin, a two-component protein exotoxin, is produced only by *Corynebacterium diphtheriae* strains infected with a tox+ temperate phage (corynephage) called beta. This property has nothing to do with plasmids. In the case of the two *Escherichia coli* enterotoxins, necessary for travelers' diarrhea, one of the plasmids encodes for both of the enterotoxins. Enterotoxins are toxins that affect the small intestine, causing fluid to flow into the intestine and subsequent diarrhea. Heat-labile enterotoxin is functionally and structurally similar to cholera toxin. The second is heat stable and apparently activates guanylate cyclase to form cyclic guanosine monophosphate, inhibiting sodium and chloride absorption. The second encodes for pili, which bring about specific adherence to mammalian epithelial cells. *(Jawetz et al, p 216; Joklik et al, pp 391, 488–489,541–542)*

412. **(D)** *Staphylococcus aureus* is not a facultative intracellular pathogen, whereas the remaining microbes are. *S. aureus* is an extracellular pathogen that typically causes acute infections. *(Joklik et al, pp 145–149,403)*

413. **(B)** *Staphylococcus aureus* does not cause erysipelas, which is a skin infection caused by *Streptococcus pyogenes*, group A. All of the other statements are true. *(Joklik et al, pp 418, 423)*

414. **(E)** Coagulase is not the sole staphylococcal virulence factor, in the manner of diphtheria toxin being the sole virulence factor for *Corynebacterium diphtheriae*. The virulence is due to a wide variety of factors which all contribute to staphylococcal virulence. All of the other statements are true. *(Joklik et al, pp 406–407)*

415. **(C)** Impetigo pyoderma, a disease characterized by blister-like multifocal pustules on the face and hands in children and adults, can be caused by *Staphylococcus aureus* and/or beta-hemolytic *Streptococcus pyogenes,* not only by *S. aureus.* All of the other statements are true. *(Joklik et al, pp 408,411,424–425)*

416. **(B)** Neonatal sepsis and meningitis is usually caused by group B streptococci (*Streptococcus agalactiae*). The organism infects the neonate from the mother's vaginal flora (about 20% of women carry group B streptococci) during vaginal delivery. Group B streptococci give a positive reaction in the cAMP test, where there is a zone of complete hydrolysis when it is inoculated perpendicular to the streak of *S. aureus. (Jawetz et al, p 204; Joklik, pp 426–427)*

417. **(B)** Acute poststreptococcal glomerulonephritis (AGN) is somewhat similar to rheumatic fever, which appears as a complication only after pharyngeal infections with group A *Streptococcus pyogenes.* AGN may occur after either pharyngeal or cutaneous infections with specific serotypes, type 12 being the most common serotype associated with cutaneous infections, usually pyodermas. *(Jawetz et al, pp 205–206; Joklik, p 423)*

418. (D) The normal pharyngeal flora includes an abundance of viridans streptococci, neisseriae, diphtheroids staphylococci, small gram-negative rods, and so forth. Although a few colonies of beta-hemolytic streptococci may indicate they are only transients, moderate or large numbers of them indicate a "strep throat" infection. *(Jawetz et al, p 205; Joklik et al, pp 423,590–593)*

419. (B) Methicillin resistance in *Staphylococcus aureus* and penicillin resistance in *Streptococcus pneumoniae* have both been shown to be caused by an altered target site. All staphylococcal clinical methicillin-resistant strains tested have been shown to produce a new penicillin-binding protein (PBP) with a low affinity for methicillin. Resistance is due to an acquired chromosomal gene, mec A, that is absent from methicillin-susceptible staphylococci. This gene has resulted in a worldwide dissemination of methicillin-resistant staphylococci in larger hospitals. Altered PBPs have also been shown to be associated with development of increased minimum inhibitory concentrations in pneumococcal pneumonia carried by *S. pneumoniae*. Altered PBPs have also been detected in clinical isolates of *Neisseria gonorrhoeae*, *Neisseria meningitidis*, and *Hemophilus influenzae* that were penicillin resistant but did not produce beta-lactamase. *(Joklik et al, pp 185,440)*

420. (C) C substance, or C polysaccharide, is a somatic antigen (not a capsular antigen), which is a species-specific teichoic acid polymer containing phosphocholine as a major antigenic determinant and precipitates with a nonspecific serum beta-globulin called C-reactive protein (CRP) in the presence of calcium. Levels of CRP, which is not an antibody, are elevated in individuals with a wide variety of acute inflammatory diseases. The C substance CRP precipitate activates complement via the classical pathway and may function as an opsonin to facilitate phagocytosis early in pneumococcal infections. *(Joklik et al, p 435)*

421. (E) *Streptococcus pneumoniae* colonies are alpha-hemolytic and sensitive to optochin (ethyl hydrocuprein). Thus, the pneumococcal colonies will not grow around a disc containing optochin, although alpha-hemolytic viridans streptococci will grow. This does not happen with any other of the bacteria listed. *(Joklik et al, pp 433–434)*

422. (D) There are 84 different pneumococcal capsular serotypes, and their antibodies do not cross-react. If the second infection is not of the same capsular serotype as the first infection, the antibodies will not be protective. Type-specific immunity to pneumococcal infection is long-lasting. Recurrent pneumococcal infections are usually caused by pneumococci of a different serologic type. *(Joklik et al, pp 436–439)*

423. (B) There is a human carrier state, in the absence of disease, for the meningococcus. The carrier state is in the nasopharynx of symptom-free people and serves as a community reservoir for the meningococcus. The carrier state is associated with development of protective antibody. Acquisition of the meningococcus in the nasopharynx of the nonimmune individual, which occurs rapidly during epidemics, may result in bacteremia and disease. Polysaccharides from types A, C, W-135, and Y are used in vaccines. *(Joklik et al, p 466)*

424. (C) The lipopolysaccharide, or endotoxin, in the outer membrane is the most likely *Neisseria meningitidis* component responsible for the production of overwhelming septicemic shock during meningococcemia. It causes intravascular activation of the complement system, the kallikrein–kinin system (hypotension) and the clotting cascade (hemorrhage). *(Jawetz et al, p 254; Joklik et al, pp 446–449)*

425. (D) In acute bacterial meningitis, age is an important factor relating the etiologic agent and the prognosis. Among adults (greater than 15 years), *Streptococcus pneumoniae* is responsible for 30 to 50% of meningitis infections, rather than *Neisseria meningitidis*, which is responsible for 10 to 35% of them. Among children (1 month to 5 years), *Hemophilus influenzae* is the most common cause of bacterial meningitis (40 to 60%), followed by *Neisseria meningitidis* (25 to 40%) and *Streptococcus pneumoniae* (10 to 20%). Among neonates (less than 1 month), meningitis caused by gram-negative bacilli (50 to 60%) is the most common bacterial cause, followed by *Streptococcus* group A and group B (20 to 40%), and *Listeria monocytogenes* (2 to 10%). The fatality rate is high among the elderly due to *S. pneumoniae*; therefore, they should be given pneumococcal vaccine as a preventative. *(Jawetz et al, pp 254–255; Joklik et al, Table 25–2, p 439)*

426.　**(D)** Tuberculous patients develop a variety of antibodies to the components of *Mycobacterium tuberculosis*. However, none of these antibodies has been associated with resistance to tuberculosis. Delayed-type hypersensitivity to tuberculoproteins develops following infection with *M. tuberculosis* and is thought to be involved in the pathogenicity of this microorganism. Yet, delayed hypersensitivity does not appear to be responsible for acquired immunity because animals rendered tuberculin-positive by the administration of wax D and tuberculoproteins do not show any increased resistance to infection with *M. tuberculosis*. Similarly, neither high levels of serum calcium nor massive proliferation of polymorphonuclear leukocytes constitute major factors of host resistance to tuberculosis. Macrophage stimulation during infection is characterized by an increase in lysosomal content of the macrophages and an enhanced ability of the macrophages to kill *M. tuberculosis*. Activation of macrophages depends upon the production of lymphokines by antigen-activated T lymphocytes. *(Joklik et al, pp 430–431)*

427.　**(D)** *Mycobacterium tuberculosis* is an acid-fast, obligate aerobic, niacin-producing bacterium, which grows slowly (it has a generation time of 1 to 6 hours) on the Lowenstein–Jensen or other artificial culture media. *(Joklik et al, pp 424–425)*

428.　**(C)** The tuberculin test constitutes an important diagnostic tool for tuberculosis. It is used to detect recent or past exposure to *Mycobacterium tuberculosis*. The infection does not

have to be active pulmonary tuberculosis or active nontubercular mycobacterial infection. Since the antigen injected intradermally in the tuberculin test is a purified protein derivative isolated from *M. tuberculosis* or other mycobacteria, a positive tuberculin test will not indicate a parasitic infection. Delayed hypersensitivity does not appear to be responsible for acquired immunity to tuberculosis, because animals rendered tuberculin-positive by the administration of wax D and the purified protein derivative (PPD) do not show any increased resistance to tuberculosis. Therefore, the tuberculin test does not indicate immunity to *M. tuberculosis*. *(Joklik et al, pp 432–433)*

429.　**(A)** The purified protein derivative is prepared by growing *Mycobacterium tuberculosis* in a chemically defined medium. It is prepared by filtration, concentration of the filtrate by ultrafiltration, and precipitation of the purified protein derivative (PPD) with 50% (NH4)2SO4. In addition to tuberculoproteins, the PPD contains polysaccharides and other molecules. The induction of delayed-type hypersensitivity requires not only the PPD but also a lipid component of *M. tuberculosis* called wax D. The PPD is usually administered intradermally in a volume of 0.1 mL containing 5 tuberculin units. *(Joklik et al, p 508)*

430.　**(E)** *Mycobacterium kansasii* causes chronic pulmonary disease indistinguishable from tuberculosis, especially in individuals who have chronic bronchitis or pulmonary emphysema. This microorganism is a photochromogen that grows slowly with an optimal temperature of 37°C. *(Joklik et al, pp 512–513)*

431.　**(A)** *Mycobacterium intracellulare*, like other mycobacteria, contains large amounts of lipids, glycolipids, polysaccharides, and peptidoglycan in its cell wall. It causes pulmonary disease clinically and is pathologically indistinguishable from tuberculosis. However, this disease cannot be easily spread by person-to-person transmission. *M. intracellulare* is not an obligate intracellular parasite because it can be cultured on such artificial media as the Jensen–Lowenstein medium. *(Joklik et al, pp 514–515)*

432. **(E)** Every attempt to culture *Mycobacterium leprae* on artificial media has failed till now. *M. leprae* responds to sulfones or rifampin. This organism is a procaryotic bacterium containing the usual 70S ribosomes. Serpentine cord formation is a characteristic of *Mycobacterium tuberculosis* and not *M. leprae*. Induction of delayed-type hypersensitivity is thought to play a role in the pathogenesis of leprosy. *(Joklik et al, pp 516–521)*

433. **(D)** Human mycobacterial pathogens other than *Mycobacterium tuberculosis* produce PPDs, which can be used in skin tests to identify the causative agent. In such differential skin tests, the homologous mycobacterial PPD gives stronger reaction than the standard tuberculin. Human mycobacterial pathogens other than *M. tuberculosis* exhibit high levels of resistance to antituberculosis drugs. They tend to have slight if any recognizable pathogenicity for guinea pigs. This group includes such rapid growers as *Mycobacterium fortuitum*, but *Mycobacterium kansasii* is not a rapid grower. *M. kansasii* is a photochromogen, which causes chronic pulmonary disease. Scrofula, or cervical adenitis, in young children is due to scotochromogen *Mycobacterium scrofulaceum*. *(Joklik et al, pp 513–515)*

434. **(D)** Exotoxins elaborated by the causative agents of these diseases are primarily responsible for their pathogenesis. Diphtheria is the only disease caused by a nonspore-forming bacterium, *Corynebacterium diphtheriae*. Tetanus toxin produced by *Clostridium tetani* is a heat-labile protein (molecular weight 70,000). The organism is introduced to wounds in the form of a spore. The three most common species of clostridia associated with gas gangrene are *Clostridium perfringens* (*Clostridium welchii*), *Clostridium novyi*, and *Clostridium septicum*. The clostridia are introduced into wounds as spores. Vegetative cells resulting from germinated spores produce a large variety of toxins and enzymes that have lethal,

necrotizing, and hemolytic properties. The causative agent of anthrax is *Bacillus anthracis*. The organism is introduced into wounds as spores. Anthrax toxin contains three distinct components (protective antigen, edema factor, and lethal factor). Antibiotic-associated pseudomembranous colitis is caused by *Clostridium difficile* that proliferates in the colon and produces a necrotizing exotoxin. *(Joklik et al, pp 615–618,636–640,643–645)*

435. **(D)** *Pseudomonas aeruginosa* is a gram-negative, highly motile organism commonly found in our environment. It produces a bluish pigment (pyocyanin) and a fluorescent pigment (fluorescein). It is an opportunistic pathogen, which causes severe infections in compromised hosts. Burn patients and pulmonary cystic fibrosis patients are especially susceptible to *Pseudomonas* infections. In addition to a variety of extracellular lytic enzymes, the organism produces an exotoxin that is very similar to diphtheria toxin. Its uniform resistance to penicillin appears to be attributed to both exclusion by the outer cell membrane and chromosomally mediated beta-lactamases. *(Joklik et al, pp 576–583)*

436. **(D)** Two distinct protein exotoxins produced by *Clostridium difficile* are responsible for a variety of gastrointestinal disorders as side effects of the administration of some antibiotics. These antibiotic-associated disorders range from the mild diarrheas to the most severe complication, pseudomembranous enterocolitis. Toxin B, or cytotoxin, produces a cytopathic effect on tissue culture cells in vitro, a procedure used to differentiate this toxin from patient feces or *C. difficile* cultures. Toxin A is a potent enterotoxin that causes severe intestinal mucosa damage. Diarrhea, which usually resolves spontaneously after discontinuing the implicit antimicrobial agent(s), is a much more frequent adverse reaction than is colitis. Only about one-third of the patients with antibiotic-associated diarrhea have been found to be positive for *C. difficile* or the cytotoxin. The antibiotics most often associated with these disorders after prolonged oral administration are ampicillin, clindamycin, and the cephalosporins. *(Jawetz et al, p 260; Joklik et al, pp 643–645)*

437. **(D)** Diphtheria toxin can be converted to diphtheria toxoid by formaldehyde treatment. Diphtheria toxoid is nontoxic, although it is still immunogenic. The specific antibody (antitoxin) produced in response to the immunization with the toxoid can neutralize the toxin, thus protecting the host from lethal action of diphtheria toxin. The antitoxin itself is neither capable of killing *Corynebacterium diphtheriae* nor facilitating their phagocytosis. Thus, the treatment of diphtheria rests largely on rapid killing of toxin-producing bacteria by antimicrobials (penicillin or erythromycin) and the early administration of specific antitoxin (antiserum) against the toxin excreted by the organisms at their site of entry and multiplication. *(Joklik et al, pp 487–493)*

438. **(D)** The skin test (Schick test) is based on the fact that diphtheria toxin produces a marked local reaction when injected intradermally unless it is neutralized by circulating antitoxin. The test should be read at 24 and 48 hours and again in 6 or 7 days. Positive reaction, characterized by a local inflammatory reaction, indicates the absence of adequate amounts of serum antitoxin; thus, the individual is not immune to diphtheria. Allergic reactions are sometimes observed in adults. All other tests listed are inadequate or too complex for routine use. *(Joklik et al, p 491)*

439. **(D)** Verotoxin is an exotoxin produced by enteropathogenic *Escherichia coli* and is cytotoxic to vero cells. Vero tissue culture cells were developed from African green monkey kidney cells. Heat-labile and heat-stable enterotoxins are produced by enterotoxigenic *E. coli* and cause diarrhea by activating adenylate cyclase and guanylate cyclase, respectively. Other strains of *E. coli* that cause diarrhea are enteroinvasive *E. coli* and enteroadherent *E. coli*. Exfoliative toxin produced by *Staphylococcus aureus* is responsible for the "scalded skin" syndrome associated with staphylococcal infections. *(Joklik et al, pp 411,546–548)*

440. **(D)** *Neisseria gonorrhoeae* colony types 1 and 2 possess pili (fimbriae) that allow the gonococcal cells to attach the body surfaces. Therefore, they are considered pathogenic. Types 3 or 4 do not possess pili and are avirulent. *Neisseria gonorrhoeae* forms indophenol oxidase and elaborates a protease which degrades IgA. It grows best at a 2 to 10% CO_2 tension. *(Joklik et al, pp 450–453)*

441. **(A)** *Chlamydia trachomatis*, a bacterial pathogen, is the most common cause of nongonococcal arthritis, which is transmitted venereally and which can be treated with tetracycline. *(Jawetz et al, pp 304–305; Joklik et al, pp 724–726)*

442. **(C)** *Neisseria gonorrhoeae* is usually cultured on the modified Thayer–Martin medium in the presence of 2 to 10% carbon dioxide. Gonococci types 1 and 2 are piliated and are regarded as virulent because they produce infection in volunteers. It is estimated that at least 30% of cases of pelvic inflammatory disease (PID) are gonococcal. Long-lasting immunity does not develop following natural infection with *N. gonorrhoeae*. This situation may be due to the heterogeneity of the gonococcal antigens. *(Joklik et al, pp 450–455)*

443. **(D)** The best way to detect congenital syphilis is by the use of fluorescent treponema antibody absorption test (IgM-FTA-ABS). All newborn infants of mothers with reactive Venereal Disease Research Laboratories or FTA-ABS tests will themselves have reactive tests whether or not they have acquired syphilis, because of passive placental transfer of maternal immunoglobulins. However, if IgM antisyphilitic antibody is present in the infant's serum, it will reflect fetal antibody production in response to intrauterine infection, because IgM maternal antibody does not penetrate a healthy placenta. *(Joklik et al, pp 663–665)*

444. **(D)** The most recently discovered venereally transmitted disease is acquired immunodeficiency syndrome. This disease, which was discovered in 1981, is caused by a retrovirus known as the human immunodeficiency

virus. *(Jawetz et al, pp 579–581; Joklik et al, pp 896–899)*

445. **(C)** Enterotoxin activity has been reported in several *Salmonella* species and in enteropathogenic *Escherichia coli*. The action of enterotoxins produced by gram-negative bacteria is to activate the membrane-bound adenyl cyclase that converts adenosine triphosphate to cyclic adenosine monophosphate (cAMP). The increase in cAMP promotes loss of electrolytes and fluid from the cells of the intestine into the lumen. Antibodies to enterotoxins have been produced. The lipid A is the toxic moiety of endotoxins and not the enterotoxins. *(Joklik et al, pp 561,568,641)*

446. **(A)** *Pseudomonas* infections often occur in patients suffering from burns or cystic fibrosis. They are difficult to treat because the causative agents are usually resistant to most of the common antibiotics. However, *Pseudomonas* infections may be successfully treated by a combination of gentamicin and carbenicillin. These infections are most frequently caused by *Pseudomonas aeruginosa*, which produces a characteristic greenish pigment. *(Joklik et al, pp 579–580)*

447. **(E)** *Pseudomonas aeruginosa* is a metabolically very active bacterium and thus cannot be classified as a fastidious microorganism. It now appears that it can grow in unsupplemented tap water. It is a motile, urease-negative, lactose-negative bacterium. At least three exotoxins (A, B, and C) that are lethal for experimental animals have been identified. *(Joklik et al, pp 577–578)*

448. **(B)** The 2-keto-3-deoxyoctonate (KDO) is a constituent of the inner core of *Salmonella* lipopolysaccharide. The toxic moiety of the liposaccharide is thought to be the lipid A. The lipopolysaccharide portion of the cell wall of Salmonella and other gram-negative bacteria is also called endotoxin. Therefore, endotoxins usually are expected to contain KDO. This compound does not undergo phase-type variation. It is the flagellar antigens of *Salmonella* or Arizona species that undergo phase one (specific) and phase two

(nonspecific) variations that are used in the Kauffman–White scheme for the serologic speciation of these genera. *(Joklik et al, pp 84–85, 358)*

449. **(D)** Bacteria belonging to genus *Salmonella* do not ferment lactose. Like other enteric organisms, they have somatic O antigens, which are part of the lipopolysaccharide components of the cell wall. They also have flagellar (H) antigens, which are proteins. The H antigens, as well as the O antigens, are used to classify and characterize the species of *Salmonella* but have nothing directly to do with virulence. *(Joklik et al, pp 559–560)*

450. **(E)** In the United States, *Salmonella typhimurium* is the most common serotype isolated from human and animal sources, and it causes a great deal of gastroenteritis in humans. The majority of human cases are acquired by the ingestion of contaminated food or water. However, salmonellosis can be transmitted by such means as direct fecal-oral transmission or by contaminated instruments. Poultry products (primarily eggs) are the most important sources of human infections. Meats and dairy products are also often implicated in epidemics. *(Jawetz et al, pp 218–221; Joklik et al, pp 562–563)*

451. **(E)** Household pets such as dogs, cats, and turtles are the reservoirs of gastroenteritis but not of typhoid fever caused by *Salmonella typhi*. The sources of infection for typhoid fever are individuals who are suffering from typhoid fever or who have become carriers of *S. typhi*. (*Salmonella* is a biochemically and serologically diverse bacterial group. Besides humans, they infect animals, but they cause enteric fevers, the most serious of which is typhoid fever. Since 1983, on the basis of DNA hybridization studies, one species, *Salmonella cholerasuis,* has been designated for the *Salmonella–Arizona* group. Reports from reference laboratories that serotype isolates include the serotype name, eg, *Salmonella* serotype *typhimurium* rather than the more taxonomically correct *Salmonella enterica* subspecies *enterica* serotype *typhimurium*.) *(Jawetz et al, pp 218–221; Joklik et al, pp 559–562)*

452. (E) The Vi antigen is located in the capsule of *Salmonella typhi*, and it frequently interferes with the agglutination of *S. typhi* by antisera containing anti-O agglutinins. This antigen is destroyed by heating for 60 minutes at 60°C. The Vi antigen may play a role in the pathogenicity of *S. typhi*. However, it is not now considered the major virulence factor of *S. typhi* because non-Vi strains are capable of producing typhoid fever in volunteers. *(Joklik et al, pp 560–561)*

453. (B) Blood cultures constitute the best specimen for analysis during the first 2 weeks of typhoid fever. In the absence of therapy, blood cultures are positive in over 80% of patients seen in the first week of illness. Bone marrow cultures may be positive for *Salmonella typhi* after the blood becomes negative. Stool or urine cultures are positive in about 25% of patients during the first week of illness. Only in the case of pulmonary abscesses may sputum yield *S. typhi*. *(Jawetz et al, p 219; Joklik et al, pp 561–562)*

454. (E) The pH of the urine is not diagnostic of urinary tract infections unless it is alkaline (indicating the involvement of urease-producing bacteria, which produce ammonia such as *Proteus* spp. or *Klebsiella*. *(Jawetz et al, p 592,600; Joklik et al, pp 418,541)*

455. (D) The vast majority of urinary tract infections are caused by Enterobacteriaceae originating from the gut. *(Jawetz et al, p 600)*

456. (D) Urinary tract infections (UTIs) acquired in the hospital are much more likely to be antibiotic resistant than are those due to bacteria from community acquired UTIs. *(Jawetz et al, pp 592,600)*

457. (C) *Neisseria meningitidis* is a gram-negative pathogen that causes 20% of meningitis cases, the second most common cause of the disease. Bacteremia produced by this organism (meningococcemia) is characterized by high fever, hemorrhagic rashes (petechiae) often culminating in disseminated intravascular coagulation, and circulatory collapse (Waterhouse–Friderichsen syndrome). Meningitis is the most common complication of meningococcemia. The endotoxin (lipopolysaccharide) associated with the outer membrane of the cell wall of this organism is responsible for these symptoms. Capsular polysaccharides and outer membrane proteins are useful antigenic markers for the classification of this organism but do not contribute to the development of septicemic shock. *(Joklik et al, pp 447–449)*

458. (A) *Campylobacter jejuni* is a curved, slender, motile, gram-negative rod. It is a common cause of gastroenteritis in children but it also occurs in all ages. Some strains of *Escherichia coli*, *Shigella sonnei*, and *Yersinia enterocolitica* cause diarrhea in humans but none of these have a curved shape. *(Joklik et al, pp 590, 676–677)*

459. (D) Fluid replacement is vitally important for the treatment of cholera. Since sodium absorption is linked to glucose, oral replacement solution must contain glucose. Oral therapy alone can be used to treat milder cases. *(Joklik et al, p 570)*

460. (D) In diarrheal infections, enterotoxins exert their essential pathogenic process by invasion of the mucosal epithelium, formation of microabscesses, and necrosis in the wall of the large intestine. All shigellae release their toxic somatic antigen (endotoxin). This endotoxin probably contributes to the irritation of the bowel wall. In *Shigella sonnei*, no enterotoxins are principally responsible for diarrhea. Several different enterotoxins are known for pathogenic strains of *Escherichia coli*. *Bacillus cereus* and *Staphylococcus aureus* exotoxin are responsible for the diarrhea due to food poisoning caused by these bacteria. Cytotoxin elaborated by *Clostridium difficile* is responsible for diarrhea associated with pseudomembranous colitis (antibiotic associated). *(Joklik et al, p 541)*

461. (C) The V and W antigens, which are always produced together, consist of a protein–lipoprotein complex that enables *Yersinia pestis* to resist phagocytosis. These antigens are considered the main virulence factors of

Y. pestis because antibodies to the V and W antigens confer immunity against plague. The V and W antigens correlate with pathogenicity and with rapid and overwhelming septicemia. *(Joklik et al, pp 584–586)*

462. **(A)** *Yersinia pestis* is a gram-negative nonmotile coccobacillus. When stained with Wayson stain, it shows marked bipolar staining, which is characteristic of this microorganism. *(Joklik et al, p 585)*

463. **(D)** The etiologic agents of relapsing fever, leptospirosis, brucellosis, and Lyme disease do not produce the F-1 antigens that possess antiphagocytic properties. *Yersinia pestis*, the causative agent of plague, elaborates F-1 antigens, which are thought to induce the production of protective antibodies against plague. *(Joklik et al, p 586)*

464. **(C)** *Yersinia enterocolitica* is the cause of human gastroenteritis and is transmitted by direct contamination of food or water by infected animals. *Y. enterocolitica* is not closely related antigenically to other species of *Yersinia*. However, the vast majority of the *Brucella* species cross-react with antisera raised against *Y. enterocolitica*. Most strains of *Y. enterocolitica* are sensitive to aminoglycosides. *(Joklik et al, pp 590–593)*

465. **(B)** Surgical therapy in the treatment of infections caused by gram-negative rods is extremely important. Because of a marked tendency to abscess formation, so characteristic of anaerobic infections, repeated drainage procedures precede antibiotic administration. Therapy with chemotherapeutic agents is not usually withheld until the causative agent has been identified, because of the technical difficulties of obtaining clinically useful specimens and the subsequent identification of the causative agent. Penicillin G is a drug of choice for most anaerobic infections caused by penicillin-susceptible organisms, although the *Bacteroides fragilis* group is most often resistant. Clindamycin is active against many anaerobic gram-negative bacilli, but it has been associated with overgrowth of *Clostridium difficile* and the subsequent development

of *C. difficile*-related enteric colitis. Since most gram-negative anaerobic bacteria are susceptible to penicillin G and clindamycin, therapeutic decisions are made before the results of antibiotic susceptibility tests are known. *(Joklik et al, pp 643–645)*

466. **(A)** Information on the mechanisms of pathogenicity of gram-negative anaerobic bacteria is limited. The production of collagenase may play a role in the spreading of organisms in tissues, and the secretion of slime may slightly hinder phagocytosis of these organisms. However, antibodies to these substances have not been conclusively shown to be protective. The single most important factor for the establishment and therefore the pathogenicity of gram-negative anaerobic bacteria is a reduced environment. *Bacteroides fragilis* has been shown to contain a low level of superoxide dismutase. However, it can only survive for a limited period of time in the presence of oxygen. *(Joklik et al, p 631)*

467. **(D)** *Bacteroides fragilis* and other species belonging to this genus are normal inhabitants of the intestinal, genital, and respiratory tracts. *Bacteroides* constitutes more than 95% of the normal fecal flora. The most commonly encountered species is *B. fragilis*, which is found particularly in the lower intestine. *Bacteroides melaninogenicus* and *Bacteroides oralis* are encountered particularly in the oropharynx. *(Joklik et al, pp 631–632)*

468. **(B)** Mycoplasmas are completely resistant to penicillin. They lack cell walls in all stages of their growth. They reproduce by binary fission. In contrast to the L forms, they do not require high salt concentrations to maintain their cellular integrity. On solid nutrient media containing serum, the center of their colonies is embedded beneath the surface of the agar, giving the appearance of a fried egg. *(Joklik et al, pp 730–732)*

469. **(D)** *Mycoplasma pneumoniae* requires sterols for growth, usually in the form of cholesterol that is incorporated into the cell membrane. Similarly, and in harmony with other species of the genus, *Mycoplasma* contains both RNA

and DNA, is completely resistant to penicillin, and lacks muramic acid because it does not possess a cell wall. *M. pneumoniae* is the causative agent of primary atypical pneumonia, which was initially described by Eaton, giving rise to the eponym Eaton agent. *(Joklik et al, pp 733–735)*

470. (A) L forms are wall-deficient bacterial variants that may occur spontaneously in a bacterial culture, or may be induced by penicillin, ultraviolet light, various salts, and other compounds. L forms can revert to the stable bacterial parental types and can produce the characteristic toxins of their parental types. In contrast to mycoplasmas, L forms do not contain sterols in their membranes. Some bacterial species produce L forms spontaneously. *(Jawetz et al, pp 22–23)*

471. (C) Amphotericin B is an antifungal agent that binds to membrane sterols and thus causes membrane damage. L forms do not contain sterols in their membrane and thus are not influenced by amphotericin B. L forms possess defective cell walls, produce the characteristic hemolysins or toxins of their parental types, require a high concentration of salt in the medium to maintain cellular integrity, and form "fried egg" colonies on suitable solid culture media. *(Joklik et al, p 1075)*

472. (A) *Leptospira interrogans* serogroup *icterohaemorrhagiae* is a tightly coiled, thin spirochete 5 to 15 mm long with very fine spirals. The ends of the organism tend to form a hook. *Borrelia recurrentis* is a spirochete with large spirals. *Treponema pallidum* has rigid spirals with acute turns and pointed ends. *Vibrio cholerae* and *Spirillum minus* are curved rods. These microorganisms are the causative agents of leptospirosis, relapsing fever, syphilis, cholera, and rat-bite fever, respectively. *(Joklik et al, pp 671–673)*

473. (D) *Campylobacter fetus* subspecies *jejuni* is one of the most common causes of bacterial diarrhea in the world. Human transmission occurs by the consumption of contaminated poultry, water, raw milk, and contact with

infected cats, dogs, sheep, or goats. Antibodies to *C. fetus* subspecies *jejuni* can be shown in patients infected with this microorganism by use of an indirect hemagglutination test. The organism is a gram-negative, microaerophilic, comma-shaped motile rod, having a unipolar or bipolar flagellum. Most strains of this microorganism are susceptible to erythromycin, which is administered when antibiotic therapy is required. This organism causes as much enteric disease in humans as do *Salmonella* and *Shigella*. *(Joklik et al, pp 666, 677–679)*

474. (C) Relapsing fever in humans occurs in two forms, the epidemic type, which is transmitted by the body louse, and the endemic type, which is tickborne. Leptospirosis is usually transmitted by rat urine that contains *Leptospira interrogans* serogroup *icterohaemorrhagiae*. Pinta and bejel are diseases that resemble syphilis but are contracted nonvenereally, usually via contact with lesions. The many microorganisms that can cause meningitis are usually introduced into the human body via the respiratory, gastrointestinal, and genitourinary tract. The body louse is not considered the chief vector in the epidemiology of meningitis. *(Joklik et al, pp 668–670)*

475. (E) The diagnosis of diarrhea caused by *Campylobacter fetus* subspecies *jejuni* can be made by inoculating fecal specimens in artificial selective media upon which this microorganism can grow when the media are incubated at 42°C for 48 hours in an atmosphere of 5% oxygen and 10% carbon dioxide. *Rickettsia rickettsii*, *Chlamydia trachomatis*, *Mycobacterium leprae*, and *Treponema pallidum* are all obligate intracellular parasites and cannot be cultivated on artificial media. They require living cells for growth. *(Joklik et al, p 677)*

476. (C) The primary virulence determinant of *Hemophilus influenzae* is a ribose- and ribitolphosphate-containing capsule that is antiphagocytic. Significant data supporting this contention are as follows: (1) the pronounced vulnerability of patients with immunodeficiencies and reversal of the condition with the administration of anticapsular antibody; (2) convalescent immune responses that tend to be correlated quantitatively with capsular antibody levels; and (3) the quantitative association of the protective activity of antiserum with anticapsular antibody and its specific absorption with purified anticapsular polysaccharide. *(Jawetz et al, pp 237–239; Joklik et al, pp 461–466)*

477. (A) *Hemophilus ducreyi* is a gram-negative rod that is transmitted sexually and is the cause of chancroid, or soft chancre. In contrast to the hard chancre produced by *Treponema pallidum*, the lesion induced by *H. ducreyi* on the genitalia consists of a ragged ulcer with marked swelling and tenderness. Furthermore, the regional lymph nodes are enlarged and painful. *H. ducreyi* does not possess axial filaments, periplasts, or large amounts of mucopolysaccharidase. These are characteristics of *T. pallidum*. *(Joklik et al, p 463)*

478. (C) Meningitis is the most serious infection that is caused usually by encapsulated *Hemophilus influenzae* type b (Hib) organisms. Meningitis due to Hib occurs rarely in infants under the age of 3 months and is uncommon in children over the age of 6 years. It has been estimated that encapsulated Hib causes over 95% of invasive disease such as meningitis. *(Joklik et al, pp 465–466)*

479. (C) Suitable specimens for the diagnosis of pertussis are either nasopharyngeal swabs, or Bordet–Gengou cough plates. The isolation rate of *Bordetella pertussis* from the respiratory tract is greatest during the catarrhal state of pertussis. Throat swabs during the convalescent phase of the disease are not appropriate because the organisms are not usually detectable during the convalescent phase of the disease. Similarly, blood cultures or skin specimens are not useful because *B. pertussis* does not invade the blood stream or cause skin abscesses. *(Joklik et al, pp 473,478–479)*

480. (D) Humans are the only known source of *Bordetella pertussis*. Phase I, but not phase IV, has fimbriae closely linked with the adherence of *B. pertussis* to the cilia of respiratory tract epithelial cells. When this attachment is

prevented, infection does not occur. Therefore, the fimbriae along with such factors as the heat-labile toxin, the lipopolysaccharide, the histamine-sensitizing factor, the lymphocytosis-promoting factor, the mouse-protective factor, the hemaglutinins, the K antigens, and possibly the islet-activating protein are closely associated in infection, pathogenesis, and immunity. *(Joklik et al, pp 478–479)*

481. (B) Although *Chlamydia* have a rigid spore-like shape, they do not possess muramic acid, a major component in the peptidoglycan cell wall, which most bacteria have. The cell shape is maintained by disulfide bonds in proteins. *(Jawetz et al, p 719)*

482. (C) Chlamydiae are not transmitted by insect vectors, as most rickettsiae are, and there are three species. *(Joklik et al, pp 701,720–722)*

483. (E) *Chlamydia psittaci* causes ornithosis, a pneumonitis contracted from birds. *Chlamydia trachomatis* infections cause nongonococcal urethritis (NGU) and a number of other diseases, including trachoma, inclusion conjunctivitis, and lymphogranuloma venereum. *C. trachomatis* is isolated from about 40% of NGU cases, and *Ureaplasma urealyticum* accounts for many of the remaining NGU cases. *(Joklik et al, pp 725,727,736)*

484. (C) Although the primary culture of *Listeria monocytogenes* from feces is difficult on ordinary bacteriologic media, its culture can definitely be enhanced using a buffered cell enrichment technique. It is not necessary to culture *Listeria* in any animal cell culture. *(Joklik et al, pp 481–482)*

485. (B) *Brucella suis* infects pigs and humans, not goats. *Brucella melitensis* infects goats and humans, and *B. abortus* infects dairy cattle and humans. The growth-enhancing properties of the four-carbon sugar alcohol erythritol, which is abundant in the placenta of dairy cattle but not in human placenta, contributes to the growth of virulent brucellae, often causing abortion. *(Joklik et al, pp 609–611)*

486. (C) It requires 4 to 8 weeks, not the normal 7 to 10 days, for the demonstration of significant rise in *Legionella* antibody titer. This delayed antibody response must be considered when attempting to diagnose or confirm *Legionella* infections using the rise in specific antibody levels in the patient's serum. (*Jawetz et al, pp 263–265; Joklik et al, p 696*)

487. (B) There have been no reported instances of person-to-person spread with *Legionella*. Therefore, patients need not be quarantined. *Legionella* is primarily a water-borne organism, spread by aerosols from contaminated water in showers, air conditioning cooling towers, and so on. (*Jawetz et al, p 264*)

488. (B) Intravenous erythromycin is the antibiotic of choice for legionellosis treatment. The newest approved test for rapid diagnosis is a specific monoclonal antibody for all *Legionella* species. This test does not depend on a specific antibody increase in the host, which often takes many weeks, but uses monoclonal antibodies to fix to the legionellae in the serum. Patients with legionellosis need not be kept in isolation since they cannot infect others. (*Jawetz, p 265; Joklik et al, pp 160,695–696*)

489. (D) *Rochalimaea quintana*, the causative agent of trench fever (shinbone fever), is distinct among rickettsiae in that it can be grown in vitro on cell-free media such as blood agar. It was first recognized in World War I by pains in the shins among trench soldiers. The other rickettsiae require living cells for propagation because they are obligate intracellular parasites. The tribe Rickettsiae contains three genera that infect humans: *Rickettsia*, *Rochalimaea*, and *Coxiella*. (*Jawetz et al, pp 294–298; Joklik et al, pp 701–708*)

490. (C) Microorganisms belonging to the genus *Rickettsia* utilize glutamate as their major carbon and energy source. On the other hand, for members of the genus *Coxiella*, pyruvate is the major source of energy. *Rickettsia* do not retain high levels of coenzyme A, nicotinamide–adenine dinucleotide, or adenosine triphosphate in their cytoplasm, which may

explain their obligate intracellular parasitism. (*Joklik et al, pp 701–707*)

491. (B) The vectors of rickettsiae are such arthropods as lice, fleas, ticks, or mites. Mosquitoes have not as yet been shown to serve as vectors for rickettsiae. (*Jawetz et al, p 295; Joklik et al, pp 702–705*)

492. (E) *Coxiella burnetii*, in contrast to other arthropod-borne rickettsial disease, can readily be transmitted to humans by contaminated aerosols or by ingestion of contaminated dairy products. Cattle, sheep, and goats have inapparent infections and may shed large quantities of *C. burnetii* in their urine, milk, feces, and especially their placental tissues. Therefore, dust may become contaminated and can serve as source of infections to humans. (*Joklik et al, p 713*)

493. (D) *Coxiella burnetii* can survive pasteurization at 60°C for 30 minutes and can survive for months in dried feces or milk. Q fever caused by *C. burnetii* resembles influenza, nonbacterial pneumonia, gastroenteritis, cardiovascular liver disease, or neurologic disease. There is neither rash nor a local lesion. There is immunologic evidence that placental transfer of *C. burnetii* may result in human fetal infection. The lack of serologic cross-reactions and cross-immunity to other rickettsial diseases places *C. burnetii* into a separate genus. (*Joklik et al, pp 713–714*)

494. (A) Trench fever is caused by *Rochalimaea quintana* and is transmitted to humans by the body louse. *R. quintana* is the only rickettsia that can be cultivated in artificial media such as blood agar. This organism is resistant to penicillin but may be susceptible to tetracycline or chloramphenicol. There are no vaccines available to prevent trench fever. Prevention and the control of trench fever rests on delousing and other sanitary measures. The diagnosis of trench fever is made by indirect immunofluorescence, complement fixation, and passive hemagglutination test. Xenodiagnosis (the feeding of uninfected lice on infected patients and the later demonstration of *R. quintana* in the tissues of lice) may also be used for the diagnosis of trench fever. (*Joklik et al, p 705*)

495. **(C)** Brill–Zinsser disease is a recrudescence, years or decades later, of an old epidemic typhus infection caused by *Rickettsia prowazekii*, which is usually susceptible to tetracycline and chloramphenicol. *R. prowazekii* is transmitted by the body louse (*Pediculus corporis*). Weil–Felix agglutinins often do not develop in patients with Brill–Zinsser disease. (*Jawetz et al, pp 296–297; Joklik et al, pp 705,710*)

496. **(D)** The Weil–Felix reaction was previously commonly used for the diagnosis of rickettsial diseases because of the presence of a common antigen on certain rickettsiae and some strains of *Proteus*. However, it lacks specificity and is no longer recommended as a diagnostic tool. For example, convalescent sera from many scrub typhus patients react most strongly with the *Proteus* strain OX-K. Scrub typhus is caused by *Rickettsia tsutsugamushi* and is transmitted by mites. There is no persisting immunity, and as with many other rickettsial diseases, it has been associated with skin rashes as well as eschars at the site of the bite of the mite. (*Joklik et al, pp 704,707*)

497 **(D)** Nocardiae are opportunistic microorganisms that cause infections in patients who received corticosteroids or other immunosuppressive therapy. *Nocardia asteroides* is a gram-positive, branching, acid-fast microorganism. The acid-fast reaction of *N. asteroides* is not as intense as that for mycobacteria; however, this microorganism is usually described as acid-fast. The sulfonamides remain the treatment of choice for nocardiosis. *N. asteroides* is widely distributed in nature and tends to enter the human body via inhalation. (*Joklik et al, pp 531–533*)

498. **(C)** *Actinomyces israelii* causes chronic, suppurative, slowly advancing granulomatous lesions in immunologically compromised hosts. Most of the infections caused by *A. israelii* are cervicofacial in nature. The lower jaw region is usually involved. From the lower jaw the infection may extend to other parts of the body to produce thoracic, abdominal, or genital actinomycosis. *A. israelii* causes disease in humans characterized by the presence of sulfur granules in the lesions. These granules represent yellow colonies of *A. israelii*. (*Joklik et al, pp 530–531*)

499. **(C)** One of the unique features of the pathology of *Actinomyces israelii* is the formation of draining sinuses within the granulomatous lesions. In contrast to nocardiosis, for which the source of infection is exogenous, in actinomycosis caused by *A. israelii*, the source of infection is endogenous. That is, this microorganism constitutes part of the normal flora of the tonsils, gums, and teeth. *A. israelii* is an anaerobic bacterium, which does not produce any well-defined virulence factors, and which does not induce effective immunity in patients who succumb to actinomycosis. (*Joklik et al, pp 528–530*)

500. **(B)** The normal flora of the pharynx includes a number of gram-positive cocci, such as viridans and other streptococci and *Staphylococcus epidermidis*. Therefore, the beta-hemolytic *Streptococcus pyogenes* (group A) could not be identified by the Gram stain alone. In the other instances listed in the question, useful information could be ascertained by Gram stain. (*Jawetz et al, p 602; Joklik, pp 401,418*)

501. **(B)** Microscopic examination of Gram-stained expectorated sputum is more useful than culture in establishing the rapid diagnosis of pneumococcal pneumonia. The cellular content of the smear should be examined first, since specimens that contain numerous squamous epithelial cells are more representative of "spit" than of the lower respiratory tract flora. The finding of typical lancet-shaped gram-positive diplococci in association with macrophages of polymorphonuclear neutrophils (PMNs) (and in the absence of other bacteria) strongly supports the diagnosis. As a generalization, in a good sample there should be more than 20 PMNs and fewer than 10 squamous cells per low-power microscopic field. (*Jawetz et al, pp 588–589*)

502. **(B)** *Salmonella* and *Shigella* are not able to ferment lactose. *(Joklik et al, pp 544–545)*

503. **(D)** There are a number of available test kits with specific antibody able to agglutinate specifically with each of the potential organisms commonly causing bacterial meningitis. Cerebrospinal fluid bacterial antigen can be detected before antibody. *(Joklik et al, pp 447–450)*

504. **(E)** A four-fold rise, versus the acute phase specific antibody titer, is the minimal standard of a significant reaction. Since twofold dilutions are used, that would mean a minimum of a two-tube change, or four-fold increase. A one-tube difference (two-fold change) is within the normal error of the system. *(Jawetz et al, pp 587–606)*

505. **(D)** *Vibrio vulnificus*, like other vibrios, are curved aerobic gram-negative rods that are motile and possess a polar flagellum. All of the other bacteria are not successfully Gram stained by ordinary techniques. *(Gilligan et al, p 132; Jawetz et al, pp 230,588–589; Joklik et al, pp 566,665)*

506. **(C)** Actinomycosis is characterized by pyogenic infections with interconnecting sinus tracts that contain granules. The gram-positive actinomycete infection is caused by any of several closely related actinomycetes species, which are part of the normal oral and gastrointestinal flora. They are anaerobic, gram-positive rods. All of the others are aerobic gram-positive rods. *(Gilligan et al, pp 131–132; Joklik et al, pp 395–398,531)*

507. **(D)** The intestine is sterile at birth, but microbes are introduced within the first 24 hours with food. In breast-fed children, their intestine contains streptococci and lactobacilli. More than 90% of the fecal flora consists of *Bifidobacterium* and *Bacteroides*, both of which are obligate anaerobes. The stool of the breast-fed infant is soft and light yellow to brown. *Lactobacillus bifidis* is a prominent microbe in these stools, which may also contain enterococci, coliforms, and staphylococci. Artificially fed infants have hard, dark-brown,

and foul-smelling stool. Diet has a marked influence on the fecal flora. Bowels of newborns in intensive-care nurseries are generally colonized heavily by Enterobacteriaceae such as *Klebsiella, Enterobacter*, and *Citrobacter*. *(Jawetz et al, pp 291–292; Joklik et al, p 397)*

508. **(A)** In spite of the stomach's acidity, there is a minimum of 103 to 105 per gram of stomach contents that is definitely not germ-free. The normal acid pH markedly protects against infection with some enteric pathogens, such as cholera. In the normal adult colon, about 96 to 99% of the resident flora consists of anaerobes, and *Bacteroides fragilis* is the major microbe, far outnumbering *Escherichia coli*. Only 1 to 4% of the bacteria are facultative aerobes. Vitamin K in humans is mainly supplied as an important by-product of biosynthesis by intestinal bacteria. That is why physicians must be careful in supplying vitamin K to patients when they have eliminated a large percentage of their normal gut bacteria by oral antibiotics. *(Jawetz et al, pp 291–293)*

509. **(C)** *Moraxella catarrhalis* is an uncommon gram-negative bacteria, which is aerobic, nonmotile, nonfermentative and oxidase-positive. On staining, they appear as small gram-negative bacilli, coccobacilli, or cocci. They are members of the normal human flora of the upper respiratory tract and occasionally cause infections. They are uniformly susceptible to penicillin. All of the other bacteria are anaerobes. *(Gilligan et al, pp 131–132; Jawetz et al, pp 228,590–593; Joklik et al, p 444)*

510. **(B)** The actinomycetes, including *Actinomyces israelii*, are filamentous bacteria related to corynebacteria and mycobacteria. They characteristically grow as gram-positive, branching organisms. All the others have special nutritional requirements, ie, they are fastidious. *(Gilligan et al, pp 131–132; Joklik et al, pp 463,526,530–531,676–677,695–696)*

511. **(E)** *Salmonella* (typhimurium) serotype *typhi* is the most common serotype isolated in the United States from human and animal sources, and it causes a great deal of gas-

troenteritis in humans. The majority of human cases are acquired by the ingestion of contaminated food and/or water. However, salmonellosis can be transmitted by such means as direct fecal–oral transmission or by contaminated instruments. Raw poultry products, and primarily eggs, are the most important sources of human infections. Meats and dairy products are also often implicated in epidemics. *(Gilligan et al, pp 54–55; Joklik et al, pp 562–563)*

512. **(B)** Lyme borreliosis (disease), although originally discovered in Lyme, Connecticut in 1975, is not limited to New England and the mid-Atlantic states. It is heaviest in the Northeast, upper Midwest (Minnesota and Wisconsin), and along the northern California coast, although it has been found in all but 5 of the 48 contiguous states. It can be cultured, but not easily. Infective arthritis of the knee, usually one of the two, is often a result of the borreliosis of Lyme disease. Late production of antibodies in quantity (more than 4 to 8 weeks after infection) complicates serodiagnosis of the disease. Tetracycline or phenoxymethyl penicillin is effective early in the disease. *(Gilligan et al, pp 120–121; Joklik et al, pp 670–671)*

513. **(B)** The vectors of rickettsiae are arthropods such as lice, fleas, ticks, or mites. Mosquitoes have not yet been shown to serve as vectors for rickettsiae. *(Joklik et al, pp 708–709)*

514. **(C)** Impetigo, a disease characterized by blister-like multifocal pustules on the face and hands in children and adults, can be caused by either *Staphylococcus aureus* and/or beta-hemolytic *Streptococcus pyogenes*, not by *S. aureus* only. Group A beta-hemolytic *S. pyogenes* has also recently been found to cause toxic shock-like syndrome (TSLS): Jim Henson, creator of the Muppets, died suddenly in May 1990, due to TSLS. *(Chapnick et al, pp 1074–1077; Joklik et al, pp 402–404,409,414,424)*

515. **(A)** Latent syphilis is defined as the absence of clinical lesions, a negative dark-field examination (no treponemes visible), a normal cerebrospinal fluid examination, and the presence of positive nontreponemal as well as treponemal serologic tests. *(Gilligan, pp 82–84; Joklik et al, pp 662–663)*

516. **(A)** *Chlamydia trachomatis* is the most common cause of nongonococcal arthritis. It is transmitted sexually and can be treated with tetracycline. *(Gilligan et al, pp 78–79; Joklik et al, pp 724–727)*

517. **(A)** Anaerobic pus often has a very foul smell. All of the other statements are true. *(Jawetz et al, p 604)*

518. **(A)** Almost all *Serratia* infections are associated with underlying disease, immunosuppressive therapy, or mechanical patient manipulations. Consequently, they have emerged as major entities in nosocomial infections, with 75 to 90% of *Serratia* infections being hospital acquired. *(Joklik et al, pp 550–551)*

519. **(D)** Ticks should be carefully removed but they should not be crushed between bare fingers since one may be infected with the *Borrelia burgdorferi* in the tick that way. At the least, a tissue, or better still, tweezers should be used to crush the tick (*Ixodes* spp). There presently is no vaccine available for Lyme borreliosis (disease). The tiny tick, which is the size of a poppy seed, can be discouraged from attaching to the skin by using insect repellent on the skin, and by using light-colored clothing over the arms and legs. Initial symptoms of the disease are flu-like chills, fever, headache, dizziness, fatigue, and/or stiff neck. Often a "bull's-eye" rash or migratory ring-like lesion (erythema chronicum migrans) appears days to weeks after a bite. *(Gilligan et al, pp 120–121; Joklik et al, pp 670–671)*

520. **(E)** *Erysipelothrix rhusiopathiae* is a nonsporogenous, nonmotile, and nonencapsulated gram-positive rod that causes erysipeloid in humans, mostly on their hands, in abattoir employees, butchers, and those handling fish, animal hides, and bones. These individuals are usually infected on the hands of those handling infected animals, fish, and so forth, and the erysipeloid is characterized by peripheral erythematous lesions on the

hand that runs a self-limiting course lasting about 3 weeks. *(Joklik et al, p 485)*

521. **(D)** *Mycobacterium kansasii* is a slowly growing photochromogen that stains unevenly with the acid-fast stain. It has a limited geographic distribution, and subclinical infections, as shown by positive skin tests, are more frequent in the Chicago, Louisiana, and Texas regions. All of the other statements are true. Acquired immunodeficiency syndrome patients are much more susceptible to *Mycobacterium avium* and *Mycobacterium intracellulare* infections. It is very difficult to separate *M. avium* and *M. intracellulare* infections, and they may be a group. *(Gilligan et al, pp 46–47; Joklik et al, pp 510–516)*

522. **(D)** In the United States, about 75% of cases are ulceroglandular and the rest are typhoidal in nature. Lymphadenopathy is often of a long duration. The ulceroglandular disease is usually acquired during the skinning of rabbits. At least 10 tick species can serve as arthropod vectors, but other bloodsucking vectors include deerflies, mites, blackflies, mosquitoes, and occasionally lice. *Streptomycin* is the recommended treatment for tularemia. *(Joklik et al, pp 595–598)*

523. **(E)** When the receptor-signal unit attaches to a G protein in a membrane, the G protein switches from a "resting state" to its active form. G proteins are known to be involved in the secretory pathways. A. G. Gilman's research clarified many of the actions of the G protein, which has many activities similar to a switchboard since it relays signals and often switches activities on and off. An activated G protein stimulates cellular activities for a few seconds or for a few minutes, like an internal timer. (Gilman's 1992 ICAAC award lecture in October will be published in *Microbiology Reviews*.) *(Joklik et al, p 865)*

524. **(D)** *Pasteurella* are small, nonmotile coccobacillary or rod-shaped, gram-negative bacteria that show bipolar staining, especially when prepared in infected animals. The tonsils of dogs are a site commonly colonized in male dogs. Many domestic cats are also colonized by *Pasteurella multocidans*, the microbe that most often infects humans. *P. multocidans* is also the species most often associated with human infections. *(Joklik et al, pp 600–601)*

525. **(C)** *Enterobacter* (formally called *Aerobacter*) infections are motile gram-negative organisms that are isolated in fairly large numbers in hospitals, although less frequently than *Escherichia coli* and *Klebsiella*. Older patients with complicating diseases are most often associated with *Enterobacter* urinary tract infections. *Enterobacter cloacae* causes the majority of infections, followed by *Enterobacter aerogenes* and *Enterobacter agglomerans*. All of the other microbial statements are true. *Actinobacillus* is part of the normal mouth flora and has been isolated in high numbers from plaque samples of patients with juvenile periodontitis. *(Joklik et al, pp 549–550,602,604,605)*

526. **(D)** Verotoxins (VTEC) are cytotoxins that are shiga-like toxins produced by *Escherichia coli*. They are called verotoxins because these toxins are assayed in vero tissue culture cells, a cell line developed from monkey kidney cells, and VTEC produce an irreversible effect on these cells. VTEC have been associated with three human syndromes: diarrhea, hemorrhagic volitis, and hemolytic uremic syndrome. The majority of VTEC isolates have been isolated from outbreaks in the United States and in Canada, not Africa. *(Joklik et al, pp 546–547)*

527. **(B)** Both the *Treponema pallidum* immobilization (TPI) and the fluorescent *Treponema* antibody absorption tests are employed as confirmative tests for syphilis. The first specific test for treponemal antibody was the TPI test. Live *T. pallidum* (Nichol's strain) extracted from infected rabbit testes is exposed to the patient's serum and to nonsyphilitic control serum. Diminution in motility of *T. pallidum* exposed to the patient's serum as compared with the control serum is a positive reaction. This test is very expensive, technically difficult, and performed in few research laboratories. *(Joklik et al, p 664)*

528. (D) Both the Mantoux and the multiple puncture test require purified protein derivative (PPD). The Mantoux test is performed by the intracutaneous injection of 0.1 mL of PPD containing 5 tuberculin units. In the multiple puncture test, PPD is introduced into the skin with an applicator containing points coated with dried PPD. Group A vaccine offers successful protection against group A meningitis for patients of all ages. The absence of household or other contact cases indicates that infections caused by *Mycobacterium kansasii* and *Mycobacterium intracellulare* are not transmitted directly from patients to healthy contacts. Both *M. kansasii* and *M. intracellulare* are relatively resistant to the routine levels of chemotherapeutic agents such as streptomycin (1 mg/mL), isoniazid (1 mg/mL), and para-aminosalicylic acid (10 mg/mL) that are effective against *Mycobacterium tuberculosis*. Individuals infected with human immunodeficiency virus are more susceptible to tuberculosis than are others. (*Joklik et al, pp 448, 507,512*)

529. (C) The pneumonia associated with Legionnaire's disease and the much milder Pontiac fever both are caused by *Legionella pneumophila*. Pontiac fever has relatively mild symptoms, similar to a mild flu but lasting 1 to 2 days. The chief symptoms are fever, myalgia, and headache. The organism is difficult to stain with the usual bacterial stains, is not acid-fast, and does not stain with hematoxylin and eosin. It can be visualized in tissue by Dieterle's silver impregnation stain and direct fluorescent antibody methods. Serologic diagnosis still plays an important role in the diagnosis of Legionnaire's disease in a number of hospitals. The problem is that seroconversion after a *Legionella* infection may take 6 to 8 weeks and antibody never develops in about 25% of patients with culture-documented legionellosis. (*Joklik et al, pp 694–696,1175*)

530. (E) There is no commonly accepted method available for preventing *Mycoplasma pneumoniae* infections other than avoiding close contact with ill patients. Formalin-inactivated vaccines have been tested, but results have been disappointing. There are no diagnostic serologic tests available to detect *M. pneumoniae* during the acute phase of the illness. Cold agglutinins, which are nonspecific antibodies that agglutinate red blood cells in the cold, appear in the convalescent serum of infected humans. (*Joklik et al, pp 733–736*)

531. (A) *Klebsiella pneumoniae* (but not *Proteus vulgaris*) produces a large, well-defined capsule composed of immunologically distinct polysaccharides. Differences in capsular types are detected by the quellung reaction (or Neufeld's reaction), but it is not used to identify *Proteus vulgaris*. In this reaction, *K. pneumoniae* cells are incubated with specific antibody against the capsular polysaccharide, causing the capsule to appear to swell and enlarge markedly. All species of *Proteus* (*Proteus vulgaris* and *Proteus mirabilis* most often isolated) produce a strong urease that hydrolyzes urea to ammonia and carbon dioxide, causing the urine to become alkaline. (*Jawetz et al, pp 208,214; Joklik et al, pp 551–552*)

532. (B) In cases of typhoid fever, chloramphenicol or ampicillin is the drug of choice. Resistance of *Salmonella typhi* to ampicillin and chloramphenicol has been encountered in only a small number of strains. Administration of antibiotics for uncomplicated gastroenteritis kills the normal flora and serves to prolong the carrier stage; thus, no antibiotic is used for uncomplicated cases. *Salmonella enteritidis* is the causative agent of gastroenteritis, whereas *Salmonella typhi* is the etiologic agent of typhoid fever. Species of *Salmonella* and of *Shigella* are unable to utilize lactose. (*Jawetz et al, pp 212–214*)

533. (A) Both Lyme disease and endemic relapsing fever are tick-borne diseases, not mosquito-borne diseases. In the United States, relapsing fever is the disease limited to individuals who have come into contact with infected ticks by vacationing in a tick-infested summer cottage. Lyme disease begins with a red area of the skin that enlarges slowly around a darker central portion where the bite occurred. This phase is accompanied by fever, headache, pain in the joints, and long-term heart problems, as well as arthritis. *Borrelia burgdorferi* causes tick-borne Lyme disease. Lyme disease is named for an eastern Connecticut town where an epidemic occurred in 1975. Tick-borne or endemic relapsing fever is caused by several species of *Borrelia*. Epidemic relapsing fever occurs in all parts of the world and is transmitted from one individual to another by the body louse. Therefore, control of the disease can be obtained by sanitary measures directed toward the eradication of lice. This is usually accomplished by delousing, as well as good personal and public standards of hygiene. (*Joklik et al, pp 668–671*)

534. **(C)** Drink pasteurized milk or cheeses made from pasteurized milk only, eg, goat cheese in some countries from uninspected animals can cause brucellosis. Be wary of eating pork, and, if you do, be sure that it is adequately cooked. Animals should be inspected by a veterinarian. There is a vaccine available for animals prepared from a virulent live *Brucella* strain 19. The successful eradication program of bovine brucellosis in the United States has markedly reduced the incidence of human brucellosis to farmers, slaughterhouse workers, and veterinarians. In other parts of the world, however, animal and human brucellosis is still widespread. (*Joklik et al, pp 611–612*)

535. **(A)** The species belonging to the genus *Actinomyces* are anaerobic or microaerophilic, whereas *Nocardia* species are aerobic. Thioglycollate is a liquid culture medium employed for the propagation of anaerobic or microaerophilic microorganisms. The microorganisms that belong to genera *Actinomyces* and *Nocardia* are prokaryotic. Therefore, according to the definition and their actual cell wall analysis, they contain peptidoglycan in their cell walls. (*Joklik et al, pp 526–527*)

536. **(D)** The gram-positive and gram-negative envelopes both contain transport proteins that mediate the passage of a limited number of solutes. The study of bacterial transporters, since their amino acid sequences are known, are strongly similar to the transporters of higher animal cells. (*Nikaido and Saier, pp 936–942*).

537. **(E)** A wide variety of clinical syndromes is caused by *Listeria monocytogenes*, ranging from a mild influenza-like illness to a fulminant neonatal listeriosis associated with mortality rates of 54 to 90%. Relatively few cases have been reported in patients with human immunodeficiency virus or acquired immunodeficiency syndrome. Listeriolysin O plays an important role in the infectious process. It is a soluble product (a hemolysin). (*Joklik et al, pp 481–484*)

538. **(E)** The short-term syndrome is frequently mistaken for staphylococcal food poisoning, because that also has about a 4-hour incubation after ingestion, and because nausea and vomiting are common to both. Fried rice is a fairly common food item causing this problem. After preparing the rice, it is usually allowed to sit at room temperature overnight until it is heated, relatively lightly, for fried rice. If the *Bacillus cereus* spores survived and the rice was not heated to a hot enough temperature for fried rice preparation, it can cause this form of *B. cereus* food poisoning. Antibiotics are not used. (*Joklik et al, pp 618–619*)

539. **(C)** In this situation, one only has to remember the coagulase-positive *Staphylococcus aureus* since all other staphylococcal species are coagulase-negative. (*Joklik et al, pp 403–404*)

540. **(D)** *Eubacterium* is an anaerobic gram-positive bacillus that is part of the normal flora of the gastrointestinal tract. All of the others listed, *Klebsiella, Citrobacter, Enterobacter*, and *Escherichia* are all genera of opportunistic Enterobacteriaceae. (*Joklik et al, pp 544,548–553,632*)

541. **(C)** Human skin responds to the pharyngitis caused by strains of group A *Streptococcus pyogenes* that elaborate the exotoxins called G streptococcal pyrogenic factors (types A, B, or C), also known as scarlet fever toxins or erythrogenic toxins. The toxins produced in the pharynx are spread via the blood and cause the red scarlet fever rash. The toxins

act in small blood vessels, causing extreme dilation and leakage. There are three serologic types of erythrogenic toxins, depending on with which temperate phage the *S. pyogenes* strain is infected. If the strain is "cured" of the phage (ie, it no longer carries the phage), it can no longer produce that toxin. Antitoxin to the other erythrogenic toxins (eg, type A) prevents the rash due to infection by type A streptococcal pyrogenic exotoxin (SPE), but does not prevent the streptococcal infection. Because there are three different types of SPE toxins, it is possible that a child might have more than one bout with scarlet fever. Scarlet fever, once a serious childhood disease, has decreased in severity during the past century with no apparent explanation. *(Gilligan et al, p 27; Joklik et al, p 422)*

542. **(E)** *Staphylococcus epidermidis* is a gram-positive bacterium that is coagulase-negative, does not contain protein A, does not contain endotoxin, ordinarily forms white colonies, and that humans ordinarily have on their skin. *(Joklik et al, pp 401–403)*

543. **(B)** Viridans streptococci are not bile soluble, as are pneumococci, and are resistant to penicillin. They are alpha-hemolytic. *(Joklik et al, pp 428–429)*

544. **(D)** Group B streptococci are associated with neonatal septicemia and meningitis. Approximately 20% of pregnant women are vaginal carriers of group B streptococci, and the organism is acquired from the mother by the neonate during vaginal delivery. None of the other diseases is associated with group B streptococci. *(Joklik et al, pp 426–427)*

545. **(C)** M proteins of *Streptococcus pyogenes* group A do produce protective antibodies, which allow the streptococci to be efficiently phagocytosed and killed. Otherwise they would be protected by the M protein. Group A streptococci do not have over 60 types of capsular polysaccharide. Many group A streptococci produce a hyaluronic acid capsule, although the antiphagocytic role of the capsule is of less importance than the M protein. All *S. pyogenes* group A strains causing a pharyngeal infection may yield sequelae that include rheumatic fever. *(Joklik et al, pp 420–422)*

546. **(D)** Virulent pneumococci are lancet-shaped diplococci and have colonies that produce alpha-hemolysis, and their growth is sensitive to optochin. However, they do not produce hyaluronic acid capsules, which many group A streptococcal pyogenes do. *(Joklik et al, pp 432,440–441)*

547. **(E)** Individuals who have undergone splenectomy, and those with sickle cell disease, nephrotic syndrome, chronic liver disease, malignancy, or primary immunodeficiency, are at increased risk of developing severe pneumococcal infections. Consequently, these individuals should be candidates for receiving the new 23-valent pneumococcal vaccine. This vaccine contains a mixture of capsular antigens of 23 of the most commonly occurring types, which account for 87% of bacteremic pneumococcal disease in the United States. Normal young adults are not at increased susceptibility to pneumococcal disease. *(Joklik et al, p 440)*

548. **(D)** *Neisseria* are gram-negative cocci, usually seen in pairs with adjacent flattened sides. All neisseriae are oxidase-positive, catalase-positive diplococci, but are not acid-fast. Humans are the only known reservoir for *Neisseria*. *(Joklik et al, pp 443–444)*

549. **(E)** Colonization by meningococci is only mediated in part by pili. It is not as closely related to virulence as are gonococcal colony types. With the gonococci, the two heavily piliated colony types are virulent for humans, whereas the three colony types that are not piliated (or only lightly) are avirulent. Household contacts of individuals with meningococcal disease are colonized to a greater extent than individuals in control households. Natural immunity to the meningococcus seems to be identified and broadened in individuals who have carried different strains of meningococci (and of other bacteria with cross-reacting antigens), at different intervals throughout life. Carriage of a meningococcus does not invariably lead to serious meningococcal infection, but it does have to be taken into consideration for treatment. *(Joklik et al, pp 447–448)*

550. (A) Capsular polysaccharide inhibits phagocytosis, pili aid in adhesion of the microbe, and the lipopolysaccharide that is attached to the outer membrane has typical endotoxic properties. Therefore, capsular polysaccharide serotype must be considered regarding virulence. Finally, all pathogenic *Neisseria* species have an IgA protease that is excreted extracellularly. It has been suggested that the destruction of IgA on mucosal surfaces contributes to meningococcal survival and virulence. There are nine serotypes that can cause meningitis, but types A, B, and C are most often involved in clinical disease. *(Joklik et al, p 447)*

551. (B) Bacillus Calmette–Guérin (BCG) vaccination involves the immunization of individuals with an attenuated strain of *Mycobacterium bovis* that has related antigenicity to *Mycobacterium tuberculosis* and that was obtained by Calmette and Guérin. An individual vaccinated with BCG will normally become tuberculin-positive. Thus, this very useful diagnostic tuberculin test can no longer be employed as evidence of recent infection in an individual, for the location of sources of infection, for the diagnosis of diseases with some clinical symptoms that are similar to tuberculosis, or as a screening device prior to x-ray examination for the diagnosis of tuberculosis. It does not, however, interfere with human immunodeficiency screening. *(Joklik et al, pp 429–434)*

552. (C) *Mycobacterium africanum* is the third mycobacterial species, in addition to *Mycobacterium tuberculosis* and *Mycobacterium bovis*, that can cause human tuberculosis. *M. africanum* has been isolated only in certain parts of Africa, but *M. bovis* remains a significant source of infection in many countries where raw milk is used. *(Joklik et al, p 510)*

553. (A) The production of diphtheria toxin by *Corynebacterium diphtheriae* is critically influenced by the concentration of iron in the environment, and it is the major pathogenic determinant. In the presence of iron, a repressor–iron complex forms that binds specifically at the phage beta-tox operator locus. The genetic information required for the synthesis of diphtheria toxin is carried in the genomes of beta phage as the gene tox. Integration of tox-containing prophages into the corynebacterial chromosome assures perpetuation of toxinogenic character. Diphtheria toxin consists of a single polypeptide chain cross-connected by two disulfide bridges with a reducing agent yielding two fragments: an N-terminal fragment A (molecular weight greater than 21,000) and a C-terminal fragment D (molecular weight 39,000). Mild treatment with formaldehyde converts the toxin into a nontoxic antigen which, when injected into animals, stimulates the production of antitoxin. *(Joklik et al, pp 487–488)*

554. (B) Anthrax is primarily a disease of domestic animals (sheep, cattle, and horses), but active immunization is the only known way of preventing anthrax infection in animals. The disease is transmitted to humans from infected animals or animal products. Spores of *Bacillus anthracis* are usually introduced into skin (neck, hand, and forearm), wounds, or pulmonary tissues. The characteristic lesions seen in cutaneous anthrax are caused by anthrax toxin and capsular materials consisting of polymers of D-glutamic acid. Skin lesions may change into necrotic ulcers from which the infection may disseminate, giving rise to septicemia, which is usually fatal. Primary pneumonia resulting from inhalation of spores from the dust of wool, hides, and hair ("wool sorter's disease") is often rapidly fatal. Sporulation usually does not take place in vivo. It occurs only after the infected animals succumb to the infection. *(Joklik et al, pp 615–618)*

555. (A) Since *Hemophilus influenzae* has an inability to synthesize hemin (factor X) and coenzyme I (factor V), these factors must be added to the growth media for their growth. *Bordetella pertussis* does not require addition of these growth factors. All of the other statements are true. *Legionella pneumophila* is associated with high fever and rigors, but brucellosis is not. *(Joklik et al, pp 462,473,612, 696–697,724–725)*

556. (B) *Staphylococcus aureus* can withstand drying well, making it a problem in hospitals if great care is not taken. It can grow both aerobically and anaerobically. All of the other statements are true (hand contamination from the nose, carriage much higher in needle-using individuals such as diabetics). The advantage of phage typing *S. aureus* is very useful to help find individuals contributing to a hospital staphylococcal outbreak. *(Gilligan et al, pp 18–19,248; Joklik et al, pp 395–396,401–402,404,409–410)*

557. (A) Diphtheria toxin is produced by toxigenic *Corynebacterium diphtheriae* strains not only in the infected host but also in proper media in vitro, so statement A is wrong. Being a soluble protein (two subunits, A and B, are known), diphtheria toxin is highly immunogenic. This immunogenicity is not lost when the toxin is converted to toxoid, which is used as a diphtheria vaccine. The toxin itself is too toxic to be used as vaccine. In the Schick test intradermal injection of a small dose of the toxin tests whether individuals have the specific antibody in their circulation. The presence of specific antibody (antitoxin) is the key element in the immunity to diphtheria. *(Joklik et al, pp 491–492; Gilligan et al, pp 33–35)*

558. (E) Humans breathing air are still susceptible to clostridial disease. For many clostridia, the most characteristic type of amino acid fermentation is the Stickland reaction, a coupled oxidation–reduction involving a pair of amino acids, one of which serves as the electron donor and the other as the electron acceptor. The growth, and in some cases the survival, of most clostridia, requires an anaerobic environment because they do not have, or have only a very low level of, enzymes that remove toxic metabolites of oxy-

gen. Superoxide dismutase and catalase are some of these enzymes required for destroying these toxic oxygen metabolites. *(Joklik et al, pp 636–640)*

559. (D) *Clostridium perfringens*, the causative agent for gas gangrene and some food poisoning, produces a number of extracellular enzymes that contribute to the pathogenicity of this anaerobe. No clostridia contain endotoxin because they are all gram-positive. *(Joklik et al, pp 639–642)*

560. (C) *Neisseria gonorrhoeae* is a gram-negative, oxidase-positive diplococcus. Some strains of gonococci produce penicillinase and thus do not respond to penicillin treatment. Gonorrhea cannot be readily diagnosed in females using Gram stains because normal gram-negative anaerobic diplococci (*Veillonella*) in the female genital tract can be confused with *N. gonorrhoeae*, which is not prevented by vaccination. *(Joklik et al, pp 455–456,622)*

561. (B) Pili (fimbriae) represent a type of adhesion agent that has been found in virulent strains of *Neisseria gonorrhoeae*. Piliated gonococci are considered pathogenic because they produce gonorrhea in volunteers. The lipopolysaccharide of *N. gonorrhoeae* is also considered a virulence factor of the gonococci, because it is thought to be responsible for some of the pathophysiologic effects observed in the disseminated gonococcal infections. The IgA protease and the outer-membrane components all contribute to its pathogenicity, but it has no axial filaments *(Jokliket al, p 453)*

562. (D) Sexually transmitted diseases are not controlled now by vaccination. It is now generally recognized that herpes simplex virus type II causes most of the genital lesions in women. It is also thought that most cases of nongonococcal urethritis are caused by *Chlamydia. Hemophilus ducreyi* is a gram-negative rod that is the causative agent of the venereally transmitted disease known as chancroid or soft chancre. In contrast to this microorganism, *Treponema pallidum* causes hard chancre. That is, the syphilitic lesions has a clean hard base due to polymerization of tissue polysaccharides and thus is called a hard chancre. *(Joklik et al, pp 469,660,726,956)*

563. **(E)** Gonorrhea is caused by a gram-negative, oxidase-positive diplococcus that may produce β-lactamase. The gonococci can infect the columnar epithelial cells of the genital tract, producing urethritis. The eyes of the newborn can also be infected by the gonococci as the infant passes through the birth canal of an infected mother. Gonorrhea is contagious. *(Joklik et al, pp 450–452)*

564. **(C)** *Neisseria gonorrhoeae* causes infections at such sites as the urethra, cervix, conjunctiva, anus, and other body locations, but not the appendix. Therefore, the proper diagnosis of gonorrhea may require pus and secretions taken from the urethra, cervix, prostate, rectal mucosa, throat, and occasional synovial fluid and blood in systemic illness. *(Joklik et al, pp 455–456)*

565. **(A)** The treponemas which cause pinta (*Treponema curateum*), bejel (*Treponema pallidum* variant strain), syphilis (*Treponema pallidum*), and yaws (*Treponema pertenue*) are serologically indistinguishable. Therefore, positive Venereal Disease Research Laboratories, rapid plasma reagin, and fluorescent treponemal antibody absorption tests will be obtained in all of the above-mentioned diseases, but not with diseases caused by viruses, fungi, and protozoa. *(Joklik et al, p 666)*

566. **(D)** Some of the distinctive properties of *Treponema pallidum* are the possession of fibrils, the inability to be grown in artificial culture media, the ability to survive for 1 to 4 days in blood stored at 4°C, and other special features. Although *Treponema pertenue* and some of the other treponemal diseases cross-react with *T. pallidum*, pinta (and the other diseases) are relatively rare in the United States. *(Joklik et al, pp 659–661)*

567. **(E)** The most widely used nontreponemal tests for syphilis are the card rapid plasma reagin (RPR) or the slide flocculation Venereal Disease Research Laboratory (VDRL)

tests. In these tests, the antigen employed is an alcoholic extract of beef heart containing cardiolipin (diphosphatidyl glycerol), which also happens to be a component of the cytoplasmic membrane of *Treponema pallidum* that causes syphilis. The VDRL and the RPR tests are employed to screen large groups of individuals. The VDRL titer reflects the activity of the disease. Such titers reach 1:32 or higher in secondary syphilis. A persistent fall in titer following penicillin or other antibiotic treatment indicates an adequate response to therapy. *(Joklik et al, pp 663–665)*

568. **(C)** Latent syphilis occurs in untreated syphilis after the healing of secondary lesions and before the beginning of the tertiary disease. The first 4 years of this period are considered early latent, and the subsequent period, up to 10 years after the primary, is the late latent. Latent syphilis develops into late or tertiary syphilis in about 30% of untreated people. The most severe aspects of late syphilis are neurosyphilis and cardiovascular syphilis. In the latent stage, the people are asymptomatic but still give evidence of the disease by the presence of specific *Treponema pallidum* antibodies. *(Gilligan et al, pp 82–84; Joklik et al, pp 661–662)*

569. **(E)** Prevention of salmonellosis demands that water sanitary standards be kept and that all food be properly cooked as well as refrigerated. The same surface should not be used to prepare raw chicken and salads. Detection and treatment of carriers particularly of *Salmonella typhi* constitutes a major control measure. *(Joklik et al, p 563)*

570. **(C)** Bacterial adherence to human uroepithelial cells is increased in *Escherichia coli*, the virulence of which can be correlated with the presence of pili on these surfaces, but not of flagella. Urease production by bacteria, such as *Proteus* spp. or *Klebsiella*, results in alkaline urine, which favors production of stones. Calculi produce obstruction and act as a locus of infection. The high pH and reduced osmolarity of the urine due to the destruction of urea also favors the increased growth of some bacteria. Beta-lactamase production

and the high content of peptidoglycan and quinones are unrelated to urinary tract infection virulence. *(Gilligan et al, pp 69–71; Jawetz et al, pp 592,680)*

571. **(B)** *Escherichia coli* is the most common cause of community-acquired urinary tract infections (UTIs), but in hospital-acquired UTIs or in individuals who have had repeated UTIs treated with antibiotics, *Proteus, Klebsiella, Pseudomonas,* and *Streptococcus faecalis* are frequently observed. Young, sexually active women frequently have UTIs with *Staphylococcus saprophyticus. Streptococcus pneumoniae* does not cause UTIs. *(Gilligan et al, pp 69–71)*

572. **(D)** Unless the urinary pH is alkaline, it is unrelated to urinary tract infections (UTIs). Alkaline urine indicates UTI with urease-producing bacteria, such as *Proteus* spp. or *Klebsiella.* All of the other statements are true. *(Gilligan et al, pp 69–71; Jawetz et al, pp 592,600)*

573. **(E)** Pus from a pseudomonal infection sometimes has a greenish cast. All of the other statements are true as written. Children's "sore throats" are due to bacterial infection only 15 to 20% of the time, and adults' sore throats are due to bacterial infections only 5 to 10% of the time. *(Jawetz et al, pp 588–589, 602,604)*

574. **(A)** Gram-negative bacterial (endotoxic) shock is seen frequently in patients with urinary tract infection, when trauma to the infected tissues causes a sudden burst of bacteremia. It is possible to detect endotoxin in the blood of patients suffering from such endotoxic shock. The fever induced by endotoxin is mediated by a protein released from neutrophils or monocytes that is designated endogenous pyrogen. Although there are some variations, the toxicity of endotoxins deriving from various gram-negative bacteria does not differ markedly. Endotoxin of gram-negative bacteria is lipopolysaccharide complex, not protein. *(Joklik et al, pp 86,391,547)*

575. **(D)** Endotoxin can activate the complement system via the alternative pathway. C3 can be activated by endotoxin in the absence

of preceding activation of C1,4,2. As a result, the various complement components (C3,5–9) are consumed and then their activity either disappears or is reduced from serum. Although most bacterial exotoxins are proteinaceous in nature, endotoxin is a lipopolysaccharide complex composed of lipid A, core polysaccharide, and "O" antigenic side chain (oligopolysaccharide side chain). *(Joklik et al, pp 288–291)*

576. **(D)** The microbe accounting for most urinary tract infections is *Escherichia coli.* Urine from normal people generally has less than 10 white blood cells (WBCs) per high-power field in the microscope. Pyuria (pus in the urine), more than 10 WBCs per high-power field in urine, and hematuria (presence of red blood cells in urine) are reasonably sensitive, although not specific indicators of urinary tract infection. Clean-catch urine is only rarely sterile; therefore, it should be analyzed quickly (within 1 hour). The lactose fermenters most often isolated from urine are the KEE organisms (*Klebsiella* spp., *E. coli,* and *Enterobacter* spp.). *E. coli* is recovered from about 70 to 80% of outpatients and 40 to 50% of inpatients with urinary tract infections. The results all agree with the *E. coli* probability except for the statement that it is an anaerobe. *(Gilligan et al, pp 70–72)*

577. **(C)** Impetigo, a disease characterized by blister-like multifocal pustules on the face and hands in children and adults, can be caused by either *Staphylococcus aureus* and/or beta-hemolytic *Streptococcus pyogenes,* not by *S. aureus* only. Group A beta-hemolytic *S. pyogenes* has also recently been found to cause toxic shock-like syndrome (TSLS), joining the previously known *S. aureus.* Jim Henson, creator of the Muppets, died suddenly in May 1990, due to TSLS. *(Joklik et al, pp 409,411,424)*

578. **(D)** Endotoxin activates C3 directly via the alternative pathway. C1q binding is the first step of the complement activation by the classical pathway. It requires the first step of the complement activation by the classical pathway, and it requires the presence of antibody (IgG or IgM). C1 esterase is not inhibited by endotoxin. Endotoxin is bound to the cell surface, not to the nucleus, since bacteria do not have nuclei. (*Joklik et al, pp 85–87*)

579. **(E)** Infections due to anaerobic gram-negative bacteria such as *Bacteroides fragilis* are invariably mixed infections (both anaerobe and aerobe are found in the wound). *Escherichia coli* is a microbe most frequently encountered in mixed infections. *B. fragilis* and *Bacteroides melaninogenicus* are the most frequently involved anaerobes found in this type of infection. Infections due to *B. fragilis* may be treated by clindamycin and metronidazole. Chemotherapy must also be directed to *E. coli* and other anaerobes that are involved in mixed infections. (*Joklik et al, pp 627–628*)

580. **(D)** *Campylobacter jejuni* infections are often associated with contact with farm and domestic animals. Water-borne outbreaks are reported. Person-to-person spreading may also occur. *Campylobacter* is not a common cause of diarrhea or food poisoning resulting from ingestion of raw seafood. (*Joklik et al, pp 676–678*)

581. **(D)** Cholera toxin causes an increase in adenyl-cyclase activity, thus increasing the level of intracellular cyclic adenosine monophosphate (cAMP). The increase in cAMP leads to the rapid secretion of electrolytes into the lumen of the small bowel. This increase is caused by increased sodium-dependent chloride secretion and prevention of sodium and chloride absorption across the brush border. Glucose-linked sodium absorption remains intact, and this system is vitally important in oral replacement of sodium. (*Joklik et al, pp 566–568*)

582. **(D)** Verotoxin is produced by enteropathogenic *Escherichia coli*. *E. coli* verotoxin is immunologically and biologically identical and genetically very similar to the shiga toxin of *Shigella dysenteriae* type 1. *E. coli* producing this toxin has been associated with food poisoning attributable to some fast-food chains in the United States and Canada. (*Joklik et al, pp 546–547*)

583. **(D)** There are four groups of *Escherichia coli* that are pathogenic to humans. The pathogenic mechanism of each group is different. Enterotoxigenic *E. coli* produces heat-labile and heat-stable enterotoxins. Enteroinvasive *E. coli* produces an invasive dysentery (*Shigella*-like). Enteropathogenic *E. coli* produces a cytotoxin (vero toxin), and enteroadherent *E. coli* has been observed to be tightly adherent to affected microvilli. (*Joklik et al, pp 546–547*)

584. **(D)** The normal pharyngeal flora may include viridans streptococci, neisseriae, diphtheroids, staphylococci, small gram-negative rods, and so on. Although a few colonies of beta-hemolytic group A streptococci may indicate they are only transients, moderate or large numbers of them indicate a "strep throat." (*Gilligan et al, pp 26–27; Jawetz et al, p 602*)

585. **(A)** Although diarrhea occurs in infections with all of the pathogens listed in the question, fecal leukocytes are observed in *Campylobacter* and *Shigella* infections. *Campylobacter jejuni* causes as much enteric disease in humans as do *Salmonella* and *Shigella*. (*Joklik et al, p 678*)

586. **(C)** Both cholera toxin and heat-labile toxin of *Escherichia coli* cause diarrhea by activating adenylate cyclase. *Clostridium difficile* toxin is a cytotoxin, and heat-stable enterotoxin of *E. coli* activates guanylate cyclase, not adenylate cyclase. (*Joklik et al, pp 546–547*)

587. **(D)** Enterotoxigenic *Escherichia coli* and *Vibrio cholerae* cause diarrhea by their enterotoxins, not by invasion of the intestinal mucosa. *Giardia lamblia* is a flagellated protozoan that attaches to the intestinal wall and causes irritation and diarrhea. *Shigella dysenteriae* invades the intestinal mucosa. (*Joklik et al, pp 546–548,550*)

588. **(C)** Gram-negative bacteria belonging to the genus *Rickettsia*, which are obligate intracellular parasites, utilize glutamate as their major carbon and energy source. *Rickettsia* do not retain high levels of coenzyme A, nico-

tinamide–adenine dinucleotide, or adenosine triphosphate in their cytoplasm, and this may explain their obligate intracellular parasitism. The tropism of rickettsiae for vascular endothelial cells and the symptoms of the disease are due in part to local damage to small blood vessels, local inflammation, and extravasation of blood (vasculitis). *(Joklik et al, pp 701–702)*

589. **(E)** *Francisella tularensis* can enter the human body through skin abrasions, tick bites, deer fly bites, or aerosol passage through the respiratory tract, but not through sexual contact. *(Joklik et al, p 595)*

590. **(A)** The usual reservoir of plague infection is various wild rodents (and their fleas), such as rats, squirrels, and guinea pigs. It produced pandemics of "black plague" with millions of fatalities. *(Jawetz et al, pp 245–246; Joklik et al, pp 586–587)*

591. **(E)** A skin test employing phenolized *Franciscella tularensis* cells produces a delayed reaction within 7 days of the disease in about 90% of persons with tularemia. The skin test is more sensitive than in most serologic tests, being reactive earlier and for a longer period of time. Tularemia can be treated with streptomycin or tetracycline. *(Joklik et al, p 595)*

592. **(C)** Anaerobic bacteria produce various gases, especially hydrogen sulfide, when they grow in tissues that then emit a foul odor. Therefore, physicians usually think of anaerobic infections whenever lesions with pus or exudates with foul odors are encountered and recommend anaerobic cultures. Anaerobic infections are caused by the gram-positive, spore-forming clostridia and gram-negative anaerobes belonging to genera *Bacteroides* and *Fusobacterium*. Anaerobic infections are usually of polymicrobial origin, involving not only the preceding genera but also Enterobacteriaceae, peptococci, peptostreptococci, or other cocci. Clinical samples should never be refrigerated and should be taken to the laboratory immediately. *(Jawetz et al, pp 257–261,604)*

593. **(D)** Lower respiratory tract infections caused by anaerobic bacteria pertain to aspiration pneumonitis and lung abscesses. Aspiration pneumonitis is a mixed infection involving *Peptococcus and* Peptostreptococcus species as the major anaerobes. The major anaerobic species isolated from lung abscesses are *Fusobacterium nucleatum, Bacteroides gingivalis, Bacteroides fragilis,* and species of *Peptococcus* and *Peptostreptococcus. Moraxella* spp. are gram-negative aerobic cocci. *(Gilligan et al, p 131; Joklik et al, p 604)*

594. **(D)** Many gram-negative, non–spore-forming, anaerobic species constitute part of the normal body flora. Under such predisposing conditions as dental surgery, neurosurgery, and gunshot and stab wounds, anaerobic gram-negative wound infection of endogenous origin can be produced. Since more than one particular species of normal flora are found in any given body surface, gram-negative anaerobic infections are polymicrobial. A reduced environment can be the single most important virulence factor for anaerobes. Therefore, gram-negative anaerobic wound infections are favored when the tissue Eh is reduced by trauma or by growth of aerobic bacteria. *(Joklik et al, pp 596–604)*

595. **(D)** Most gram-negative anaerobes associated with infections are also present on mucous membrane or other areas as part of the indigenous flora. Therefore, special collection procedures must be used to obtain reliable and useful clinical specimens. For urinary tract and pulmonary infections, bladder aspiration and transtracheal needle aspiration are recommended, respectively. *(Joklik et al, pp 625–627)*

596. **(E)** Anaerobic gram-negative bacteria may be beneficial to their hosts. For example, *Bacteroides fragilis* is involved in the synthesis of vitamin K and other gram-negative anaerobic bacteria are involved in dehydroxylation and conjugation of bile acids. Bile acids play essential roles in bile formation, fat absorption, and the metabolism of cholesterol. Similarly, the presence of the gram-negative anaerobic

bacteria hinders the establishment of such virulent bacteria as *Shigella*, *Salmonella*, or other pathogens by bacterial interference. (*Joklik et al, p 604*)

597. **(B)** Neonatal sepsis and meningitis is usually caused by group B streptococci (*Streptococcus agalactiae*). The organism infects the neonate from the mother's vaginal flora (about 20% of pregnant women carry group B streptococci) during vaginal delivery. (*Joklik et al, pp 424,426*)

598. **(E)** *Mycoplasma pneumoniae*, the causative agent of primary atypical pneumonia, which was first described by Eaton, is usually susceptible to tetracycline. A useful serologic test for the diagnosis of primary atypical pneumonia is the cold agglutinin test. The patient's serum, obtained during the acute and convalescent stage of the disease, is mixed with washed type O red blood cells and the mixture is incubated overnight at 4°C and observed for hemagglutination. There is no hot coagulation test. (*Joklik et al, pp 730–731*)

599. **(E)** Pertussis vaccine is effective for individuals who are under 4 years of age. Primary immunization is usually initiated at 2 months of age. The vaccine is divided into three doses, 4 to 8 weeks apart. It is given in combination with diphtheria and tetanus toxoids. The phase I killed *Bordetella pertussis* cells act also as adjuvants. Vaccine-associated encephalopathy is estimated to occur once in 310,000 immunizations in the United States. (*Joklik et al, pp 479–480*)

600. **(D)** Obligately intracellular bacteria only grow in living cells; they cannot grow on artificial media. Of the bacteria listed, all *Legionella*, including *Legionella micdadei*, can also grow on special laboratory media. Therefore, the legionellae are facultative intracellular bacteria. *Mycobacterium leprae* still cannot be grown on artificial media. (*Joklik et al, pp 694–696*)

601. **(E)** All of the clinical infections listed may be caused by *Chlamydia trachomatis* except for leptospirosis. (*Joklik et al, pp 724–727*)

602. **(A)** In pasteurization of milk, which consists of heating to a temperature of 62°C for 30 minutes followed by rapid cooling, the milk is not sterilized, but pasteurization does kill all disease-producing bacteria commonly found in milk that do not produce spores. Flash pasteurization uses a higher temperature for a fraction of a minute. All of the bacteria listed are known to be transmitted to humans via unpasteurized milk or cheeses prepared from the milk. Lactobacilli do not cause disease and are present in unpasteurized milk. (*Joklik et al, pp 96,396*)

603. **(D)** *Listeria monocytogenes* is not resistant to all beta-lactam antibiotics. Benzylpenicillin (penicillin G) or ampicillin are the recommended treatments for *Listeria* infections. The ability of *L. monocytogenes* to grow at temperatures as low as 2.5°C is the basis for the cold-enrichment technique used in the clinical laboratory to isolate it from specimens containing a mixed bacterial flora, such as are present in feces. (*Joklik et al, pp 481,484*)

604. **(D)** *Legionella* do not readily stain gram-negative (or with hematoxylin and eosin) under the usual staining conditions. That is one of the reasons the microbe was overlooked during the initial outbreak in 1976. Modified staining procedures are used. Also, the legionellae are not fast-growing bacteria forming visible colonies after 1 day. It takes 3 to 5 days of incubation for growth. (*Joklik et al, pp 694–696*)

605. **(E)** All of the statements are correct except E. (*Joklik et al, pp 694–697*)

606. **(C)** The causative intracellular organisms for legionellosis, brucellosis, and tuberculosis are facultative intracellular pathogens, whereas all viruses, including acquired immunodeficiency syndrome (human immunodeficiency virus), are obligate intracellular pathogens. Staphylococci causing blood infection are primarily extracellular. (*Jawetz et al, pp 263–265; Joklik et al, pp 609–611*)

607. **(D)** Rickettsiae contain both types of nucleic acids (RNA and DNA), and they divide by transverse binary fission. *Rickettsia akari, Rickettsia rickettsii, Rickettsia tsutsugamushi,* the respective causative agents of rickettsial pox, Rocky Mountain spotted fever, and scrub typhus, infect mites and ticks, which may in turn pass their infection to their progeny transovarially. Little is known about the determinants of virulence of rickettsiae. They obtain most of their energy from the oxidation of glutamate. *(Joklik et al, pp 701–703)*

608. **(D)** Rocky Mountain spotted fever (RMSF) was originally reported in the Rocky Mountain region. However, since that time this disease has been encountered in the 48 contiguous United States. In 1988, 615 cases were reported in the United States, with 32% from the South Atlantic region and 245 from the West South Central region. Oklahoma had the highest rate, followed by North Carolina, Arkansas, Missouri, and Kansas. Q fever, in contrast to other rickettsial diseases, does not produce a rash and is essentially a pneumonitis. Trench fever, or 5-day fever, is caused by *Rochalimaea quintana,* which is unique in that it can be cultured on artificial culture media such as blood agar. Brill–Zinsser disease is a relapse of a prior epidemic typhus infection, not RMSF. Penicillin is not the antibiotic of choice for RMSF. Tetracycline should be used. The Weil–Felix test is no longer recommended for diagnosis of RMSF. *(Joklik et al, pp 705–708)*

609. **(D)** Diagnosis of Rocky Mountain spotted fever can be confirmed by the Weil–Felix tests employing *Proteus vulgaris* strains OX-2 and OX-9, which share antigens with *Rickettsia rickettsii,* the causative agent of this infection. Agglutinins to *Proteus* OX-2 and/or OX-9 usually appear 5 to 8 days after infection. Type-specific complement fixation tests can also be performed by most state health departments. Finally, indirect fluorescent antibody tests (immunofluorescence tests) have become useful diagnostic tools. The Weil–Felix test lacks specificity and sensitivity and is no longer recommended as a diagnostic test. *(Jawetz et al, p 295; Joklik et al, p 707)*

610. **(D)** The Weil–Felix reaction was formerly employed primarily for the diagnosis of rickettsial diseases due to the sharing of some common antigens between *Proteus vulgaris* strains OX-2, OX-9, or OX-K and certain pathogenic rickettsiae. Also, patients suffering from epidemic relapsing fever, but not endemic relapsing fever, may develop agglutinins to *Proteus* OX-K. *(Jawetz et al, p 295; Joklik et al, p 707)*

611. **(E)** Rocky Mountain spotted fever was originally reported in the Rocky Mountain region. However, since that time this disease has been encountered in all of the 48 contiguous United States, including the eastern seaboard and other sections. Q fever, in contrast to other rickettsial diseases, does not produce a rash and is essentially a pneumonitis. Trench fever, or 5-day fever, is caused by *Rochalimaea quintana,* which is unique in that it can be cultured, or artificial culture media such as blood agar. Brill–Zinsser disease is a relapse of a prior epidemic typhus infection. *Rickettsia* do contain both RNA and DNA. *(Joklik et al, pp 705–707)*

612. **(E)** There is a spectrum of fundamental properties that establish the actinomycetes as bacteria. That is, in common with the prokaryotic bacteria, actinomycetes do not have nuclear membrane, they do not contain sterols in their membranes, they have muramic acid as well as diaminopimelic acid in their cell walls, and finally, they are resistant to antifungal antibiotics. They are normal inhabitants of the mouth and gut. *(Joklik et al, pp 526–527)*

613. **(A)** *Actinomyces israelii* is found in tissues as branching gram-positive filaments forming yellow colonies known as sulfur granules. Coloration of these colonies is due to production of yellow pigment by *A. israelii.* Sulfur granule formation is not a usual finding in nocardiosis. *(Joklik et al, pp 531–533)*

614. **(D)** Differentiation of *Actinomyces israelii* from *Mycobacterium tuberculosis* can be made on the basis of various physiologic characteristics. For example, *A. israelii* is not acid-fast, while

M. tuberculosis is acid-fast. On solid media, *A. israelii* forms white, spidery colonies in 2 to 3 days. *M. tuberculosis* forms scaly, small, dry, yellowish colonies after 10 to 20 days at 37°C. *A. israelii* is not known to be able to elaborate measurable quantities of niacin. *M. tuberculosis* was shown to be a good producer of niacin. *A. israelii* is a member of the normal mouth and gut flora, while *M. tuberculosis* is not. *(Joklik et al, pp 528–530)*

615. (B) *Neisseria gonorrhoeae* requires CO_2 for its primary isolation (note that *Brucella abortus* also requires CO_2 for its primary isolation). *Treponema pallidum* cannot be grown in vitro, and *Mycobacterium tuberculosis*, *Staphylococcus aureus*, and *Actinomyces israelii* do not require CO_2. *(Joklik et al, p 443)*

616. (A) Only *Hemophilus influenza* readily stains gram-negative. *Listeria monocytogenes* is gram-positive, as are *Bacillus cereus* and *Staphylococcus saprophyticus*. *Legionella pneumophila* does not stain well using the usual staining procedures; that is why it was not originally detected in the 1976 outbreak. Using modified staining procedures, *Legionella* does stain gram-negative. *(Joklik et al, pp 694–695)*

617. (C) All of the bacteria listed except *Neisseria gonorrhoeae* may cause meningitis in neonates or children. *(Joklik et al, pp 449–450)*

618. (C) Recombinant DNA technology has enormous application to basic science as well as to applied areas of science and medicine. Gene manipulation is being exploited to create microbial strains to make such products as hormones (insulin), vaccines (influenza virus, hepatitis virus), pharmaceuticals (interferons and other lymphokines) and diagnostic reagents (microbial DNA probes). *(Joklik et al, p 151)*

619. (E) Although most of these methods (except for pyocin typing) may be used for the purpose indicated, the most useful and reliable method is to analyze the plasmid profiles of isolated strains. Pyocin (bacteriocin) is useful for typing of *Pseudomonas aeruginosa* only. *(Joklik et al, p 562)*

620. (A) Antimicrobial prophylaxis of exposed persons remains a controversial issue and is usually limited to the persons at greatest risk, such as children (usually under age 6) who have a household-type intimate contact with the index case (also recruits in an army camp). Close observation, even after prophylaxis, is important. Rifampin, minocycline, and cipro-floxin have all been reported to be effective. Penicillin, to which the organism is sensitive, fails to eliminate the carrier state, so it should not be used. It is usually not necessary to use prophylactic therapy for hospital personnel exposed to meningococcal disease unless they have had intimate contact with an untreated patient. *(Joklik et al, p 450)*

621. (C) *Staphylococcus saprophyticus* is a gram-positive, coagulase-negative staphylococcus that can be distinguished from *Staphylococcus epidermidis*, also a coagulase-negative staphylococcus, by its resistance to novobiocin and its failure to ferment glucose anaerobically. It occurs on normal skin and in the urethral flora transiently and in small numbers. More recently, its pathogenic potential has been discovered in sexually active young women, and it is secondary only to *Escherichia coli* as the most frequent cause of urinary tract infections. *(Joklik et al, p 414)*

622. (B) Groups A, C, Y, and W-135 meningococcal vaccines are licensed and available. The immunogenicity of these polysaccharides is age dependent. Although infants can respond well as early as 3 months of age to group A vaccine, responses to the other groups are more variable for children under age 2. Other patients of all ages respond well to all of these vaccines. These vaccines are also available for use in military populations in which epidemic disease is otherwise likely. Group B meningococci continue to be a problem because the polysaccharide is a very poor immunogen and no group B vaccines are presently available. *(Joklik et al, p 450)*

623. (E) The family Enterobacteriaceae contains two genera, *Salmonella* and *Shigella*, which are both among the leading causes of bacterial diarrhea. Both genera ferment glucose but not lactose. They can penetrate the epithelial lining of the small bowel, although *Shigella* rarely spreads to other body parts. *(Joklik et al, pp 556–559)*

624–628.   (624-D, 625-B, 626-C, 627-A, 628-D) Gilligan has a list of all the medically important gram-negative and gram-positive aerobic bacteria. *(Gilligan et al, p 131)*

629. (B) Gilligan has a list of medically important bacteria that cannot be Gram stained and also Enterobacteriaceae. *(Gilligan et al, p 132)*

630. (A) Gilligan has a list of medically important bacteria that cannot be Gram stained and that are oxidase-positive, glucose-fermenting, gram-negative rods. *(Gilligan et al, p 132)*

631. (D) Gilligan has a list of medically important glucose-nonfermenting, gram-negative rods and oxidase-positive, glucose-fermenting, gram-negative rods. *(Gilligan et al, p 132)*

632. (E) The high prevalence of UTIs in women represents a very large reservoir of patients afflicted by the distressing symptoms of urinary infection, which is often recurrent. Even in a woman with multiple recurrent UTIs, provided there is no anatomic or functional abnormality of the urinary tract, there is no increased incidence of renal failure or hypertension. Copious fluid intake is extremely effective if used at the onset of symptoms, probably by mechanically flushing out organisms in nonpregnant women. Cranberry juice is a current favorite therapy and is usually effective, but recent indications are that single 7- to 14-day courses are not as effective as once thought to be. *(Rubin et al, p 1085)*

633. (E) All of the answers are correct. *(Jawetz et al pp 289–293)*

634. (B) The patient has bacterial meningitis. This is supported since the patient has an extremely high white blood cell count (normal is only 0 to 3 cells/mm^3) as well as a low CSF glucose level. These CSF parameters are not consistent with viral and fungal infections. Children aged 2 months to 5 years old are most commonly infected with *Hemophilus influenzae* type b. Other important bacterial agents affecting children of this age and causing meningitis are *Streptococcus pneumoniae*, which is a gram-positive coccus, and *Neisseria meningitis*, which is a gram-negative diplococcus. *(Gilligan et al, pp 85–87)*

635. (A) Although non–spore-forming, gram-negative rods that are a clinically important part of the normal human colonic flora include *Fusobacterium* and *Bacteriodes* genera, *Bacteriodes fragilis* is the most important of the *Bacteriodes* species, and it is often involved in forming intra-abdominal and intra-pelvicabscesses. At laparotomy, the patient was found to have a gangrenous appendix. *Blastomyces* is a fungus, and of the bacteria, only *Clostridium* is anaerobic but spore-forming. Chemoprophylaxis is in order for those clinically exposed to this microbe who have an extremely high white-cell count. *(Gilligan et al, p 87)*

636. (D) Medically important infections due to anaerobic bacteria are fairly common. The infections are usually polymicrobial, that is, they are mixed infections with other anaerobes, facultative anaerobes, and aerobes. Anaerobic bacteria are present throughout the human body—on the skin, on mucosal surfaces, and in very high concentrations in the mouth and the gastrointestinal tract—but they are not normally found in the blood.

The mucous membranes of the mouth (and pharynx) are usually sterile at birth but may be contaminated by passage through the birth canal. Within 4 to 12 hours after birth, viridans streptococci are established as the major resident flora members, and they remain that way for life.

At birth, the intestine is sterile; however, organisms are soon introduced with food. In breast-fed infants, the intestine contains large numbers of streptococci and lactobacilli. The bifidobacteria produce acid for carbohydrates and tolerate acidic pH (5.0).

In the normal adult colon, 96 to 99% of the resident bacterial flora consists of anaerobes. Normal flora of the vagina initially after birth has aerobic lactobacilli, which persist as long as the pH remains acid (several weeks). When the pH becomes neutral (which lasts until puberty) there is a mixed flora of cocci and bacilli. At puberty, aerobic and anaerobic lactobacilli come back again in large numbers. The normal vaginal flora includes beta-hemolytic streptococci, anaerobic *Bacteriodes* species, and clostridia. *(Jawetz et al, pp 289–293)*

637. **(A)** Rocky Mountain spotted fever occurs most often in children and adolescents, whereas most fatalities occur in adults. RMSF accounts for more than 95% of the reported cases and for most of the deaths due to rickettsial disease to humans in the United States most, but not all, individuals with RMSF give a history of a recent tick bite. Infection can, and often does, occur through contamination of fingers while removing ticks feeding on humans or animals.

Both chloramphenicol and tetracycline are effective antibiotics for rickettsia, but because the clinical presentation of meningococcemia and RMSF overlap, chloramphenicol is the drug of choice when these two diseases cannot be distinguished clinically. *(Joklik et al, pp 705–707; Gilligan et al, pp 1251–125)*

638. **(B)** A false response was requested, and B is the false response. The name of the microbe that causes Lyme disease is *Borrelia burgdorferi*. *(Gilligan et al, pp 119–12529; Joklik et al, pp 670–671)*

639. **(D)** Spontaneous abortion in pregnant women with brucellosis does not occur. It occurs with pregnant cows. *(Joklik et al, pp 609–614,363,700–712, Gilligan et al, pp 99–101)*

640. **(B)** Gonorrhea is the most common of the classic sexually transmitted diseases. The current pandemic began in the early 1960s. When compared with many other infectious diseases, gonorrhea is not highly contagious. Acute gonorrhea in humans has an incubation period of 2 to 8 days, while most cases occur within 4 days of infection. Laboratory diagnosis of gonococcal infection is based mainly on the identification of *Neisseria gonorrhea* in infected sites by microscopic examination and culture. In urethral smears from men with symptoms of urethritis, the Gram stain is considered positive for gonorrhea when gram-negative diplococci of typical morphology are found or closely associated with polymorphonuclear leukocytes (PMNs).

Physicians must be aware of the local prevalence of penicillinase-producing *N. gonorrheae* (PPNG). Although penicillin was once the standard treatment, there are significant numbers of PPNG around, and resistant strains must be treated differently. Some of the alternatives for penicillin are ceftriaxone, spectinomycin, and trimethoprin-sulfamethoxazole. *(Joklik et al, pp 454–459; Jawetz et al, pp 603–604)*

641. **(E)** Many people are surprised to learn that there is a vaccine that protects against some, but not all, strains of pneumococcal bacteria which are responsible for most cases of pneumonia in this country. That may be one reason why fewer than 30% (not 10%) of those who get the shots do get them. The vaccine has few side effects, usually nothing more than a sore arm. Those over 65, as well as anyone at high risk, should get the pneumonia vaccine. Individuals who have undergone splenectomy, and those with sickle cell anemia, HIV, nephrotic syndrome, chronic liver disease, malignancy, or primary immunodeficiency are at increased risk of developing severe pneumococcal infections. Consequently, these individuals should be candidates for receiving the relatively new 251-valent pneumococcal vaccine. This vaccine contains a mixture of capsular antigens of 251 of the most commonly occurring pneumococcal types, which account for 87% of bacteremic pneumococcal disease in the United States. Normal young adults are not at increased susceptibility to pneumococcal disease. *(Joklik et al, p 440)*

642. **(E)** An immediate application for research on genome structure has come from the discovery of repetitive DNA elements, which al-

lows identification of strain-specific fingerprint patterns. DNA fingerprinting has provided the first epidemiologically useful tool for monitoring the spread of individual strains of *Mycobacterium tuberculosis.*

Infection with HIV is associated with increased susceptibility to TB and with accelerated progression of disease and mortality, prompting fears of a new era of uncontrolled increases of TB worldwide.

Repetitive elements have provided an important target in the development of tests for the detection of mycobacteria in clinical specimens. *(Young and Cole, pp 1–6)*

643. **(E)** Cholera is endemic in the Bengal region of India and Bangladesh, and has spread to other parts of India from this region. The taxonomy of *Vibrio cholerae* has been confusing because of attempts to link the nomenclature to various ecologic and pathologic entities. Classic epidemic cholera is caused by organisms that agglutinate in antisera against the OH antigen and produce disease primarily by means of a specific enterotoxin.

Epidemics of cholera-like illnesses caused by a previously unrecognized organism occurred recently in southern Asia, and a recent report documented the first case of cholera imported into the United States by this organism. The newly described organism was referred to as toxigenic *V. cholerae* 0139 strain.

Recent advances have reduced the mortality of cholera to less than 1%. Prompt replacement of fluid and electrolyte losses causes a rapid response of reversal of the patient's condition within a matter of hours. After initial recovery from shock, fluid and electrolyte balance can be maintained with oral electrolyte solutions and glucose. Oral therapy alone can be used to treat milder cases.

Tetracycline lowers the number of infecting organisms and thereby lowers the fluid loss by 60%. Trimethoprin-sulfomethoxazole (TS) and other antibiotics are sometimes used, although some strains are resistant to TS. *(Joklik et al, pp 566–570)*

644. **(D)** There are only three (not five) exotoxins produced by GAS—A, B, and C. These substances produce fever and enhance suscepti-

bility to endotoxic shock. While the A and C endotoxins are variable in their expression, B is an enzyme that degrades fibronectin and has the property of cleaving inactive interleukin-1 beta to an active form which is important in the inflammation process. *(Morrow, p 15)*

645. **(E)** In 1993, there was a resurgence of pertussis in the United States. Altogether, 6,335 cases were reported, the most in 16 years. The epidemic of pertussis in greater Cincinnati was investigated using active microbiologic surveillance. The population of 1.7 million in this area is served by a single children's hospital and pertussis laboratory. They prospectively followed patients given a new diagnosis of pertussis during July through September to determine the characteristics of the epidemic. From 1979 to 1992, there was a cumulative total of 642 pertussis cases. In 1993 alone, 352 cases were diagnosed, an increase of 259% over the 1992 total. The outbreak began in the suburbs of during the 1992 summer and spread through greater Cincinnati. Of 255 cases diagnosed from July to September (195 excess cases over the maximum base-line level of 20/month in the previous 14 years), 75% were in white patients. As compared with 1979 to 1992, there was a shift of incidence from younger infants to older children. Immunization records showed 74% of the children with pertussis were 19 months to 12 years old and had received 4 or 5 combined diphtheria–pertussis–tetanus (DPT) vaccine, and that 82% of those 7 to 71 months had received at least three doses of DPT vaccine. Whole-cell vaccines came from both of the major manufacturers. Disease was not severe, but 31% of the children were hospitalized during that period. It was concluded that the 1993 pertussis epidemic in Cincinnati occurred primarily among children who had been appropriately immunized. It is clear that the whole-cell pertussis vaccine failed to give full protection against the disease. *(Christie et al, p 16)*

646. **(E)** Diarrheal illnesses represent a major cause of morbidity throughout the world, with over 5 million people dying from diarrheal disease annually. The Leuko-Test procedure is rapid, simple, and can be performed by anyone familiar with latex agglutination tests. Lactoferrin is a very stable protein that serves as a marker for leukocytes. The test is standardized and rapid (under 5 minutes).

The current method of distinguishing inflammatory from noninflammatory leukocytes must be performed within minutes of specimen collection because fecal leukocytes are not stable and this microscopic method is one of the most unpopular tests in the clinical lab. The Leuko-Test can be performed on refrigerated and frozen stool samples. *(Guerrant et al, pp 12518–12522)*

647. **(D)** There is not just one phage type of *E. coli* 0157:H7. In 1994, there were at least 62 known phage types of *E. coli* 0157:H7. That is why it is important to do subtyping to distinguish outbreak strains from those present in the community. Hemolytic uremic syndrome (HUS) is a common cause of acute renal failure in children, and children and the elderly are at highest risk for clinical manifestations and complications.

E. coli 0157:H7 may be present in the intestines of healthy cattle and may contaminate the meat during slaughter. Home-cooked hamburgers can be a source of infection and underscores the need to cook the beef thoroughly until the interior is no longer pink and juices run clear. *(Joklik et al, pp 544–548)*

648. **(D)** Q(query) fever is a zoonosis caused by *Coxiella burnetii*. It is a respiratory disease that may be severe enough to develop into interstitial pneumonia. The microorganism is a natural parasite of cattle and sheep, and humans are incidental hosts, being infected by inhalation of infected excreta or contact with animal tissues. *C. burnetii* is spread from animal to animal by ticks and remains as an inapparent infection in the mammalian host until parturition. The organisms multiply readily in the placenta and other birth tissues and are found in the urine and stool. These wastes contaminate the soil and serve as the source of infection for humans. *(Joklik et al, pp 713–714; Ryan, pp 436–437)*

649. **(C)** Since *Helicobacter pylori* was first isolated from biopsy specimens derived from patients with acute and chronic gastritis, gastric and duodenal ulcers, and other gastrointestinal disorders, there have been studies of the efficacy of *H. pylori*-associated gastritis that have shown a significantly better response in the antibiotic-treated group.

The spirochaetal *H. pylori* strains have a number of characteristics that distinguish them from the spirochaetal *Campylobacter* organisms. In tissue sections, *H. pylori* can be easily seen with silver stain, but often can also be seen directly in Gram stains. *Campylobacter* organisms have a single polar flagellum, while *H. pylori* has a tuft of polar flagella that are sheathed. *(Joklik et al, pp 679–681)*

650. **(D)** *Staphylococcus aureus* is coagulase-positive, while *Staphylococcus saprophyticus* is coagulase-negative. Therefore, a positive coagulase test would differentiate these microbes. *(Jawetz et al, pp 196–197)*

651. **(E)** *Streptococcus agalactiae* is a group B streptococcus that is part of the normal female genital tract flora and an important cause of neonatal sepsis and meningitis. They are typically beta-hemolytic streptococci and give a positive response in the so-called cAMP test. This test is characterized by an accentuated zone of complete hemolysis when the group B streptococci is inoculated perpendicular to a streak of *Staphylococcus aureus*. *(Jawetz et al, p 204; Joklik et al, pp 426–427)*

652. **(A)** *Helicobacter pylori* has a tuft of polar flagella that are sheathed. *H. pylori* has often been isolated from gastric and duodenal ulcers. Of special interest is the susceptibility of *H. pylori* to bismuth, a component of some over-the-counter remedies for gastritis and gas, but it is not susceptible to cimetidine. *(Joklik et al, pp 679–680)*

653. **(B)** *Pseudomonas aeruginosa* is a gram-negative rod in which most cells have a single po-

lar flagellum. It produces an extracellular slime layer, similar to a capsule, which is referred to as the glycocalyx or mucoid substance. This is composed of alginate, a polymer of D-mannuronate and L-gulonate. *(Joklik et al, p 576)*

654. **(N)** *Shigella* is the most likely organism. The presence of fecal leukocytes indicates an inflammatory diarrhea due to an invasive enteropathogen. The bacterial agents most likely to cause inflammatory diarrhea are *Salmonella* spp., *Shigella* spp., *Campylobacter* spp., *Yersinia* spp., and enteroinvasive *Escherichia coli* (that produce verotoxin). Biologic reactions indicate that the microbe is most likely to be a *Shigella* since it is lactose-negative and all *Shigella* are nonmotile and do not produce H₂S. Its ability to grow on MacConkey agar eliminates *Campylobacter*; its inability to produce H₂S and its nonmotility eliminate *Salmonella*. Since the microbe is nonmotile at 25°C and is urea-negative, *Yersinia* is eliminated. Dairy farmers are not at increased risk for *Shigella* infections since humans represent the only reservoir of *Shigella*. There is no effective vaccine, to date, that prevents shigellosis. The shiga toxin, which interferes with protein synthesis, has cytotoxic properties. As with other diarrheal diseases, the immediate concern in shigellosis is the patient's state of hydration. *Shigella*, in contrast to *Salmonella* gastroenteritis, responds to antibiotic treatment by a decrease in fever and diarrhea, and a decrease of the duration of the carrier state. Ampicillin is the drug of choice for sensitive bacteria. *(Gilligan et al, pp 61–63; Joklik et al, pp 556–559,677)*

655. **(B)** The child had a classic presentation for whooping cough (pertussis), whose etiologic agent is *Bordetella pertussis*. This infection is usually limited to the upper pathways, and pneumonia due to this organism or secondary bacterial agents is not common. Normal chest radiograms are usual. These children often have paroxysms (sudden recurrences or intensification) of coughing, followed by gasps for breath. The sound of this inspiration is the whoop of whooping cough.

The microbe binds to ciliated epithelial cells. Since the nasopharynx is lined with ciliated epithelial cells, culture of this site has a higher yield than other sites. There is a striking lymphocytosis in pertussis. *(Gilligan et al, pp 29–31; Joklik et al, pp 477–478)*

656. **(F)** *Mycobacterium tuberculosis* is the most likely organism. The fact that he is HIV-positive, along with a low absolute CD4⁺ lymphocyte count, should not alter this decision. Being HIV-positive is now recognized as an important risk factor for the development of tuberculosis (TB). TB in HIV-infected individuals is a major reason for the reversal in the long-term trend in a steady decline in the number of TB cases in the United States. *(Gilligan et al, pp 45–47; Joklik et al, pp 507–508)*

657. **(P)** The etiologic agent is *Vibrio vulnificus*. The major family of microbes that grows on MacConkey agar that is oxidase-positive, glucose-fermenting, gram-negative rods is Vibrionaceae. This family consists of three genera, *Vibrio*, *Aeromonas*, and *Plesiomonas*, all of which are associated with gastrointestinal diseases. Systemic infections, as were seen in this case, are rare. *Vibrio vulnificus* has been isolated from oysters. Most individuals can consume oysters contaminated with *V. vulnificus* with impunity since it causes septicemia only in individuals with hepatic cirrhosis or underlying immunocompromised states. *(Gilligan et al, pp 127–129; Joklik et al, p 572)*

658. **(E)** The most likely etiologic agent is *Corynebacterium diphtheriae*. This child seemed to have a strep throat that did not get better. After physical examination, the classic pseudomembrane observed in diphtheria cases was seen, and *C. diphtheriae* is the etiologic agent. It is an aerobic, club-shaped, gram-negative rod composed of fibrin, dead epithelial cells, and red and white blood cells. Aspiration of the pseudomembrane can cause death by suffocation. It is important to notify the clinical laboratory when diphtheria is being considered since isolation of *C. diphtheriae* does not often occur. The disease is rare and hard to discern because nonpatho-

genic diphtheroids are found in most throat cultures and are almost indistinguishable by colony and Gram-stain morphology. However, a selective medium, cysteine tellurite agar, greatly aids *C. diphtheriae* isolation as black colonies. The tellurite also inhibits the growth of normal pharynx inhabitants. The pathogenic potential of any clinical isolate must be proven by its ability to produce the diphtheria toxin. The diphtheria toxoid is protective for this disease. Diphtheria is treated using both antibiotics and diphtheria antitoxin (prepared in horses) in an attempt to neutralize any circulating diphtheria toxin. Antibiotics eradicate the microbe so that no more toxin is produced. *(Gilligan et al, pp 33–35; Joklik et al, pp 491–493)*

659. **(S)** The microorganism most likely to be responsible for this illness is *Francisella tularensis.* This is a zoonotic infection, and tularemia is sometimes called "rabbit fever" and is strongly associated with this animal. The laboratory must be notified since *F. tularemia* is highly infectious (it must be handled in biological safety hoods) and because serology is often used in diagnosing tularemia. She had an eight-fold rise in her titer against *F. tularemia,* and a four-fold rise in titer over a 2-week period would be considered diagnostic with an acute tularemia infection. This patient obtained the infection via direct contact with an infected rabbit. Tularemia may also be obtained from the bite of an infected tick, mosquito, or deerfly. *(Gilligan et al, pp 103–105; Joklik et al, pp 597–598)*

660. **(C)** The most likely etiologic agent is *Streptococcus pneumoniae.* The patient had a community-acquired bacterial pneumonia on the basis of his physical examination and the chest radiograph. The extraordinarily high white blood cell count of 52,400 with elevated numbers of neutrophils supports this diagnosis. Although the sputum Gram stain was nondiagnostic, as it is on many patients with bacterial pneumonia and bronchitis, it can be valuable in guiding initial empirical therapy. The most common cause of community-acquired pneumonia, ie, *S. pneumoniae* and the finding

of gram-positive diplococci in the blood culture was consistent with this conclusion. Patients with sickle cell anemia are at a greatly increased risk of infection with encapsulated bacteria such as pneumococci. About 25 to 30% of patients with pneumococcal pneumonia will have positive blood cultures. Although the *Streptococcus pyogenes* group A is also possible, in a blood culture the group A streptococci are likely to present as gram-positive cocci in chains. Also, the two streptococci are easily separated with *S. pyogenes* being beta-hemolytic and bacitracin susceptible, while pneumococci are alpha-hemolytic and are bacitracin nonsusceptible. *(Gilligan et al, pp 3–5; Joklik et al, pp 438–440)*

661. **(H)** This woman had a septic arthritis due to *Neisseria gonorrhoeae.* Gram-stained smears of urethral or subcervical exudate revealed many gram-negative diplococci within pus cells. Since the etiologic agent grew from the vaginal discharge, and since she had multiple sexual partners, the indication was that she likely had a sexually transmitted disease (STD). Arthritis is often a complication of one of the STD agents, *N. gonorrhoeae.* Estimates are that 0.5 to 3% of infected patients develop systemic infection, and septic arthritis is the most common result. This woman should also be examined for *Chlamydia trachomatis* and *Treponema pallidum,* since these other STD agents also coinfect at the same time. Because of the common occurrence of gonococci and chlamydiae, a combination of tetracycline for the chlamydia therapy and ceftriaxone for the gonorrhea therapy is routinely used at STD clinics. Because she is more likely to acquire human immunodeficiency virus (HIV) infection with multiple sex partners, she should also be screened for HIV and counseled regarding safer sexual practices. Both of her sexual partners should be notified, and, if possible, treated. *(Joklik et al, pp 450–458)*

662. **(A)** *Staphylococcus aureus* is the most likely microbe to have caused this illness. The use of two separate blood cultures and the presence of a foreign body (needle) as on the end of a line definitely points toward a line-related sepsis. Since coagulase-negative staphylococci, such as *Staphylococcus epidermidis*, are normal skin inhabitants, one of the cultures was taken through the line and the other from a peripheral site. Since the same *S. aureus* coagulase-positive culture was obtained from both sites, the *S. aureus* is infecting the blood. *(Gilligan et al, pp 21–23; Joklik et al, pp 402–403)*

663. **(D)** Erysipelas (cellulitis) is usually highly suggestive, but not pathognomonic, for group A beta-hemolytic *Streptococcus pyogenes*. *Staphylococcus aureus* also causes cellulitis occasionally. Cellulitis (erysipelas) infections generally yield little purulent material, so it is more difficult to obtain a diagnostic specimen. A specimen can usually be obtained by aspirating the rapidly advancing border, usually the most active areas, with a needle attached to a syringe containing a small amount of sterile saline (without preservative). If no specimen is obtained by the initial aspiration, inject 0.1 to 0.2 mL of the saline and aspirate again, using one drop for a Gram stain, and culture the remainder. The Gram-stained smear alone does not differentiate between the staphylococci and streptococci since they are both gram-positive cocci. Diligently search for the site of entry of the infecting organism. A culture of pus from the primary site of entry, whether it be a crack between the toes or a purulent sinusitis, will give some clue to the organism causing the infection. Benzylpenicillin is universally, with rare exceptions, effective against group A *S. pyogenes*. Therefore, it is appropriate, after taking samples for a blood culture, to inject that antibiotic for therapy for the hospitalized patient. Oral therapy should not be given in serious infections because you are not as sure of immediate absorption and so forth. Erysipelas was often fatal before the development of antibiotics. *(Joklik et al, p 424)*

664. **(I)** The biggest suspicion is of *Borrelia burgdorferi*, and a serum test for antibodies would be used in an effort to detect a posi-

tive, but weak, test for Lyme borreliosis. The major diagnostic problem is that Lyme borreliosis antibodies do not appear in quantity for 4 to 6 weeks after infection. The serum antibody tests for Lyme disease are almost useless in the earliest phase. If the patient has taken any antibiotics for any reason, false-negative tests may occur. Also, cross-reactions occur between other spirochetes and *B. burgdorferi*, leading to false-positive tests. If Lyme borreliosis is not treated promptly, the disease may move into the progressive stage, with more distressing, less common symptoms such as heart arrhythmia, weakness in legs, facial paralysis, and numbness. The major symptoms of Lyme disease are flu-like chills, fever, headache, dizziness, fatigue, and stiff neck. A "bull's-eye" rash (erythema chronicum migrans) may appear days to weeks after a bite, though not in all cases (about 25% never get the rash). Swelling and pain, usually in one joint, may lead to arthritis. However, the disease does not follow set rules, and there are many different sets of symptoms that are intermediate and change. After being first identified in Lyme, Connecticut, in 1975, the Lyme borreliosis has spread rapidly throughout the Northeast and upper Midwest and has been found in almost all of the 48 contiguous United States. *(Gilligan et al, pp 120–121; Joklik et al, pp 670–671)*

665. **(N)** The most probable causative organism is *Chlamydia trachomatis*, which is causing urethritis. The organism has two forms, elementary bodies and reticulate bodies. The elementary body is the infectious extracellular form. *C. trachomatis* is believed to be the most common agent of sexually transmitted disease in the United States, causing over 3 million cases per year, compared to about 750,000 per year of new gonorrhea cases and about 100,000 new cases per year of syphilis. A definite diagnosis of *C. trachomatis* can be made by one of three ways: culture, antibody-based technique and DNA hybridization. *(Gilligan et al, pp 77–79; Joklik et al, pp 724–726)*

666. **(C)** *Staphylococcus aureus* strains producing toxic shock syndrome toxins are responsible for toxic shock syndrome in adults and children of both sexes. Clinical features include fever, marked hypotension, diarrhea, and a fine scarlatiniform (sunburn-like rash followed by desquamation). Group A *Streptococcus pyogenes* was recently shown to cause toxic shock syndrome in a boy with streptococcal pharyngitis and no streptococcal blood infection. *(Chapnick et al, pp 1074–1077; Gilligan et al, p 130; Joklik et al, pp 350,409,412)*

667. **(E)** Tetanus toxin blocks the functioning of the inhibitory transmitter in the spinal cord. Once the inhibitory synaptic function is blocked, only the excitatory synaptic function continues to control the nervous function. Once the toxin binds to the receptor of synapses, the harmful action of the toxin cannot be neutralized by the antitoxin. This is the reason why the therapy with the specific antitoxin should be initiated as soon as tetanus is suspected by clinical symptoms. *(Joklik et al, p 391)*

668. **(A)** Botulinum toxin inhibits the release of acetylcholine at the myoneural junction, causing flaccid paralysis of the affected muscle. *(Joklik et al, p 391)*

669. **(B)** Cholera toxin activates adenylate cyclase resulting in an increased level of cyclic adenosine monophosphate (cAMP). This increased level of cAMP causes secretion of ions and fluid into the intestinal lumen (severe diarrhea). *(Joklik et al, pp 391,568)*

670. **(B)** *Listeria monocytogenes* is a small gram-positive coccobacillus. All the others listed in the question are gram-negative. *(Joklik et al p 481)*

671. **(A)** Undulant fever is an older but still used name for brucellosis, which may be caused by *Brucella abortus*. Undulant fever is characterized by symptoms including malaise, anorexia, fever, and profound muscular weakness. *(Joklik et al, p 609)*

672. **(A)** *Rickettsia prowazekii* is transmitted to humans by lice and is the causative agent of epidemic typhus. *(Joklik et al, p 701)*

673. **(D)** *Coxiella burnetii* differs from the other rickettsiae in that it is resistant to drying; thus, the parturition products of infected cows or other animals can contaminate the environment and infect humans via aerosols to produce pneumonitis without skin rashes. *(Joklik et al, pp 701,703)*

674. **(B)** *Rickettsia rickettsii*, the causative agent of Rocky Mountain spotted fever, is transmitted to humans by ticks. Most patients with spotted fever present evidence of recent tick bites. However, infection may also be acquired by fingers that were contaminated during tick removal. *Rickettsia prowazekii* and *Rochalimaea quintana*, the causative agents of epidemic typhus and trench fever, respectively, are transmitted to humans by the body louse. *Rickettsia akari* and *Coxiella burnetii*, the etiologic agents of rickettsialpox and Q fever, are transmitted to individuals by mites and aerosols, respectively. *(Joklik et al, pp 701–703)*

REFERENCES

Chapnick EK, et al. Streptococcal toxic shock syndrome due to noninvasive pharyngitis. *Clin Infect Dis* 1992;14(5):1074–1077.

Christie CDC, et al. *New Engl J Med* 1994: 331:16–2529.

Gilligan PH, Shapiro DS, Smiley ML. *Cases in Medical Microbiology and Infectious Diseases*. Washington, DC: American Society for Microbiology; 1992.

Jawetz E, Melnick JL, Adelberg EA, et al. *Medical Microbiology*, 19th ed. Norwalk, CT: Appleton & Lange; 1991.

Joklik WK, Willett HP, Amos DB, Wilfert CM. *Zinsser Microbiology*, 20th ed. Norwalk, CT: Appleton & Lange; 1992.

Morrow KJ Jr. *Genetic Engineering News* 1994.

Nikaido H, Saier MH. *Science* 1992;258:936–942.

Rubin RH, Tolkoff-Rubin NE, Cotran RS. Urinary tract infection, pylonephritis and reflux neph-ropathy. In *The Kidney*, 3rd ed. Brenner, Rector FC Jr, eds. Philadelphia: WB Saunders, 1986.

Young DB, Cole ST. Leprosy, tuberculosis, and the new genetics (minireview). *J Bacteriol* January 1993.

CHAPTER 6

Medical Mycology
Questions

DIRECTIONS (Questions 675 through 730): Each of the numbered items or incomplete statements in this section is followed by answers or by completions of the statement. Select the ONE lettered answer or completion that is BEST in each case.

675. Fungi

   (A) are prokaryotic cells
   (B) are susceptible to certain antibacterial antibiotics
   (C) are gram-positive microorganisms
   (D) are, in general, smaller than bacteria
   (E) contain either DNA or RNA, but not both

676. Dimorphism in fungi refers to

   (A) the ability of fungi to produce two types of spores
   (B) the characteristic of certain fungi to develop male and female hyphae in one colony
   (C) the ability of fungi to grow in two different forms, yeast and mycelial, depending on environmental conditions
   (D) the ability of fungi to undergo mitosis as well as meiosis
   (E) the property of fungi to develop spherical and elongated forms of nuclei

677. All of the following statements about fungal growth are true EXCEPT

   (A) hyphae result from continuous apical extension

   (B) all fungi, except for those belonging to the class zygomycetes, are septated
   (C) budding is a common reproductive mechanism of yeast cells
   (D) entangled masses of individual hyphae are called mycelium
   (E) only the yeast form of fungi produces sexual spores

678. All of the following statements concerning fungal spores are true EXCEPT

   (A) a conidium is an asexually formed fungal spore
   (B) in the majority of fungi pathogenic to humans, sexual cycles of spore formation are not demonstrated
   (C) morphologic characteristics of conidia are a useful aid for the identification of fungi
   (D) fungal spores are as resistant to heat as bacterial spores
   (E) fungal spores cause allergies in some people

679. The cell walls of most fungi

   (A) are the target of penicillin action
   (B) contain teichoic acid and peptidoglycan
   (C) contain chitin and β-1:3-linked glucan
   (D) lack antigenicity
   (E) contain sterols

680. Mycotic infections

   (A) can be diagnosed without isolation of a causative agent.
   (B) usually need no medication because they tend to heal spontaneously
   (C) are opportunistic infections
   (D) do not resemble to bacterial infecitons in their clinical manifestions
   (E) are one of the most frequent complications that kill AIDS patients

681. All of the following statements are true EXCEPT

   (A) aflatoxins are produced by *Aspergillus flavus* and have been implicated in human liver cancer
   (B) amatoxins and phallotoxins are produced by poisonous mushrooms
   (C) amatoxins and phallotoxins interfere with messenger RNA functions in the liver
   (D) mycotoxicosis can be treated with sera containing specific antitoxins
   (E) heating has essentially no effect on reducing the toxicity of mycotoxins

682. Dermatophytosis is a fungal skin infection that

   (A) is caused by one specific species of fungus
   (B) often spreads to the subcutaneous tissues or deep-seated organs
   (C) should be treated with amphotericin B
   (D) is transmitted from human to human
   (E) is often fatal

683. The characteristics of zygomycoses (synonyms: mucormycosis and phycomycosis) include all of the following EXCEPT

   (A) the causative fungi often invade capillary blood vessels, producing occlusion of the vessels
   (B) they are highly transmissible from person to person
   (C) infections occur mostly in compromised hosts

   (D) septa are absent in hyphae of the causative agents
   (E) the central nervous system is often involved

684. Conditions often underlying opportunistic fungal infections include all of the following EXCEPT

   (A) use of broad-spectrum antibacterial antibiotics for extended periods
   (B) therapeutic use of immunosuppressive drugs
   (C) therapeutic use of radiation
   (D) loss of T-helper-cell functions due to human immunodeficiency virus infections
   (E) all of the above

685. Which of the following statements concerning *Coccidioides immitis* and coccidioidomycosis is NOT correct?

   (A) infections usually occur through the inhalation of arthroconidia
   (B) spherules are formed in infected tissues and are considered to be of diagnostic value
   (C) the coccidioidin test is useful in the diagnosis of the infection
   (D) amphotericin B is the drug of choice in the treatment
   (E) arthroconidia are found in the soil of any state in the United States

686. Coccidioidomycosis is

   (A) transmitted from person to person via airborne spherules
   (B) by and large an inapparent and self-limited infection in endemic areas
   (C) best treated with griseofulvin
   (D) most prevalent in the southeastern region of the United States
   (E) diagnosed by demonstrating arthroconidia formed in vivo

687. Acquired resistance to coccidioidomycosis is demonstrated by

(A) elevated levels of humoral antibody

(B) an immediate wheal reaction following an intradermal injection of coccidioidin

(C) a positive tuberculin reaction

(D) delayed hypersensitivity to coccidioidin

(E) a negative reaction to coccidioidin

688. A leukemic patient complains of respiratory symptoms including frequent coughs. X-ray examination of the left lung reveals the presence of a coin-sized lesion characterized by the presence of an air space surrounding the cavity. Sputa of the patient show the presence of thick and uniformly septate hyphae. The culture of sputa yields hairy colonies firmly adhering to the agar surface. The patient's tuberculin test is negative. The most likely cause of the respiratory problem of this patient is

(A) tuberculosis

(B) mucormycosis

(C) aspergillosis

(D) histoplasmosis

(E) candidiasis

689. The binding of polyene antibiotics to the cytoplasmic membrane of fungi initially causes

(A) the initiation of cell division

(B) blocking of protein synthesis

(C) accumulation of intracellular K^+

(D) loss of mitochondria

(E) loss of intracellular K^+

690. All of the following statements concerning the pathogenicity of fungi are true EXCEPT

(A) only a small number of fungi are able to cause diseases in previously healthy persons

(B) most fungi are readily killed by neutrophils

(C) no exotoxin or endotoxin is involved in fungal pathogenesis

(D) T-cell–mediated responses are not important in the development of immunity to fungal infections

(E) for some fungi, the capsule is an important pathogenic factor

691. *Pneumocystis carinii*

(A) infection should be treated with trimethoprim-sulfamethoxazole

(B) is a strict pathogen

(C) in infected tissues cannot be detected by any stains

(D) can be cultured on blood agar

(E) can be treated effectively by ketoconazole

692. Azole antifungal agents such as ketoconazole and itraconazole

(A) are metabolites of bacteria

(B) interfere with the biosynthesis of ergosterol in susceptible fungi

(C) should never be given orally

(D) are similar to polyene antibiotics in their mode of action

(E) are indicated only for dermatophytosis

693. A female patient who participated in an archeological excavation of Indian ruins in the southwestern region of the United States complains of severe systemic and respiratory symptoms. Her skin coccidioidin test is positive. The titers of complement-fixing antibody are as follows: Day 15 after exposure, 1:8; Day 21 after exposure, 1:16; Day 28 after exposure, 1:64. You may predict that she

(A) will recover soon because high complement fixation does not correlate with the severity of infection

(B) may have active disseminated coccidioidomycosis

(C) can be released soon because high levels found in the complement fixation test mean high immunity

(D) may not need amphotericin B treatment

(E) none of the above

694. A healthy middle-aged construction worker who engaged in a demolition task 10 days ago complains of respiratory symptoms similar to those of pneumonia. No causative agents are successfully isolated from his sputa. The patient does not respond to any antibacterial antibiotics and dies before a definitive diagnosis is established. Microscopic examination of specimens taken from granulomatous and suppurative lesions of the lung obtained during necropsy reveal the presence of large budding yeast cells. The bud is attached to the parent cell by a broad base. Based on this data, you diagnose the disease of this patient as

(A) histoplasmosis

(B) coccidioidomycosis

(C) cryptococcosis

(D) blastomycosis

(E) sporotrichosis

695. A male gardener sustains a minor scratch on his forearm while working in a thorny rose garden. A couple of weeks later, the wound progressively develops into granulomas involving the draining lymphatics. Although the wound does not spread beyond the subcutaneous tissues, it fails to respond to antibacterial antibiotic treatments. Microscopic examination of the exudates obtained from infected areas reveals the presence of yeast cells that assume a cigar shape. Cultures of aspirated fluids from the infected areas result in the isolation of a dimorphic fungus that grows yeast at 35°C and hyphae at 25°C. The most likely diagnosis of this infection is

(A) chromomycosis

(B) histoplasmosis

(C) sporotrichosis

(D) coccidioidomycosis

(E) blastomycosis

696. All of the following statements concerning chromomycosis are correct EXCEPT that it

(A) is caused by a group of dematiaceous fungi that produce melanin-like pigments

(B) is a deep-seated systemic mycotic infection

(C) is most often caused by traumatic implantation

(D) is characterized by granulomatous nodules and epithelial hyperplasia

(E) affects both immunocompetent and immunocompromised individuals

697. Flucytosine

(A) is effective against filamentous fungi

(B) cannot be administered orally

(C) can be used without worrying about the development of resistance to the drug

(D) is converted to 5-fluorouracil, which can be incorporated into fungal RNA or serves as inhibitors of thymidylate synthetase

(E) should not be used in combination with amphotericin B

698. Histoplasmosis and tuberculosis share the following characteristics EXCEPT

(A) causative agents can survive within resident macrophages

(B) infection elicits a delayed-type hypersensitivity skin reaction to appropriate antigens

(C) pulmonary infections often leave calcified lesions

(D) most infections are lethal

(E) they can be treated by rifampin, streptomycin, and pyrazinamide

699. A 65-year-old female patient is admitted to an intensive care unit because of a sudden swelling of the right side of the face and an episode of bleeding from the right nostril. According to her daughter, these signs were not apparent a few days ago. She has a long history of diabetes and high blood pressure and recently developed clinical signs of ketoacidosis and renal insufficiency. Her blood sugar level at the time of admission is 700 mg/dL. The facial lesion becomes partially necrotic and shows slight protrusion of the right eye and facial paralysis. The patient dies on the second day. Histopathologic examination of the lesions reveals occlusion of small vessels and the presence of unseptate hyphae. This is most probably caused by

(A) candidiasis

(B) nocardiosis

(C) mucormycosis

(D) erysipelas

(E) gas gangrene

700. A 20-year-old high school graduate, a resident of a rural town in Kentucky, is seen in a local hospital with fever, cough, and enlargement of the lymph nodes. Radiologic examination reveals a pattern similar to primary tuberculosis, but his tuberculin test was negative. A histoplasmin skin test is positive. Serologic tests fail to detect heterophil antibodies against Epstein–Barr viruses. Cultures of the sputum, however, reveal mycelial growth when incubated at room temperature. Microscopic examination of the isolates shows abundant tuberculate chlamydospores along the hyphae. This infection is

(A) histoplasmosis

(B) listeriosis

(C) infectious mononucleosis

(D) blastomycosis

(E) coccidioidomycosis

701. A 50-year-old female is brought to an emergency room because of fever and severe headache. She had complained of malaise, cough, and mild chest pain several days earlier. At the time of examination, she is conscious but nuchal rigidity is present. Kernig and Brudzinski signs are also positive. A lumbar puncture yields clear spinal fluid with opening pressure of 300 mm, protein of 70 mg/dL, and glucose of 80 mg/dL. Microscopic examination of India-ink–stained sediments of the spinal fluid reveals the presence of some leukocytes and encapsulated yeast cells. The most likely diagnosis of this patient is

(A) candidiasis

(B) sporotrichosis

(C) cryptococcosis

(D) blastomycosis

(E) histoplasmosis

702. A 20-year-old male homosexual complains of dysphagia, malaise, and loss of body weight. Physical examination shows extensive oral thrush and bilateral swelling of neck lymph nodes. There are no records showing that the patient has been under antibiotic medication or other drug treatment. Appropriate measures that you should take immediately do NOT include

(A) amphotericin B treatment

(B) anti-human immunodeficiency virus antibody titer

(C) T4/T8 ratio

(D) microscopic examination and culture of oral plaque

(E) routine blood cell counts and differential

703. An 8-year-old child develops a coin-sized, round, itchy skin lesion on the right side of her cheek. The peripheral area of this lesion is slightly elevated and clearly demarcated from the healthy skin. Her mother tells the dermatologist that this child keeps two cats. The first measure that the physician should take is to

(A) microscopically examine KOH-digested scales taken from peripheral areas of the lesion

(B) treat the patient with cortisone ointment

(C) treat the patient with antibacterial ointment

(D) wait until the result of the culture test comes back

(E) refer this patient to an infectious disease specialist

704. An outdoor construction worker presents with a grossly swollen foot. The ulcerous lesion shows cording of the local lymphatics. Biopsy shows the presence of large yeast cells that are dividing by splitting instead of budding. From this finding, you must suspect

(A) sporotrichosis
(B) chromomycosis
(C) actinomycosis
(D) dermatophytosis
(E) blastomycosis

705. A male chronic drug abuser is brought to a local hospital with symptoms compatible with endocarditis. Repeated blood cultures yield white, creamy colonies containing noncapsulated yeast-like cells. Although the general characteristics of this isolate match those of *Candida albicans*, it does not form "germ tubes" when incubated at 37°C in human sera. The most likely identification of this yeast is

(A) *Candida stellatoidea*
(B) *Cryptococcus neoformans*
(C) *Saccharomyces cerevisiae*
(D) *Candida parapsilosis*
(E) *Rhodotorula* spp.

706. The major effector cells or host cell products that control *Candida albicans* within the host are

(A) specific antibodies against the fungus
(B) natural killer cells
(C) neutrophils
(D) macrophages
(E) complement

707. *Microsporum rubrum*

(A) is an anthropophilic dermatophyte
(B) causes nail infections that are difficult to treat
(C) is sensitive to griseofulvin
(D) produces red pigments when cultured on appropriate media
(E) all of the above

708. All of the following are considered to contribute to the pathogenesis of *Candida albicans* EXCEPT

(A) acid protease production
(B) complement receptors on the cell surface
(C) cell-surface adhesin molecules
(D) dimorphism, especially the ability to grow in a hyphal form
(E) all of the above

709. Griseofulvin

(A) is an antibacterial agent
(B) is taken up by susceptible fungi and interferes with cell divisions and possibly other cell functions associated with microtubule
(C) is effective in the treatment of all forms of mycotic infections
(D) accumulates in the blood cells
(E) should not be given orally

710. A 30-year-old woman complains of vaginal discharge. From clinical findings, you suspect that she has vaginal candidiasis. You must do all of the following EXCEPT

(A) perform a microscopic search for budding yeast or pseudohyphae in the discharge
(B) obtain a history of antibiotic usage
(C) test the urine for glucose
(D) culture the discharge on Sabouraud glucose agar
(E) ask the patient to stop exercising

711. The main reason that individuals taking tetracycline often develop candidiasis (caused primarily by *Candida albicans*) is that

(A) the antibiotic is nutritionally favorable for the growth of *Candida albicans*
(B) the antibiotic damages the host mucous membrane
(C) the antibiotic stimulates the biosynthesis of ergosterol of *C. albicans*
(D) *C. albicans* degrades the antibiotic
(E) the normal bacterial flora is drastically altered by tetracycline

712. Griseofulvin is the drug of choice for

(A) candidiasis

(B) chromomycosis

(C) histoplasmosis

(D) dermatomycosis

(E) actinomycosis

713. All of the following drugs can be used in the treatment of dermatophytosis EXCEPT

(A) tolnaftate

(B) naftifine

(C) griseofulvin

(D) ketoconazole

(E) flucytosine

714. All of the following statements about mycotic infections are true EXCEPT

(A) most mycotic infections are rarely transmitted from person to person

(B) clinical symptoms of most mycotic infections are indistinguishable from those of other microbial infections

(C) the diagnosis of mycotic infections can only be established by microbiologically demonstrating causative fungi

(D) except for the histoplasmin and coccidioidin tests, most skin tests are not reliable for the diagnosis of mycotic infections

(E) all mycotic infections can be treated by amphotericin B

715. All of the following statements are true concerning *Candida albicans* and candidiasis EXCEPT that

(A) *C. albicans* is a dimorphic fungus, and its yeast-form cells transform into hyphae when incubated in human sera at 37°C

(B) *C. albicans* is considered to be a member of the normal flora of human mucous membrane

(C) candidiasis is one of the most common opportunistic mycotic infections

(D) candidiasis occurs only in alcoholics and drug addicts

(E) systemic candidiasis should be treated with amphotericin B

716. In infected tissue, yeast cells of *Histoplasma capsulatum* are found within

(A) erythrocytes

(B) B cells

(C) T cells

(D) mast cells

(E) macrophages

717. Polyene antibiotics have high affinity for sterols in the cytoplasmic membrane of eukaryotic cells. When susceptible cells are exposed to a polyene antibiotic, the cells

(A) initiate the accumulation of K^+

(B) begin to clump

(C) cease protein synthesis immediately

(D) start to lose intracellular K^+

(E) rapidly transform to protoplasts

718. A 15-year-old high school student who lives in Wisconsin complains of chills, fever, cough, and headache. Two weeks prior to this, he visited his uncle who owns a farm in western Tennessee. While in Tennessee, the patient helped his uncle to clean up an old barn which was covered with starling droppings. He was healthy when he returned from Tennessee. The patient remembered that considerable dust stirred up when the ground and the roof were raked. Chest x-ray examination revealed patchy infiltrates in his lung and enlargement of mediastinal lymph nodes. Which of the following tests is most appropriate for the patient at this point?

(A) coccidioidin test

(B) histoplasmin test

(C) tuberculin test

(D) HIV test

(E) Schick test

719. Benign, self-limited pulmonary histoplasmosis is most prevalent in persons residing in

(A) Canada
(B) southern California
(C) the central Mississippi Valley
(D) the northeastern United States
(E) the northwestern United States

720. Tuberculate macroconidia are diagnostically useful structures formed by the causative agent for

(A) histoplasmosis
(B) candidiasis
(C) aspergillosis
(D) coccidioidomycosis
(E) all of the above

721. Histoplasmin is a(n)

(A) antibody against *Histoplasma capsulatum*
(B) killed *H. capsulatum* cell
(C) protease produced by *H. capsulatum*
(D) culture filtrate (supernatant) of old *H. capsulatum*
(E) extract of *H. capsulatum*-infected tissue

722. A 30-year-old diabetic man presented with fever, bifrontal headache and other symptoms compatible with meningitis. He had noted glucosuria despite continuing his usual insulin dose and special diet. Physical examination recorded a temperature of 100°F rectally, pulse of 90/min, normal respiration rate, and blood pressure of 120/80. A lumbar puncture was performed. The fluid was clear, but there were 55 white cells/mm^3 and 90% lymphocytes. India ink test of the spinal fluid failed to demonstrate microscopically any encapsulated yeast cells. This patient may have

(A) neisserial meningitis
(B) pneumococcal meningitis
(C) viral meningitis
(D) crypotococcal meningitis
(E) all of the above

723. The dermatophytid reaction is a manifestation of

(A) secondary bacterial infection
(B) hypersensitivity to dermatophytic antigens
(C) susceptibility to exotoxin from dermatophytes
(D) mixed infections by both fungal and bacterial agents
(E) invasion of the dermis with dermatophytes

724. A 50-year-old professional gardener was admitted for evaluation of fever and weight loss noted over the past 6 months. He had noted a nonhealing skin ulcer on the left forearm. Although moderately ill, he showed no signs of distress. His vital signs were within normal limits. A chest x-ray revealed a fibronodular infiltrate in the right lower lung field. A punch biopsy of the ulcer showed histologic evidence of chronic inflammation with polymorphonuclear leukocytes and monocytes infiltrating the tissue. In addition, stains for acid-fast bacteria were negative. But fungal stains revealed yeast which had broad-based budding. This patient should be treated initially with

(A) kanamycin
(B) penicillin
(C) griseofulvin
(D) tetracycline
(E) amphotericin B

725. A 20-year-old woman was a victim of a traffic accident. Her cervical spinal cord trauma resulted in quadriplegia. She required an indwelling urinary catheter, which led to multiple urinary tract infections. These were treated with a variety of broad-spectrum antibiotics. At the time of the present admission to the hospital, there was again evidence of urinary tract infection manifested by cloudy urine and fever. On the third hospital day, urography revealed a large left kidney with delayed function and poor urine concentration. Microscopic examination of sediment obtained by centrifuging urine samples and specimens of tissue obtained surgically showed budding yeast cells, pseudohyphae, and hyphal elements. The most likely diagnosis of her disease is

(A) cryptococcosis

(B) aspergillosis

(C) candidiasis

(D) zygomycosis

(E) actinomycosis

726. *Trichophyton rubrum*

(A) is a geophilic dermatophyte

(B) causes infections of deep-seated organs in humans

(C) is an anthropophilic dermatophyte

(D) infection tends to heal spontaneously

(E) is a zoophilic dermatophyte

727. The morphological characteristic that is useful in the diagnosis of mucormycosis is

(A) spherule

(B) large budding yeast

(C) encapsulated yeast

(D) coenocytic hyphae

(E) pseudohyphae

728. Fungi and bacteria share which of the following morphological and physiological characteristics?

(A) adenosine triphosphate (ATP) is generated in the mitochondrion

(B) the nucleus is surrounded by the nuclear membrane

(C) the cytoplasm is surrounded by the cell wall

(D) the cell wall contains cross-linked peptidoglycan

(E) they are susceptible to polyene antibiotics

729. A 21-year-old male college student who was born, raised, and living in Minnesota developed headache, chills, fever, weakness, severe substernal chest pain, and a cough productive of scanty amounts of sputum. Several weeks previously, he and several of

his friends had explored a cave in Kentucky. This cave is known for the inhabitation of a large number of bats. Physical examination revealed that he was in mild respiratory distress with a temperature of 40°C, and a palpable liver and spleen. The chest x-ray film showed a diffuse interstitial pneumonitis. Laboratory tests, including a Gram stain examination of sputum, were unremarkable. At the time, a histoplasmin skin test was strongly positive. A tuberculin test was found to be negative. He learned later that two of his friends who participated in the trip also developed similar clinical symptoms. The diagnosis of this patient is

(A) tuberculosis

(B) coccidiomycosis

(C) blastomycosis

(D) cryptococcosis

(E) histoplasmosis

730. The following fungus is responsible for an occupation disease of gardner, farmer, miner, and timber worker.

(A) *Histoplasma capsulatum*

(B) *Trichophyton mentagrophytes*

(C) *Coccidioides immitis*

(D) *Sporothrix schenckii*

(E) *Aspergillus fumigatus*

DIRECTIONS (Questions 731 through 744): Each group of items in this section consists of lettered headings followed by a set of numbered words or phrases. For each numbered word or phrase, select the ONE lettered heading that is most closely associated with it. Each lettered option may be selected once, more than once, or not at all.

Questions 731 and 732

(A) *Blastomyces dermatitidis*

(B) *Coccidioides immitis*

(C) *Histoplasma capsulatum*

(D) *Nocardia asteroides*

(E) *Phycomyces* spp.

731. Large budding yeast with broad base

732. Gram-positive, weakly acid-fast rod

Questions 733 and 734

    (A) cryptococcosis

    (B) candidiasis

    (C) dermatophytosis

    (D) blastomycosis

    (E) chromomycosis

733. Causative agent often found in pigeon droppings

734. Causative agents produce melanin-like pigments

Questions 735 and 736

    (A) sporotrichosis

    (B) aspergillosis

    (C) chromomycosis

    (D) histoplasmosis

    (E) candidiasis

735. Opportunistic endogenous mycotic infection

736. Dimorphic and grows predominantly as hyphae in infected tissues

Questions 737 and 738

    (A) griseofulvin

    (B) ketoconazole

    (C) amphotericin B

    (D) 5-fluorocytosine

    (E) nystatin

737. Drug of choice for chromomycosis

738. Polyene antibiotic that is too toxic to be administered intravenously

Questions 739 through 741

    (A) sterols in the membrane

    (B) glucans in the cell wall

    (C) chitin in the cell wall

    (D) reparatory enzymes in mitochondria

    (E) DNA polymerase

739. Target of fluconazole

740. Positively stained by periodic acid Schiff stain

741. Fluoresces when stained with calcofluor dye

Questions 742 and 743

    (A) arthroconidia of *Coccidioides immitis*

    (B) conidia of *Histoplasma capsulatum*

    (C) conidia of *Aspergillus fumigatus*

    (D) macroconidia of *Trichophyton mentagrophytes*

    (E) chlamydospore of *Candida albicans*

742. Characteristically formed on cornmeal agar

743. Multiseptate

Question 744

    (A) *Coccidioides immitis*

    (B) *Histoplasma capsulatum*

    (C) dermatophytes

    (D) *Candida albicans*

    (E) *Aspergillus fumigatus*

    (F) *Sporothrix schenkii*

    (G) *Cryptococcus neoformans*

    (H) *Mucor* spp.

    (I) *Blastomyces dermatitidis*

    (J) *Actinomyces bovis*

    (K) *Saccharomyces cerevisiae*

    (L) *Amatia*

    (M) *Paracoccidioides brasiliensis*

744. Prokaryotic microorganism

Medical Mycology
Answers and Explanations

675. (C) Fungi are not prokaryotic cells which lack the nuclear membrane. They are eukaryotic cells which are, in general, larger than most bacteria. They contain both DNA and RNA and are completely insensitive to antibacterial antibiotics. All fungi are gram-positive. *(Ryan et al, pp 571–577)*

676. (C) All other definitions are incorrect. Many medically important fungi such as *Candida albicans* and *Histoplasma capsulatum* characteristically display this property. Temperatures, oxygen, carbon dioxide, and certain carbon and nitrogen sources are known to affect the morphogenesis of dimorphic fungi. *(Joklik et al, p 1072; Ryan et al, p 577)*

677. (E) Both yeast and mold produce sexual spores. For example, *Saccharomyces cerevisiae*, which is a yeast, produces sexual spores known as ascospores, and *Neurospora crassa*, which normally grows in mycelial form, also produces sexual spores known as ascospores. Some sexual spores formed by mold are known as zygospores. All other statements listed in A through D are correct. *(Joklik et al, pp 1071–1079; Ryan et al, pp 572–573)*

678. (D) Unlike bacterial spores, which are highly resistant to heat, chemicals, and other deleterious agents, all types of fungal spores are not so resistant to various physical and chemical agents. For example, most fungal spores are completely killed when heated at 80°C for 30 minutes. Such heat treatment does not inactivate bacterial spores. Fungi in which no sexual cycles have been discovered are called "fungi imperfecti" or *Deuteromycetes* or *Deuteromycotina*. Interestingly, many fungi that infect humans belong to this group. All other statements are true. *(Joklik et al, p 1079; Ryan et al, pp 573–574)*

679. (C) Unlike bacterial cell walls, fungal cell walls do not contain peptidoglycan or teichoic acid. The lack of penicillin target (peptidoglycan) make all fungi insensitive to penicillin or related antibiotics. Most fungal cell walls contain chitin (a polymer of β-1:3-linked N-acetylglucosamine), glucans (or mannan or galactan), and proteins. Calcofluor white is a highly sensitive fluorescent stain that binds chitin and cellulose (some fungi have cellulose in the cell wall). Because of the presence of glucans, fungal cell walls react positively to the periodic acid-Schiff reagent. They are all immunogenic when introduced to animals. Sterols are localized in the cytoplasmic membrane, not in the cell wall. *(Joklik et al, pp 1073–1076; Ryan et al, p 571)*

680. (E) Mycotic infections are one of the leading causes of death in AIDS patients. Not all mycotic infections are opportunistic infections. Some mycotic infections (coccidoidomycosis) occur in both compromised hosts and apparently "normal" individuals. Symptoms of mycotic infections often mimic those of bacterial infections; thus, isolation of a causative agent is essential for establishing the diagnosis of any mycotic infection. *(Ryan et al, pp 575–577,579–582)*

681. **(D)** Some fungi generate substances with direct toxicity for humans and animals. Such toxins are secondary metabolic products of fungi. These toxins are collectively called mycotoxins. Mycotoxicoses (mycetismus) occur after their inadvertent ingestion. Heating of mycotoxins has little effect on reducing the toxicity. The anatoxins and phallotoxins represent two important families of mycotoxins produced by poisonous mushrooms such as *Amania*. The liver is a target organ for these toxins. Alpha amtanitin (anatoxin) binds to a subunit of RNA polymerase II and consequently interferes with messenger RNA and protein synthesis. Phalloidin binds to and stabilizes F actin. Treatment of mushroom poisoning is largely supportive as specific antidotes are not available. Aflatoxins are tumorigenic for animals. *(Joklik et al, pp 1082–1083)*

682. **(D)** Essentially all fungi responsible for dermatophytosis belong to these three genera: *Trichophyton, Epidermophyton,* and *Microsporum*. These fungi infect only the skin, nail, and hair and rarely infect the subcutaneous tissue or deep-seated organs. The disease can be transmitted from person to person by direct contact or via fomites. Dermatophytosis is common among people who live in communities where a high standard of sanitation is difficult to maintain. Dermatophytosis is a nuisance disease and rarely threatens life itself. The most effective antibiotic is griseofulvin. Dermatophytoses of the skin may be treated with topical antibiotics such as tolnaftate, miconazole, or clotrimazole. *(Joklik et al, pp 1125–1131; Ryan et al, pp 585–589)*

683. **(B)** All of the statements listed in the question except B are correct. Phycomycoses are opportunistic mycoses. Patients with diabetic ketoacidosis, leukemias, and immunodeficiencies are particularly at risk from these mycoses. These infections are usually caused by inhalation of sporangiospores that germinate and thrive in environments such as the nasal, oropharyngeal, or respiratory mucosa of compromised patients. Mucormycosis typically begins in the nasal region and progresses rapidly to involve the sinuses, eyes,

brain, and the meninges. The disease is not transmissible from person to person. *(Joklik et al, pp 1151–1152; Ryan et al, p 599)*

684. **(E)** All of the conditions listed in the question predispose individuals to opportunistic mycotic infections. Candidiasis, cryptococcosis, and aspergillosis are common fungal infections associated with acquired immunodeficiency syndrome. Prolonged use of broad-spectrum antibiotics may alter the normal microbial flora promoting the growth of opportunistic pathogens. Radiation damages or kills various types of cells that are essential for normal immune response. *(Joklik et al, p 1136; Ryan et al, pp 815–820)*

685. **(E)** *Coccidioides immitis* is a dimorphic fungus that causes coccidioidomycosis. This fungus lives in the soil of a highly restricted geographic area: the southwestern United States, contiguous regions of northern Mexico, and specific areas of Central and South America. The fungus and the infection it causes are almost entirely limited to this endemic area. Infection usually occurs through contact with or inhalation of arthroconidia formed in soil. All other statements are correct. *(Joklik et al, p 1092; Ryan et al, pp 607–611)*

686. **(B)** Although *Coccidioides immitis* can cause severe and fatal infection, by far the most common form of coccidioidomycosis in the endemic area is a mild respiratory ailment, called valley fever or San Joaquin Valley fever. Virtually everyone who inhales the arthroconidia of *C. immitis* becomes infected and acquires a positive delayed-type hypersensitivity response. Disseminated infection occurs in only 1% of the infected individuals. Many of the patients in whom disseminated coccidioidomycosis develop have depressed cell-mediated immunity. Spherules, which are pathohistologically diagnostic, are formed in the infected host but do not transmit infection to others. Griseofulvin is the drug of choice for dermatophytosis. Amphotericin B is the drug of choice for coccidioidomycosis. *(Joklik et al, pp 1092–1097; Ryan et al, pp 607–611)*

687. (D) A delayed-type hypersensitivity reaction is elicited when a mycelial culture filtrate (coccidioidin) is injected cutaneously. The skin test becomes positive within 2 weeks after the onset of symptoms and before the appearance of precipitins and complement-fixing antibodies and often remains positive indefinitely. A positive test in healthy subjects implies immunity to symptomatic reinfection. All other reactions or findings cannot be correlated to acquired resistance to coccidioidomycosis. *(Joklik et al, p 1095; Ryan et al, pp 607–611)*

688. (C) Both clinical symptoms and cultural characteristics of the causative agent suggest that the diagnosis of this patient is aspergillosis, a common opportunistic infection seen in compromised hosts. Tuberculosis is unlikely because the patient's tuberculin skin test is negative. The causative fungus for mucormycosis (phycomycosis) produces characteristic nonseptate hyphae in vivo. *Histoplasma capsulatum*, which causes histoplasmosis in humans, grows in yeast form in the infected person. *Candida*, the causative agent for candidiasis, does not produce hairy colonies on the agar surface. *(Joklik et al, pp 1135–1152; Ryan et al, pp 697–599)*

689. (E) The cytoplasmic membrane of fungi contains ergosterol and other sterols as its integral components. When polyene antibiotics, which have a high affinity to sterols, bind to membrane sterols, the membrane loses its normal permeability control. This loss results in the leakage of intracellular components. Because of its relatively small size and high concentration in the cytoplasm, K^+ is the first component that leaks out of the cell when the cytoplasmic membrane is damaged by polyene antibiotics. Polyene antibiotics do not cause other events immediately or at all. *(Joklik et al, pp 164–166,1088–1089; Ryan et al, pp 582–583)*

690. (D) Although many thousands of fungal species are known, only a handful of fungi can cause infections in healthy persons. *Histoplasma capsulatum* and *Coccidioides immitis* are such examples. Fungi that enter the host are usually killed nonspecifically by neutrophils and other phagocytes. No exotoxin or endotoxin similar to those of bacteria are found in fungi, although a few toxins produced in certain fruiting bodies of fungi (mushroom) are responsible for often fatal food poisoning. For developing immunity to fungal infections, T-cell–mediated cellular immunity is very important, and individuals who have defective cell-mediated immunity may develop severe fungal infections (chronic mucocutaneous candidiasis, for example). Although specific pathogenic factors are not identified for the majority of pathogenic fungi, the capsule of *Cryptococcus neoformans* is known as the major pathogenic factor in this fungus. *(Ryan et al, pp 579–581; Roitt et al, pp 17.11–17.12)*

691. (A) Although the taxonomic position of *P. carinii* still remains uncertain, recent evidence suggests that this organism is a fungus instead of a parasite as previously believed. Human strains of this organism has not yet been successfully cultured. The organism causes a highly lethal pneumonia in immunocompromised patients and premature infants. It is an opportunistic pathogen. The cystic form of this organism in the tissue can be stained only with special stains such as methenamine silver, but not with Gram stain. Sporozoid and trophozoid forms can be stained with Gram stain. The drug of choice is trimethoprim-sulfamethoxazole. *(Ryan et al, pp 619–622)*

692. (B) Ketoconazole, itraconazole, and other azole antifungal agents are chemically synthesized, not microbial products. Its mode of action is the interference of ergosterol biosynthesis in fungi. In contrast to this, the mode of action of polyene antibiotics is the disturbance of the normal function of the fungal cytoplasmic membrane due to their specific binding to ergosterol in the membrane. Some azole antifungal agents such as ketoconazole can be given orally, significantly reducing the cost of treatment of severe systemic mycoses. Azole antifungal agents are effective against a variety of pathogenic fungi. *(Ryan et al, pp 582–584)*

693. (B) The complement fixation (CF) test for antibodies (IgG) to coccidioidin is a powerful diagnostic and prognostic tool. Because the CF test becomes positive more slowly and persists longer, the presence of CF antibodies may reflect either active infection or the recovery stage. In coccidioidomycosis, the CF titer correlates with the severity of disease. A critical titer of 1:32 or higher reflects active disseminated disease, because many patients, such as those with single extrapulmonary lesions, do not develop high titers. *(Joklik et al, p 1096; Ryan et al, pp 610–611)*

694. (D) The key diagnostic finding is the morphology of the yeast isolated from granulomatous and suppurative lesions of the lung. *Blastomyces dermatitidis*, which causes blastomycosis, grows in yeast form in infected tissues. The bud of growing yeast is attached to the parent cell by a broad base. Although the fungi that cause all other diseases listed in the question grow in yeast form in infected tissues, most buds are attached to the parent cell by a narrow base. *(Joklik et al, pp 1103–1108; Ryan et al, pp 606–607)*

695. (C) Both clinical symptoms and mycologic findings indicate that the patient has sporotrichosis. This infection is caused by the dimorphic fungus *Sporothrix schenckii*. The infection is, as in this case, initiated by traumatic inoculation of the organisms into the skin. Secondary spread may follow, with involvement of the draining lymphatics, lymph nodes, and rarely, the underlying tissues. Antibacterial antibiotics are useless in the treatment of fungal infections since no fungi are susceptible to such antibiotics. The yeast-form cells found in smears of biopsy materials or exudates from ulcerative lesions are usually spherical or cigar-shaped. Chromomycotic lesions contain spherical, pigmented cells (4 to 12 mm) that exhibit transverse septation. Involvement of the lymphatics is rare in histoplasmosis, blastomycosis, and coccidioidomycosis. *(Joklik et al, pp 1113–1116; Ryan et al, pp 613–614)*

696. (B) Chromomycosis is not a deep-seated systemic mycotic infection. The infection usually occurs on the exposed lower extremities. It is primarily a cutaneous and subcutaneous infection caused by traumatic implantation of any one of several dematiaceous fungal species into the subcutaneous tissues. The pathology typically consists of granulomatous nodules and epithelial hyperplasia. The infection is often complicated by secondary bacterial infections. Dematiaceous fungi are imperfect fungi that produce varying amounts of melanin-like pigments. Species generally recognized as agents of chromomycosis are *Fonsecaea pedrosoi*, *Phialophora verrucosa*, *Cladosporium carrionii*, *Rhinocladiella aquaspersa*, and *Fonsecaea compacta*. The natural reservoir of these fungi is soil and plant debris. Both immunocompetent and immunocompromised individuals are susceptible to these fungi. Flucytosine has achieved the most success in the treatment of this infection. *(Joklik et al pp 1117–1119; Ryan et al, pp 614–615)*

697. (D) Flucytosine was originally developed as an anticancer drug. Its effectiveness is limited to certain yeast form fungi (*Cryptococcus neoformans*). This drug is usually given orally in combination with parenteral amphotericin B injection. This is because (1) these two drugs work synergistically, and (2) this minimizes the development of drug resistance by susceptible fungi. The drug works as an inhibitor of RNA and DNA synthesis as described in D. *(Ryan et al, p 583)*

698. (E) Histoplasmosis should be treated with amphotericin B, not with streptomycin, which is an antituberculous drug. Both histoplasmosis and tuberculosis are caused by facultative intracellular pathogens (*Histoplasma capsulatum* and *Mycobacterium tuberculosis*, respectively), which can survive in resident macrophages. The majority of individuals infected with these organisms do not develop clinical diseases but elicit delayed-type hypersensitivity skin reaction to specific antigens (histoplasmin and tuberculin, respectively) contained in cultural filtrates. Calcification often occurs in healed pulmonary lesions of both diseases. These drugs listed in the question are antituberculous drugs and are not effective for histoplasmosis. *(Joklik et al, pp 498–510,1097–1103)*

699. **(C)** This description is a typical clinical picture of mucormycosis occurring in a diabetic patient. *Mucor* is a member of *Phycomycetes*, which forms unseptate hyphae. In candidiasis, septate hyphae and budding yeast are seen in infected tissues. Nocardiosis, erysipelas, and gas gangrene are not mycotic infections. They are caused by bacteria (*Nocardia asteroides*, *Streptococcus pyogenes*, and *Clostridium perfringens*, respectively). *(Joklik et al, pp 1151–1152)*

700. **(A)** The clinical picture and laboratory test results are compatible with histoplasmosis caused by *Histoplasma capsulatum*. Histoplasmosis is the most prevalent pulmonary mycosis of humans and animals caused by the dimorphic fungus *H. capsulatum*. Infection is initiated by inhalation of the fungus or conidia it produces. Ninety-five percent of the infections are inapparent and are detected only by the manifestation of residual lung calcifications, and delayed-type hypersensitivity to histoplasmin. Yeast-form cells are usually found in macrophages. When cultured, the fungus forms mycelial colonies that produce characteristic tuberculate conidia (chlamydospores) along the hyphae. In infectious mononucleosis, heterophil antibodies against Epstein–Barr viruses can be detected. Fungi causing blastomycosis and coccidioidomycosis do not produce tuberculate chlamydospores. The drug of choice is amphotericin B. *(Joklik et al, pp 1097–1103; Ryan et al, p 599)*

701. **(C)** The patient is clearly showing the meningeal symptoms: headache, nuchal rigidity, positive Kernig and Brudzinski signs, and elevated spinal fluid pressure (normal is about 100 mm H_2O). Unlike spinal fluid obtained from bacterial meningitis patients, spinal fluid from cryptococcosis patient is not markedly turbid. The presence of encapsulated yeast cells in the sediment of spinal fluid confirms the diagnosis. Although some of the fungi that cause the diseases listed in the question grow in yeast form in infected tissues, only *Cryptococcus neoformans*

is encapsulated. The presence of cryptococcal capsular polysaccharides in the spinal fluid can be detected serologically by a latex agglutination test, which uses latex particle coated with the specific rabbit immunoglobulin (anticapsular antibodies). *C. neoformans* is considered an opportunistic pathogen and is not dimorphic. The natural reservoir of this fungus is the soil and avian feces, and infection follows airborne exposure and inhalation of the yeast. The yeast may infect virtually any organ in the body, but they preferentially invade the central nervous system. *(Joklik et al, pp 1144–1147; Ryan et al, pp 601–603)*

702. **(A)** Considering the background of this patient, one must immediately suspect the possibility of human immunodeficiency virus (HIV) infection. This diagnosis can be established by observing increased anti-HIV antibody titer and decreased T4/T8 ratio (T-helper cells characterized by CD4 marker are preferentially affected by HIV). Oral thrush (oral candidiasis) is one of the most common secondary infections seen in acquired immunodeficiency syndrome (AIDS) patients. A routine blood cell count and differential are required for all cases showing these symptoms. Amphotericin B treatment is appropriate once the diagnosis of AIDS and candidiasis is established. *(Joklik et al, pp 337,1136–1144; Ryan et al, pp 591–596)*

703. **(A)** From the clinical symptoms and her frequent contacts with cats, dermatophytosis must be suspected. Microscopic examination of KOH-digested scales or hairs should reveal dermatophytic hyphae. The confirmation of diagnosis can be made by identifying the etiologic fungus isolated from the scales or hairs obtained from the lesions. To use cortisone ointment for skin lesions of unknown origin is a dangerous and inappropriate practice of medicine. Antibacterial antibiotics are not effective for the treatment of any fungal infections including dermatophytosis. *(Joklik et al, pp 1125–1132; Ryan et al, pp 585–589)*

704. **(B)** The most likely diagnosis of this patient is chromomycosis. The most characteristic

finding is the demonstration of large yeast cells that were dividing by splitting rather than budding. *(Joklik et al, pp 1116–1119; Ryan et al, pp 614–615)*

705. **(D)** *Candida parapsilosis* often causes endocarditis in drug abusers. Unlike *Candida albicans* and some *Candida stellatoidea*, *C. parapsilosis* does not form germ tubes when incubated in human sera at 37°C. All other fungi listed in the question are yeasts, but they are all not dimorphic fungi. *Saccharomyces cerevisiae* is a baker's yeast and rarely causes infections in humans. *Rhodotorula* is a yeast that produces pink pigments and occasionally infects compromised hosts. *(Joklik et al, pp 1136–1144; Ryan et al, pp 596–597)*

706. **(C)** The resistance to *Candida albicans* is predominantly cell mediated. Humoral antibodies play no major roles in the resistance of the host to this fungus. Although macrophages contribute significantly to the host resistance to this fungus, neutrophils are the primary cell type that provide protection against *C. albicans* infection. Thus, neutropenic patients are particularly susceptible to systemic candidal infection. Chronic mucocutaneous candidiasis is often associated with defective T-cell functions. Natural killer cells do not kill *C. albicans* directly. *(Joklik et al, pp 1136–1144; Ryan et al, p 595)*

707. **(E)** All of the statements listed in this question are correct. Dermatophytosis caused by *Trichophyton rubrum* is one of the hardest mycotic infections to cure completely. *(Joklik et al, pp 1125–1132; Ryan et al, p 587)*

708. **(E)** Although the pathogenic mechanisms of *Candida albicans* are not completely understood, four of the properties of this fungus listed in this question are claimed to contribute to its pathogenesis. Proteases, particularly one acid protease, is thought to be critical in initiating infections because mutants defective in protease production are avirulent. Cell-surface adhesion molecules are essential for establishing colonization. Complement receptors on candidal cells increase the pathogenicity by several different mecha-

nisms including molecular mimicry and competition with phagocyte receptor for ligand. Some believe that hyphae penetrate tissues more easily than yeast form cells. *(Joklik et al, pp 1139–1140; Ryan et al, pp 593–595)*

709. **(B)** Griseofulvin is useful for the treatment of dermatophytosis. This drug is not indicated for any other mycotic or bacterial infections. When taken orally, it accumulates in keratinous tissues and kills dermatophytes by interfering with the normal functions of fungal microtubulus. *(Ryan et al, p 583)*

710. **(E)** Exercise does not cause or aggravate vaginal candidiasis. It must first be determined whether vaginal discharge contains *Candida*. This can be done by microscopic search for yeast or pseudohyphae in the discharge and by isolating *Candida* from the discharge on appropriate mycologic agar media (Sabouraud dextrose agar is the most common medium). Vaginal candidiasis (vaginal thrush) occurs more often in pregnant women, diabetics, and women receiving antibacterial or hormonal treatment, including birth control pills. *(Joklik et al, pp 1140–1141; Ryan et al, pp 595–596)*

711. **(E)** In humans, the microflora of the oral cavity and other parts of the body is made up of hundreds of species of microorganism, which include opportunistic pathogens. Each species controls and is controlled by the environment in which it is harbored. Under normal conditions, no one species of microorganism dominates others, and a state of coexistence is maintained. The use of broad-spectrum antibacterial antibiotics, such as tetracycline, results in the selective killing of susceptible bacteria, thus disturbing this balance maintained by the normal microbial flora. As a result, certain microorganisms, such as *Candida albicans*, resistant to tetracycline initiate abnormal growth resulting in the development of candidiasis. *C. albicans* neither degrades nor utilizes tetracycline. Tetracycline has no stimulatory activity for the biosynthesis of ergosterol. *(Joklik et al, pp 1136–1144; Ryan et al, pp 138–139)*

712. (D) Griseofulvin is useful in all forms of dermatophyte infection. It is given orally, and the drug is rapidly deposited in the epidermis and subsequently in the stratum corneum. The treatment of growing cells with griseofulvin causes morphologic abnormalities, such as swelling and branching in the growing tip, whereas old cells distant from the growing point are not affected. It inhibits mitosis in the metaphase, causing multipolar mitosis and abnormal nuclei. The molecular basis for the antimitotic action of this drug is attributed to an interference with the assembly process of tubulin into microtubules. Griseofulvin is not used for other mycotic infections. *(Joklik et al, pp 175,1131; Ryan et al, pp 583,588)*

713. (E) All drugs except flucytosine are used in the topical or oral treatment of dermatophytosis. Flucytosine is indicated for the treatment of cryptococcosis. *(Ryan et al, pp 588,603)*

714. (E) Although amphotericin B is effective for the treatment of most of the deep-seated and subcutaneous mycoses, the drug is not indicated for superficial mycotic infections caused by dermatophytes. All other statements listed in this question are correct. *(Joklik et al, p 1089; Ryan et al, pp 579–584)*

715. (D) Candidiasis is not limited to alcoholics and drug addicts. Candidiasis usually occurs in individuals whose normal defense mechanisms are temporarily or permanently compromised. Candidal vaginitis is common among pregnant women. Thrush (oral candidiasis) occurs often in the elderly or in the newborn who may not be able to maintain good oral hygiene. All other statements listed in the question are correct. *(Joklik et al, pp 1136–1144)*

716. (E) *Histoplasma capsulatum* is a facultative intracellular pathogen. It is usally introduced into the host in a form of conidium (asexual spores formed in soil). Within the host, the fungus becomes yeast form which is eventually engulfed by macrophages. Phagocytosed yeast cells of *H. capsulatum* are not killed by resident macophages or neutrophils. They can remain viable and even multiply within the macrophages. Only activated macrophages can kill such intracellular pathogens. *(Ryan et al, pp 603–606)*

717. (D) Polyene antibiotics (amphotericin B and nystatin) specifically bind to sterols (ergosterol in the case of fungi and cholesterol in the case of host cells) of the cytoplasmic membrane (cell membrane). As a result, the cell loses its permeability control causing leakage of its intracellular potassium ions. Further damage of the membrane causes the leakage of amino acids, nucleotides, and other larger intracellular molecules culminating in the death of the cell. All other statements listed in the question are incorrect. Although the protein synthesis of affected cells ceases eventually, the main target of polyene action is not the protein-synthesizing system. *(Joklik et al, p 165; Ryan et al, pp 582–583)*

718. (B) Considering the past history of this patient, the most likely infection that must be considered here is histoplasmosis. Although other diseases cannot be eliminated at this stage, he should be immediately tested for *Histoplasma capsulatum* infection. *H. capsulatum* grows and sporulates in soil under humid conditions, particularly soil containing bird or bat droppings. In the United States, the greatest concentrations are areas along the Ohio and Mississippi Rivers. Like tuberculosis and coccidioidomycosis, infection with *H. capsulatum* results in the development of delayed-type hyersensitivity to an antigen of the causative agent (histoplasmin). Histoplasmin does not cross-react with *Mycobacterium tuberculosis* antigen (tuberculin) or *Coccidioides immitis* antigen (coccidioidin). For firmly establishing the diagnosis of histoplasmosis, the isolation of *H. capsulatum* from this patient is essential. HIV test for AIDS and Schick test for diphtheria toxin susceptibility appear to be inapproriate for this case. *(Ryan et al, pp 603–606)*

719. (C) The central Mississippi Valley is one of the endemic areas for histoplasmosis. Soils in the endemic region are often infested with spores (conidia) of *Histoplasma capsulatum*, and the people living in this region may develop subclinical histoplasmosis due to the inhalation of spores. Eighty to ninety percent of the population living in the area may be histoplasmin skin test positive by the age of 20 years. Most such infections are, however, benign and self-limited without developing into active infections. Calcium deposition is often observed in old healed lesions of pulmonary histoplasmosis. Other regions listed in this question are not known as endemic areas for histoplasmosis. *(Joklik et al, p 1100; Ryan et al, pp 603–606)*

720. **(A)** The most useful diagnostic structure that is produced in vitro by *Histoplasma capsulatum* is the tuberculate macroconidium. No other pathogenic fungi produce morphologically similar conidia although many fungi produce conidia that are diagnostically useful. Arthoconidia of *Coccidioides immitis* is such an example. *(Ryan et al, pp 603,608)*

721. **(D)** Histoplasmin is an immunologically active material extracted from the culture filtrate of *Histoplasma capsulatum*. It causes a delayed-type hypersensitivity skin reaction in the individuals who have been exposed to or infected with *H. capsulatum*. The positive reaction to the histoplasmin test does not necessarily indicate the presence of an active infection. The negative reaction, however, is useful for excluding histoplasmosis. *(Joklik et al, pp 1102–1103; Ryan et al, p 605)*

722. **(E)** With the information provided, one cannot eliminate any type of meningitis. Although positive India ink test of the spinal fluid for encapsulated yeast cells helps establish the diagnosis (cryptococcal meningitis), a negative result does not necessarily exclude cryptococcal meningitis because roughly 50% of cryptococcal meningitis cases show a positive India ink test. The spinal fluid should be further tested for crypotococcal capsular antigens using the latex agglutination test or enzyme immunoassay method. From the information provided, the patient may have meningitis that is caused by any other viral, bacterial, or fungal agent. *(Ryan et al, pp 783–789,603)*

723. **(B)** The dermatophytid reaction ("id" reaction) is the dermal reaction to the fungal antigens occurring in areas removed from the infected lesions. This is an allergic manifestation of infection at a distal site, and the lesions are devoid of organisms. The dermatophytid reaction is unrelated to any known bacterial infections. *(Joklik et al, pp 1129–1131)*

724. **(E)** Yeast cells with broad-based budding are diagnostically useful characteristics of *Blastomyces dermatitidis*, which causes blastomycosis. This system fungal infection should be treated with amphotericin B. Antibacterial antibiotics such as kanamycin, penicillin, and tetracycline are absolutely useless for the treatment of blastomycosis. Griseofulvin is used only for the treatment of dermatophytosis. *(Ryan et al, pp 582–583,606)*

725. **(C)** Among the causative fungi that are responsible for the mycoses listed, the only fungus that produce yeast cell, pseudohyphae, and hyphal cell is *Candida albicans*. *Cryptococcus neoformans* that causes human cryptococcosis grows as yeast form both in vitro and in vivo. Aspergilli, which are responsible for human aspergillosis, *Zygomycetes* that cause zygomycoses, and *Actinomyces*, the causative agent for actinomycosis (incidentally, this is a bacterial infection), are not dimorphic and do not become yeast form at any stages of their life cycle. *(Ryan et al, pp 591–599)*

726. **(C)** This dermatophyte is an anthropophilic dermatophyte unabale to survive in soil or in animals (except for humans). This dermatophyte is responsible for chronic, recurrent dermatophyhtosis that is difficult to cure. Dermatophytosis due to *Trichophyton rubrum* rarely heals spontaneously. Like any other dermatophyte infection, *T. rubrum* infection is confined to the superficial keratinous tissues. *(Ryan et al, pp 585–589)*

727. **(D)** Mucormycosis is a form of zygomycosis (phycomycosis) that affects compromised hosts only. All fungi resonsible for zygomycosis are morphologically characterized by

the absence of septa in their hyphae (coenocytic hyphae). Multiple nuclei are shared by one hypha. Hyphae of other fungi are usually septated. Spherules are diagnostically useful structures seen in coccidioidomycosis. Encapsulated yeast cells are seen in *Cryptococcus neoformans* infection. Pseudohyphae are produced by *Candida albicans* when it invades the host tissues. *(Ryan et al, p 599)*

728. **(C)** Although most bacteria generate their own ATP, its synthesis occurs on the cytoplasmic membrane (bacteria have no mitochondira). Bacterial nuclei are not surrounded by the nuclear membrane, whereas fungal nuclei are surrounded by the distinct nuclear membrane. Essentially all bacterial cell walls contain cross-linked peptidoglycan. In fungi, peptidoglycan is replaced with chitin and glucans. Only fungi are susceptible to polyene antibiotics because they possess ergosterol in their cytoplasmic membrane. Thus, the only characteristic that is shared by both bacteria and fungi is the presence of the cell wall outside of their cytoplasmic membrane. *(Ryan et al, pp 571–577)*

729. **(E)** Clinically all of these diseases may present similar symptoms. This patient inhaled *Histoplasma capsulatum* conidia while exploring the cave. *H. capsulatum* grows well and forms conidia in moist soil enriched with bird droppings. In the United States, infestation of *H. caspulatum* is commonly seen in southeastern states drained by the Ohio and Mississippi Rivers. The fact that two of his friends who participated in this journey also developed similar symptoms suggests they all inhaled large doses of *H. capsulatum* conidia while exploring the cave resulting in active infection. When infected with *H. capsulatum* conidia, they usually develop a positive delayed-type hypersensitivity to histoplasmin (an *H. capsulatum* antigen) regardless of whether they develop active infection or not. The past history of this patient and his positive reaction to the histoplasmin test support the conclusion. It should be kept in mind, however, that more cautions are necessary in interpreting the result of the histoplasmin test if the patient is from the Ohio–Missis-

sippi Valley areas because more than 50% of residents in these areas are histoplasmin positive. *(Ryan et al, pp 603–606)*

730. **(D)** *Sporothrix schenkii* is a ubiquitous fungus found in soil, decaying organic matter, and on the surface of plants. Thus, sporotrichosis occurs predominantly in those people who are exposed to soil, trees, and plants. Infection is acquired by traumatic implantation of conidia. Although other mycotic infections listed in this quesitons are transmitted through conidia, they are usually not limited to any particular types of occupation. *(Ryan et al, pp 613–615)*

731. **(A)** *Blastomyces dermatitidis* is a dimorphic fungus that causes blastomycosis. It grows as yeast in infected tissues. The organism produces the characteristic yeast form with broad-based buds, which is of use diagnostically. Broad-based buds are not formed by the organisms that cause the other infections listed in the question. *(Joklik et al, pp 1103–1108; Ryan et al, pp 606–607)*

732. **(D)** Nocardia (*Nocardia asteroides*) is not a fungus although it grows filamentously and forms a colony that resembles a fungal colony. It is classified as prokaryote (bacterium). Nocardiosis due to *N. asteroides* is characterized by the formation of multiple and confluent abscesses and intense suppuration. In contrast to actinomycosis, a similar disease caused by *Actinomyces israelii*, the nocardial lesions show less fibrosis, burrowing, and cavity formation. Sulfur granules are never present. *(Joklik et al, p 534; Ryan et al, pp 419–421)*

733. **(A)** The most common natural reservoir for *Cryptococcus neoformans* is the soil and avian feces, and infection follows airborne exposure and inhalation of the yeast. *Candida* is not commonly found in bird droppings. *(Joklik et al, p 1144; Ryan et al, pp 601–603)*

734. **(E)** Chromomycosis and phaeohyphomycosis are caused by dematiaceous fungi, which are imperfect fungi that produce varying amounts of melanine-like pigments. These pigments are found in the conidia or hyphae or both and give the organism an olive green, brown, or black color. Among the fungi that cause chromomycosis, *Fonsecaea pedrosoi* is the most common. The pathology of chromomycosis typically consists of granulomatous nodules and epithelial hyperplasia. *(Joklik et al, p 1118; Ryan et al, p 615)*

735. **(E)** Among the mycotic infections listed in the question, aspergillosis and candidiasis are considered as opportunistic infections. Aspergilli, though abundantly growing in the environment surrounding us, are not members of the normal microbial flora in humans. Thus, aspergillosis is not an endogenous opportunistic mycotic infection. Aspergillosis usually occurs as a result of inhalation of or exposure to air-borne conidia. *Candida* species, particularly *Candida albicans*, are members of the normal microbial flora of the skin, mucous membranes, and gastrointestinal tract. Thus, candidiasis is considered an endogenous infection. *(Joklik et al, pp 1136,1147; Ryan et al, pp 591–599)*

736. **(E)** *Sprothrix schenckii*, causative agent for sporotrichosis; *Fonsecaea pedrosoi* and related fungi, which cause chromomycosis; *Histoplasma capsulatum*, which causes histoplasmosis; and *Candida albicans*, causative fungus for candidiasis, are all dimorphic fungi. Of these dimorphic fungi, only *Candida albicans* grows in mycelial form in infected tissues. Aspergilli are not dimorphic fungi. *(Joklik et al, pp 1071–1153; Ryan et al, p 693)*

737. **(D)** This drug (5-fluorocytosine or flucytosine) is useful in the systemic treatment of some deep-seated fungal infections in humans, particularly candidiasis, cryptococcosis, and chromomycosis. Only in chromomycosis, however, is this the drug of choice. Since flucytosine-resistant strains may emerge rapidly if the drug is used alone, it is usually used in combination with amphotericin B in candidiasis and cryptococcosis. Griseofulvin is the drug of choice for dermatophytosis. Ketoconazole is used for the treatment of candidiasis, dermatophytosis, and systemic mycoses. *(Joklik et al, p 1089)*

738. **(E)** Both amphotericin B and nystatin are polyene antibiotics. Because of its high toxicity, nystatin cannot be administered intravenously. Nystatin is clinically useful. Its most important use is in the treatment of cutaneous or superficial infections caused by *Candida*. *(Joklik et al, p 165; Ryan et al, p 582)*

739. **(A)** Fluconazole is a new class of antifungal agent. It is N-substituted imidazole with an antifungal spectrum and mechanism of action similar to that of the imidazole derivatives (ketoconazole, miconazole, and clotrimazole). Fluconazole is better tolerated when administered orally than the imidazole derivatives. It interferes with the synthesis of fungal ergosterol. *(Joklik et al, pp 165–166; Ryan et al, pp 583–584)*

740. **(B)** Periodic acid Schiff (PAS) is a useful stain to demonstrate fungi in pathohistologic specimens. The fungal cell wall is specifically stained by the PAS reagent. The other stain often used in staining fungal elements in pathohistologic preparations is the methenamine silver stain. *(Joklik et al, p 1075)*

741. **(C)** Calcofluor stains chitin and cellulose. Since chitin is one of the common components of fungal cell walls, this fluorescent dye is a useful stain to demonstrate fungi microscopically. *(Joklik et al, p 1075; Ryan et al, p 576)*

742. **(E)** Cornmeal agar is a special medium deficient in readily metabolizable substrates. When *Candida albicans* is cultured on cornmeal agar, it produces characteristic chlamydospores at the tip of pseudohyphae. No other candidal species produce similar chlamydospores. Conidia of other types listed in the question are not formed on cornmeal agar. *(Joklik et al, p 1137)*

743. **(D)** The dermatophyte *Trichophyton mentagrophytes* produces two types of conidia, microconidia and macroconidia. Macroconidium is a multicellular spore with multiple septa. The morphology of these conidia, when combined with other morphological and biochemical characteristics, helps iden-

tify species of dermatophytes. *(Joklik et al, p 1127; Ryan et al, p 587)*

744. **(J)** Of all the microorganisms listed, *Actinomyces* is the only prokaryotic cell. All others are fungi, which are eukaryotic cells. The common feature of all actinomycetes is their tendency to form filaments. Actinomycetous filaments become quite long and branched extensively. These filaments are often termed (wrongly) hyphae or mycelia because of their resemblance to mold. All actinomycetes are bacteria, not mold, despite their superficial morphologic resemblance. *(Joklik et al, p 526; Ryan et al, pp 417–419)*

REFERENCES

Joklik WK, Willett HP, Amos DB, Wilfert CM. *Zinsser Microbiology*, 20th ed. Norwalk, CT: Appleton & Lange; 1992.

Roitt I, Brostoff J, Male D. *Immunology*, 4th ed. London: Mosby; 1996.

Ryan KJ, Champoux JJ, Drew WL, et al. *Sherris Medical Microbiology*, 3rd ed. Norwalk, CT: Appleton & Lange; 1994.

CHAPTER 7

Medical Parasitology
Questions

DIRECTIONS (Questions 745 through 770): Each of the numbered items or incomplete statements in this section is followed by answers or by completions of the statement. Select the ONE lettered answer or completion that is BEST in each case.

745. The egg (ovum) shown in the sketch is diagnostic of

Figure 7–1

(A) *Strongyloides stercoralis*
(B) *Enterobius vermicularis*
(C) *Ascaris lumbricoides*
(D) *Ancylostoma duodenale*
(E) *Trichuris trichiura*

746. An 18-month-old child passed a "big worm" that resembles an earthworm. The most likely diagnosis is

(A) *Trichuris trichiura*
(B) *Enterobius vermicularis*
(C) *Ascaris lumbricoides*
(D) *Strongyloides stercoralis*
(E) *Necator americanus*

747. A 37-year-old man who had been in excellent health visited Tanzania where he was bitten on the leg by tsetse flies. He developed in that leg an indurated skin lesion. A few days later, he had a fever of 40°C, lymphadenopathy, a tendency to sleep frequently, apathy, and mental depression. Microscopic examination of lymph node aspirates showed actively motile organisms 5 to 15 μm long that were shaped like a curved, flattened blade with a free flagellum to the posterior end. The most likely etiologic agent responsible for this illness is

(A) *Trichomonas vaginalis*
(B) *Pneumocystis carinii*
(C) *Trypanosoma cruzi*
(D) *Entamoeba histolytica*

748. Which of the following statements is NOT true about the treatment of echinococcosis?

(A) most chemotherapeutic agents are relatively ineffective
(B) praziquantel or bendozole may be useful for the treatment of early echinococcosis
(C) treatment is basically surgical
(D) care must be exercised not to break hydatid cysts during surgical removal
(E) all cysts need to be surgically removed

749. The following infected erythrocyte is characteristic for the ring stage of

Figure 7–2

(A) *Plasmodium vivax*
(B) *Plasmodium ovale*
(C) *Plasmodium malariae*
(D) *Plasmodium falciparum*
(E) *Plasmodium latum*

750. A 43-year-old woman has been brought to a local clinic where it was established that she had filariasis. This was likely based on

(A) visible microfilaria on blood smears
(B) presence of eosinophilia
(C) presence of antibody to the pinworm
(D) positive complement fixation tests

751. Onchocerciasis is acquired by bite of an infected

(A) tsetse fly (*Glossina*)
(B) blackfly (*Simulium*)
(C) sandfly (*Lutzomyia*)
(D) sandfly (*Phlebotomus*)
(E) mosquito (*Anopheles*)

752. A skin biopsy taken from the lesion of an individual with mucocutaneous leishmaniasis is most likely to show

(A) flagellated promastigotes in polymorphonuclear neutrophils
(B) schizonts
(C) amastigotes undergoing binary fission
(D) eosinophilic granuloma formation
(E) extensive tissue necrosis with only rare protozoan forms

753. The scolex (head) shown in the sketch is diagnostic of

Figure 7–3

(A) *Taenia saginata*
(B) *Diphyllobothrium latum*
(C) *Leishmania donovani*
(D) *Toxoplasma gondii*
(E) *Balantidium coli*

754. A patient had a history of cyclical fever of 102°F, with drowsiness, marked jaundice, headache, some disorientation, anemia, thrombocytopenia, and hyperbilirubinemia. Blood smears show plasmodium parasitemia of 28%. Diagnosis of malaria was confirmed on the basis of finding

(A) lemon-shaped cysts in striated muscles
(B) developing organisms in spleen biopsies
(C) parasitized red blood cells
(D) free-swimming flagellate forms of the parasite

755. The main attribute of *Entamoeba histolytica* that is responsible for its worldwide distribution may be due to

(A) extreme antigenic variation
(B) unusual stability of its cyst in the environment
(C) unusual motility of trophozoites in contaminated water
(D) widespread distribution by mosquitoes

756. A cestode that competes with its definitive host for dietary vitamin B_{12} is

(A) *Taenia saginata*
(B) *Taenia solium*

(C) *Diphyllobothrium latum*

(D) *Hymenolepis nana*

(E) *Echinococcus granulosus*

757. The insect vector of *Trypanosoma cruzi* is the

(A) sandfly (*Phlebotomus*)

(B) tsetse fly (*Glossina*)

(C) sandfly (*Lutzomyia*)

(D) kissing bug (*Reduviid*)

(E) blackfly (*Simulium*)

758. Which organism is associated with blood in the urine and chronic urinary tract obstruction?

(A) *Schistosoma mansoni*

(B) *Schistosoma haematobium*

(C) *Schistosoma japonicum*

(D) *Dracunculus medinensis*

(E) *Paragonimus westermani*

759. Involvement of the liver, lungs, and eyes in humans (usually children) occurs after ingestion of the ova of the dog ascarid, known as

(A) *Ascaris lumbricoides*

(B) *Onchocerca volvulus*

(C) *Loa loa*

(D) *Toxocara canis*

(E) *Strongyloides stercoralis*

760. The developmental form of *Leishmania* transmitted to humans is the

(A) trypomastigote

(B) epimastigote

(C) promastigote

(D) amastigote

(E) nomastigote

761. The form of the hemoflagellates (*Leishmania* or *Trypanosoma*) seen within mammalian cells is the

(A) amastigote (leishmanial stage)

(B) promastigote (leptomonad stage)

(C) epimastigote (crithidial stage)

(D) trypomastigote (trypanosomal stage)

(E) none of the above

762. Humans may acquire *Toxoplasma gondii* by

(A) the venereal route

(B) ingestion of cysts in poorly cooked meat

(C) sustaining a cat bite

(D) swimming (wading) in contaminated water

(E) penetration of the skin of the lower extremity by the oocyst

763. A 28-year-old woman with acquired immunodeficiency syndrome (AIDS) who has had five cats in her small apartment for the past 18 months has episodes of confusion and seizures. A computed tomography scan indicates three ring-enhancing cavitary brain lesions. The most likely cause of these brain lesions is

(A) *Plasmodium ovale*

(B) *Entamoeba coli*

(C) *Toxoplasma gondii*

(D) *Cryptosporidium parvum*

764. A homosexual patient developed a sudden and explosive diarrhea. The stools were foul-smelling, greasy, and devoid of blood or mucus. Microscopic examination of the stools showed sting-ray–shaped trophozoites 9 to 15 μm long, with four pairs of flagella. The most likely cause of diarrhea in this patient is

(A) *Giardia lamblia*

(B) *Trichomonas vaginalis*

(C) *Leishmania donovani*

(D) *Trypanosoma brucei*

765. The event that correlates with the presence of fever paroxysm in *Plasmodium vivax* malaria is

(A) inoculation of sporozoites by the mosquito
(B) invasion of hepatocytes by sporozoites
(C) invasion of new red blood cells by merozoites
(D) schizont rupture
(E) gametocyte formation

766. The adult stage of the cestode life cycle does NOT take place in humans infected with

(A) *Taenia saginata*
(B) *Taenia solium*
(C) *Diphyllobothrium latum*
(D) *Echinococcus granulosus*

767. Disease is acquired by the oral route and the major site of pathology is the hepatobiliary system in humans infected with

(A) *Schistosoma mansoni*
(B) *Schistosoma haematobium*
(C) *Schistosoma mekongi*
(D) *Opisthorchis sinensis*

768. Natural resistance to malaria caused by *Plasmodium vivax* has been demonstrated in populations who are

(A) Duffy blood group antigen positive
(B) glycophorin A positive
(C) glucose 6-phosphate dehydrogenase deficient
(D) Duffy blood group antigen negative

769. A nonflagellated protozoan that causes gastroenteritis in humans is

(A) *Entamoeba histolytica*
(B) *Trichomonas vaginalis*
(C) *Balantidium coli*
(D) *Giardia lamblia*

770. Diagnosis cannot usually be established by examination of the stool in persons infected with

(A) *Ascaris lumbricoides*
(B) *Strongyloides stercoralis*
(C) *Taenia saginata*
(D) *Schistosoma mansoni*
(E) *Onchocerca volvulus*

DIRECTIONS (Questions 771 through 781): Each group of items in this section consists of lettered headings followed by a set of numbered words or phrases. For each word or phrase, select the ONE lettered heading that is most closely associated with it. Each lettered heading may be selected once, more that once, or not at all.

Questions 771 and 772

(A) *Toxoplasma gondii*
(B) *Trypanosoma cruzi*
(C) *Naegleria fowleri*
(D) *Cryptosporidium*
(E) *Plasmodium falciparum*

771. Congenital blindness and central nervous system involvement

772. Coccidian protozoan restricted to production of intestinal disease and especially in AIDS patients

Questions 773 and 774

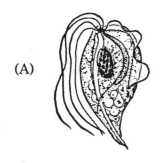

(A)

Figure 7–4

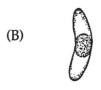

(B)

Figure 7–5

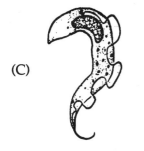

(C)

Figure 7–6

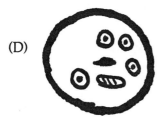

(D)

Figure 7–7

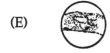

(E)

Figure 7–8

773. Causative agent of Chagas' disease

774. Sexually transmitted urogenital tract protozoan

Questions 775 through 777

(A) *Wuchereria bancrofti*
(B) *Onchocerca volvulus*
(C) *Enterobius vermicularis*
(D) *Trichinella spiralis*
(E) *Necator americanus*
(F) *Taenia solium*
(G) *Diphyllobothrium latum*
(H) *Taenia saginata*
(I) *Hymenolepis nana*
(J) *Schistosoma japonicum*
(K) *Schistosoma haematobium*
(L) *Clonorchis sinensis*
(M) *Paragonimus westermani*

775. Skeletal muscle, cardiac, and central nervous system involvement

776. Generally humans are infected by eating raw beef

777. Adult parasites are usually in the parenchyma of the human lung

Questions 778 and 779

(A) sporozoan intestinal disease in AIDS patients
(B) interstitial pneumonitis in an immunosuppressed patient
(C) fulminant hemorrhagic meningoencephalitis after swimming
(D) flatulent diarrhea after travel to Moscow
(E) hepatic abscess

778. *Entamoeba histolytica*

779. *Pneumocystis carinii*

Questions 780 and 781

(A) *Wuchereria bancrofti*

(B) *Trichinella spiralis*

(C) *Plasmodium malariae*

(D) *Enterobius vermicularis*

(E) *Entamoeba coli*

780. Over the past 3 months, a 12-year-old boy heated slightly homemade pork sausage and had dinner on many occasions; now he has developed periorbital eosinophilia and severe muscular pains

781. A 5-year-old girl who spent a year attending school in West Africa returned to the United States because of poor sleeping and intense itching in her anal area; anal swab samples showed the presence of symmetrical ova, flattened on one side and containing a larvae

Medical Parasitology
Answers and Explanations

745. **(E)** The ovum shown in the sketch is produced by the nematode *Trichuris trichiura*. Malnourished children are most commonly infected by ingesting food or water containing embryonated eggs. Diagnosis is easily made by the demonstration in feces of eggs with polar plugs. The eggs produced by *Enterobius vermicularis* are asymmetrical and are flattened on one side. *Ascaris lumbricoides* produces ova with several layers, and the outermost egg layer has characteristic nipple-like projections. Finally, the hookworm *Ancylostoma duodenale* produces symmetrically oval, thin-shelled eggs. (*Joklik et al, pp 1191–1197*)

746. **(C)** *Ascaris lumbricoides* is the largest intestinal roundworm, measuring 15 to 35 cm, and it is passed in stools. Adult *Trichuris trichiura* is seldom found in stools because the worms are attached firmly to the intestinal wall. *Enterobius vermicularis* ova (50 to 60 μm) containing larvae are usually not found in the stools. They are recovered from the perianal area with cellophane tape or swabs. Definitive diagnosis of *Strongyloides stercoralis* is based on the demonstration of larvae in the feces. These larvae usually are less than 1 cm long. *Necator americanus* intestinal infections are diagnosed by finding 50- to 60-μm thin-walled ova in the stools. (*Joklik et al, pp 1187–1197*)

747. **(C)** Key features which suggest *Trypanosoma cruzi* as the etiological agent include the bites of tsetse flies that serve as the biological vectors of trypanosomiasis, the visit to Tanzania where trypanosomosis is prominent, the detection of trypanosomes in lymph node aspirates, and the encephalitis which caused this 37-year-old man to sleep frequently and be apathetic and mentally depressed. *Entamoeba histolytica* is a spherical organism which usually causes gastroenteritis or liver abscesses and is transmitted by the fecal oral route. *Pneumocystis carinii* is the cause of diffuse pneumonitis in immunocompromised individuals. *Trichomonas vaginalis* may induce vaginitis; it is a pear-shaped organism 7 to 30 μm in diameter with five flagella, and it is transmitted by sexual intercourse. (*Ryan et al, pp 619–622,659–663,668–670,679–683*)

748. **(E)** Most chemotherapeutic agents are relatively ineffective for the treatment of echinococcosis. Praziquantel, or bendazole, has been reported to be useful for the treatment of early echinococcosis. However, treatment is purely surgical. If it is impossible to remove the intact hydatid cyst, marsupialization and sterilization of the cyst contents with 2% formalin in 30% sodium chloride and 2% iodine may be effective. Not all cysts need to be surgically removed. Removal is indicated when they appear to cause symptoms and are likely to compromise host organ function. Care must be exercised not to break the hydatid cysts during surgical removal, because release of the hydatid cyst contents may cause anaphylaxis. (*Ryan et al, pp 716–717*)

749. **(D)** Malaria is considered to be a destructive and economically wasteful protozoan disease. It is caused by various species of the genus *Plasmodium*. Four species of *Plasmodium* are capable of causing malaria in man. One of these, *P. ovale*, is very rare. The other three recognized species are *P. falciparum*, *P. vivax*, and *P. malariae*. The organisms are strictly parasitic and have two hosts—humans and the *Anopheles* mosquitoes. In humans, they live mainly inside red blood cells in which they undergo a number of characteristic microgametocyte and macrogametocyte stages. The ring stages of *P. vivax*, *P. malariae*, and *P. ovale* are coarse, one-third to one-half of the diameter of the red blood cell, and there is usually one ring per red blood cell. *P. falciparum* (shown in Fig. 7–2) forms two fine rings about one-sixth to one-fifth of the diameter of the red blood cell. Blood smears stained with the Giemsa stain clearly show these two fine rings, which are used to diagnose malaria caused by *P. falciparum*. *(Brooks et al, pp 347–351)*

750. **(A)** Eosinophilia may be present during the acute inflammatory stage of filariasis. However, definitive diagnosis of this parasitic disease, which is caused by *Wuchereria bancrofti*, rests upon the demonstration of *W. bancrofti* microfilaria in the blood, lymph, or pleural fluids. Various serologic tests have been developed for the diagnosis of filariasis, but they generally lack specificity and sensitivity. The presence of antibody to *Enterobius vermicularis* (pinworm) cannot be of any value in the diagnosis of filariasis. *(Ryan et al, pp 704–705)*

751. **(B)** Onchocerciasis caused by *Onchocerca volvulus* is acquired by bites of infected female blackflies belonging to genus *Simulium*. Infective larvae are deposited when the blackflies bite. Then an inflammation develops, followed by pruritic papules and nodules due to a response to *O. volvulus* proteins. Microfilaria then migrate and concentrate in the eyes and cause lesions that can lead to blindness. *Trypanosoma gambiense* is transmitted from person to person by the tsetse flies. The sandfly *Phlebotomus* transmits *Leishmania donovani*, and the sandfly *Lutzomyia* is the chief vector of *Leishmania tropica* or *Leishma-*

nia braziliensis. *(Ryan et al, pp 706–707; Joklik et al, pp 1177–1178)*

752. **(C)** A skin biopsy taken from the lesion of an individual with cutaneous leishmaniasis is most likely to show amastigotes undergoing binary fission. This is so because the life cycle of *Leishmania donovani*, the causative agent of leishmaniasis is as follows: The amastigotes of *L. donovani* are ingested from human tissues by the small biting sand flies. Then the amastigotes develop into the promastigotes in midgut of the sandflies and migrate to the mouth and pharynx of the sandflies. Now, the promastigotes of *L. donovani* are ready for injection into human and other hosts by the sandflies and upon injection change to amastigotes in human tissues. Therefore, diagnosis of leishmaniasis depends on the demonstration of amastigotes in stained smears of biopsy material. Schizonts are morphologic forms of the parasites causing malaria. The pathology of leishmaniasis is basically a hyperplasia. *(Joklik et al, pp 1178–1179)*

753. **(A)** The scolex (head) shown in the sketch belongs to the cestode (tapeworm) *Taenia saginata*. The diagnosis of taeniasis is based on the recovery of the typical thomboidal head with its four suckers without hooks. The scolex of *Diphyllobothrium latum* resembles a spatula and it has in its center ventral and dorsal grooved suckers. *Leishmania donovani*, *Toxoplasma gondii*, and *Balantidium coli* lack scoleces. *(Joklik et al, pp 1205–1208)*

754. **(C)** The diagnosis of malaria is confirmed on the basis of finding red blood cells that contain malarial parasites. Usually capillary or venous blood is used to prepare and stain with Giemsa or Wright stains thick and thin blood smears. Thick smears are useful for the detection of light parasitemia, which may not be detected with thin blood smears. The malaria parasites do not form cysts or flagellated organisms. *(Ryan et al, pp 641–650)*

755. **(B)** The main attribute of *Entamoeba histolytica* that is responsible for its worldwide distribution may be due to the extreme stability of its cyst in the environment. Extreme antigenic variation has not been documented in *E. histolytica* and certainly there is no evidence that shows clearly that antigenic variation can explain the worldwide distribution of *E. histolytica*. Amebiasis is usually acquired by direct person to person contact via the fecal–oral route. The trophozoites of *E. histolytica* die rapidly in the external environment. *(Ryan et al, pp 659–665)*

756. **(C)** *Diphyllobothrium latum* is the fish tapeworm (cestode). This tapeworm resides in the small intestine and absorbs large quantities of vitamin B_{12}. If the parasite is located in the proximal portion of the jejunum, hyperchromic changes and even pernicious anemia may occur. *(Joklik et al, pp 1206–1208)*

757. **(D)** Infective forms of *Trypanosoma cruzi* pass to humans by inoculation of infected *Reduviid* bug feces into the conjunctiva or a break in the skin, *not* by the bite of the insect. *Trypanosoma gambiense* is transmitted from person to person by the tsetse fly (*Glossina palpalis*). The sandfly (*Phlebotomus*) transmits *Leishmania donovani*, and *Lutzomyia* sandfly is the chief vector in the transmission of leishmanias *Leishmania braziliensis*, *Leishmania tropica*, and *Leishmania mexicana*) in the New World. *(Joklik et al, pp 1177–1178)*

758. **(B)** *Schistosoma haematobium* occurs predominantly in Africa and the Middle East regions. This fluke may produce obstructive uropathy and genital elephantiasis. *(Joklik et al, pp 1211–1215)*

759. **(D)** *Toxocara canis* or *Toxocara catis* is an ascarid worm of the dog or cat. Embryonated eggs are ingested, usually by children. The larvae hatch, penetrate the intestinal mucosa, and wander in the viscera (liver, brain, eye, spinal cord, lungs, cardiac muscle, kidneys, and lymph nodes), causing fever, hepatomegaly, eosinophilia, and ocular manifestations. *(Joklik et al, pp 1194–1196)*

760. **(C)** The genus *Leishmania* includes four species: *Leishmania tropica*, *Leishmania dono-*

vani, *Leishmania mexicana*, and *Leishmania braziliensis*, all of which occur as promastigotes in the phlebotomine sandfly. Leishmaniasis is transmitted to humans by the promastigotes. *(Joklik et al, pp 1178–1179)*

761. **(A)** The amastigote is the form of hemoflagellate seen within mammalian cells. *(Joklik et al, pp 1178–1179)*

762. **(B)** Many animals, both wild and domestic, are infected with *Toxoplasma gondii*. Humans become infected primarily by eating poorly cooked or raw meat containing cysts. Contamination of food or drink with oocysts from cat feces also occurs, but the actual transmission of the disease by the latter route is questionable. *(Joklik et al, pp 1183–1184)*

763. **(C)** A variety of opportunistic infections occur usually in patients with AIDS. The most frequently encountered parasitic organisms are *Pneumocystis carinii*, *Toxoplasma gondii*, and *Cryptosporidium parvum*. The diseases these three parasitic organisms cause are pneumonia, encephalitis, and enteritis, respectively. Infection of humans with *T. gondii* begins from contact with cat feces which contain cysts of *T. gondii*. Domestic cats and other felines are the definitive hosts of *T. gondii*. *Plasmodium ovale* causes malaria, the chief clinical manifestation of which is reduction of red blood cells with subsequent jaundice. *Entamoeba coli* is a nonpathogenic parasite that can be found in the human intestinal tract. Since our patient had five cats in her apartment, had AIDS, and developed encephalitis, the most likely cause of her illness from the four parasites listed in this question is *T. gondii*. *(Ryan et al, pp 641–655; Joklik et al, p 1164)*

764. **(A)** The most likely organism that caused diarrhea in this patient is *Giardia lamblia*. This organism is a sting-ray–shaped trophozoite 9 to 21 μm long, 5 to 15 μm wide, and 2 to 4 μm thick. The parasite appears as a face with two bespectacled eyes and a slanted mouth. *G. lambia* has four pairs of flagella and resides in the alkaline environment of the duodenum and jejunum. In the descending colon, the flagella are drawn into the cytoplasm and a cyst wall is produced. The cysts that are formed are oval and smaller than the trophozoites. The cysts are the infective forms of *G. lamblia*, may survive in cold water for 2 months, and are resistant to the levels of chlorine found usually in municipal water. They are transmitted from host to host by the fecal–oral route and may cause a sudden, explosive diarrhea, in which the stools are foul-smelling, greasy, and devoid of blood or mucus. Direct person-to-person transmission of *G. lamblia* appears to be responsible for the high infection rate in male homosexuals. *Trichomonas vaginalis* causes vaginitis, *Leishmania donovani* causes cutaneous ulcers or visceral infection (kala-azar), and *Trypanosoma brucei* is the cause of sleeping sickness, skin lesions, lymphadenitis, and vasculitis. *(Ryan et al, pp 668–680)*

765. **(D)** Periodic fever paroxysms of malaria are closely related to events in the bloodstream. An initial chill, lasting 15 minutes to 1 hour, begins as a generation of parasites (mature schizonts) rupture their host red cells and escape into the blood. The succeeding febrile stage, lasting several hours, is characterized by a spiking fever. During this period, the parasites (merozoites) invade new erythrocytes. Certain merozoites that entered red cells become differentiated as male or female gametocytes. These gametocytes are taken up and ingested by blood-sucking female *Anopheles*. *(Joklik et al, pp 1180–1182)*

766. **(D)** *Echinococcus granulosus* is a dog tapeworm in which sheep are the usual intermediate host. Humans, when closely involved with dogs and sheep, may accidentally ingest eggs from dog feces and become intermediate hosts. *(Joklik et al, pp 1210–1211)*

767. **(D)** Ova of the parasite (fluke) *Opisthorchis sinensis* pass through the freshwater snail and encyst in fish flesh. Ingested raw or poorly cooked fish releases the metacercaria, which migrates luminally to the biliary tree. *(Joklik et al, p 1215)*

768. **(D)** *Plasmodium vivax* (but not *Plasmodium ovale*) requires Duffy group receptors on erythrocytes in order to penetrate the erythrocyte membrane, and these receptors are lacking in many Africans, particularly West Africans. *(Joklik et al, pp 1180–1182)*

769. **(A)** *Entamoeba histolytica* is a nonflagellated protozoan that infects the cecum and colon (dysentery). Bloodstream invasion results in dissemination to the liver and then to other organs. *Trichomonas vaginalis*, which is a flagellated protozoan, causes vaginitis. *Balantidium coli* is a nonpathogenic, nonflagellated protozoan. *E. histolytica* and *Giardia lamblia* may be transmitted sexually, especially among homosexual males. *Giardia lamblia* is a flagellated protozoan that causes diarrhea. *(Joklik et al, pp 1164,1170–1173)*

770. **(E)** The detection of ova or larvae in feces is essential for the diagnosis of infection with *Ascaris lumbricoides*, *Strongyloides stercoralis*, *Taenia saginata*, and *Schistosoma mansoni*. The diagnosis of *Onchocerca volvulus* is made by demonstrating microfilaria in a thin skin sample taken from an involved area. When the eye is involved, the organism may be seen in the anterior chamber. *(Joklik et al, pp 1192,1208,1211–1213)*

771. **(A)** *Toxoplasma gondii* is a protozoan that produces crescentic cells in the brain, eye, and other tissues, causing congenital blindness and central nervous system syndromes. Fatal infections occur in AIDS patients and immunosuppressed individuals. *T. gondii* may cause retinitis, chorioretinitis, encephalitis, and pneumonitis. *Trypanosoma cruzi* is the causative agent of trypanosomiasis or sleeping sickness. *Plasmodium falciparum* is a malarial protozoan that is involved in the production of the most severe form of malaria. *Naegleria fowleri* is a free-living ameba that has been associated with amebic meningoencephalitis. *(Joklik et al, pp 1174–1185)*

772. **(D)** *Cryptosporidium* species are coccidian protozoa which are related to toxoplasmas. However, they differ from toxoplasmas in that they cause infections restricted to the epithelial cells of the intestine. In AIDS patients, they produce severe diarrhea. See previous answer as to why the other choices are incorrect. (*Joklik et al, pp 1171–1185*)

773. **(C)** Chagas' disease, or American trypanosomiasis, is caused by *Trypanosoma cruzi*, which is a typical flagellate protozoan. As shown in sketch C, it is a curved, stumpy trypanosome about 20μ long with a pointed posterior end, an elongated nucleus, and a long flagellum. Sketches A, B, D, and E represent *Trichomonas vaginalis*, the macrogametocyte of *Plasmodium falciparum*, *Entamoeba histolytica*, and the developing schizont of *Plasmodium malariae*, which are the etiological agents of trichomoniasis, malignant tertian malaria, amebiasis, and quartan malaria, respectively. (*Joklik et al, pp 1164–1182*)

774. **(A)** *Trichomonas vaginalis* is a protozoan that is sexually transmitted. It causes discomfort, purulent urethritis, itching, and irritation of the urogenital tract. The trichomonas are all spindle or pear-shaped organisms easily recognized by their three-to-five free anterior flagella and their undulating membrane. The protozoa also contain stiff axostyle, a nucleus, and in many cases a sausage-shaped parabasal body. See previous answer as to why the other choices are incorrect. (*Joklik et al, pp 1171–1185*)

775. **(D)** Individuals with trichinosis caused by *Trichinella spiralis* acquire this protozoan by ingesting infective larvae, which become adults in the tissues. Following the initial gastrointestinal phase, the parasite has a tendency to cause damage in skeletal muscle in such vital tissues as nervous and cardiac tissue. This damage leads to neurologic symptoms and myocarditis with congestive heart failure. *Wuchereria bancrofti* and *Onchocerca volvulus* are the etiologic agents of lymphadenitis. *Enterobius vermicularis*, *Necator americanus*, *Taenia solium*, *Taenia saginata*, *Diphyllobothrium latum*, and *Hymenolepis nana* are

primarily associated with infections characterized by abdominal discomfort, itching, diarrhea, weight loss, anorexia, and vomiting. *Schistosoma japonicum* and *Schistosoma haematobium* cause infection of the urinary bladder or occasional lung lesions. *Clonorchis sinensis*, the liver fluke, causes biliary hyperplasia, connective tissue hyperplasia, fatty degeneration of liver parenchyma, portal liver cirrhosis, and pancreatitis. *Paragonimus westermani* causes a tuberculosis-like illness characterized by low-grade fever, weight loss, hemoptysis, and cough. (*Joklik et al, pp 1187–1215*)

776. **(H)** *Taenia saginata*, also known as the beef tapeworm, is transmitted to humans by the ingestion of raw or improperly cooked beef. *Taenia solium*, the port tapeworm, enter the human body by eating raw pork. *Wuchereria bancrofti* and *Onchocerca volvulus* infections are the results of infected mosquito and blackfly bites, respectively. Eating infected raw or improperly cooked fish may lead to infection by *Clonorchis sinensis* or *Diphyllobothrium latum*. Consumption of raw, infected, freshwater crabs and crayfish is the means by which *Paragonimus westermani* is acquired by individuals. *Schistosoma japonicum* and *Schistosoma haematobium* transmission to humans is via ingestion of metacercaria or penetration of the human skin by cercaria (the larval forms of *S. japonicum* and *S. haematobium*). *Hymenolepis nana*, *Enterobius vermicularis*, and *Necator americanus* infections result from the ingestion of ova produced by these microorganisms. (*Joklik et al, pp 1164–1215*)

777. **(M)** *Paragonimus westermani* adult flukes tend to live in the parenchyma of the human lung and cause pulmonary infection, resembling tuberculosis. *Necator americanus* larvae, but not adult parasites, may also be found in the human lungs, and thus be the cause of pneumonitis. Adult *Schistosoma japonicum* and *Schistosoma haematobium* are found in the mesenteric veins and vesicular vein on the outside wall of intestine or the urinary bladder. *Clonorchis sinensis* adult worms live in the distal bile ducts, the biliary passages, the gallbladder, and the pancreatic duct.

Wuchereria bancrofti and *Onchocerca volvulus* adult parasites are localized in the lymphatic system where they produce lymphadenitis. Finally, adult *Enterobius vermicularis, Necator americanus, Taenia solium, Taenia saginata, Diphyllobothrium latum,* and *Hymenolepis nana* are usually attached to the wall of the intestine. *(Joklik et al, pp 1187–1215)*

778. **(E)** *Entamoeba histolytica* is the etiologic agent of amebic dysentery. Contaminated water is the most common mode of the spread of this infection, which is usually a mild gastrointestinal disease. However, *E. histolytica* can burrow into the mucosa of the large intestine and cause ulceration. Furthermore, it can also enter the bloodstream through the capillaries of the portal system and cause secondary foci of infection, particularly in the liver, where it produces hepatic abscesses. *(Joklik et al, pp 1164–1168)*

779. **(A)** *Pneumocystis carinii* is a sporozoan parasite of worldwide distribution that causes pneumonia in immunosuppressed individuals. Lately, an increased number of cases of pneumonia due to this parasite has been encountered in AIDS patients. Sporozoa are obligate intracellular parasites that lack organs of locomotion. *(Joklik et al, pp 1179,1184)*

780. **(B)** Trichinosis caused by the nematode (roundworm) *Trichinella spiralis* is transmitted to individuals by ingesting infected raw pork meat, or improperly cooked infected pork and pork sausage. Following the initial gastrointestinal phase of the disease, which lasts for approximately one week, the second phase sets in. Now the larvae of *T. spiralis*

enter the circulation and the patients develop fever up to 41°C, periorbital edema, eosinophilia, and severe muscular pains. *Wuchereria bancrofti* and *Plasmodium malariae* infections are the results of mosquito bites and are characterized by lymphadenitis and destruction of the red blood cells, respectively. *Entamoeba coli* has not been shown to be pathogenic. *(Joklik et al, pp 1164,1180,1187,1201,1203)*

781. **(D)** The outstanding symptoms of *Enterobius vermicularis* infection are severe itching in the anal region, which in children is usually accompanied by insomnia or fretful sleep and irritability. The disease has worldwide distribution. Seventy percent of schoolchildren in West Africa are infected. In the United States, *E. vermicularis* (pinworm) is the most common parasitic disease caused by a nematode. Diagnosis of the disease rests on the demonstration in cellophane tape preparation or anal swabs of asymmetrical ova flattened on one side and containing larvae. *(Joklik et al, pp 1187–1189)*

REFERENCES

Joklik WK, Willett HP, Amos BD, Wilfert CM. *Zinsser Microbiology,* 20th ed. Norwalk, CT: Appleton & Lange; 1992.

Brooks GF, Butel JS, Ornston LN, et al. *Medical Microbiology,* 19th ed. Norwalk, CT: Appleton & Lange; 1991.

Ryan KJ, Champoux JJ, Drew WL, et al. *Sherris Medical Microbiology,* 3rd ed. Norwalk, CT: Appleton & Lange; 1994.

Medical Virology
Questions

782. A 20-year-old man is suffering from nonsuppurative enlargement of the parotid glands and painful swelling of the testicles. He also has had slight fever and anorexia, and complains of pain during eating. Administration of antibiotics commonly used to control other than viral diseases did not alter the symptoms of this patient, who recovered completely in 2 weeks. These findings are consistent with

(A) measles
(B) German measles
(C) chickenpox
(D) mumps
(E) shingles

783. The effectiveness of interferon as an antiviral agent lies in the fact that it

(A) prevents the entry of viruses into cells
(B) destroys the host cell DNA polymerase
(C) prevents the uncoating of the viruses by the host cell enzyme
(D) inhibits the translation of viral mRNA
(E) neutralizes extracellular virions

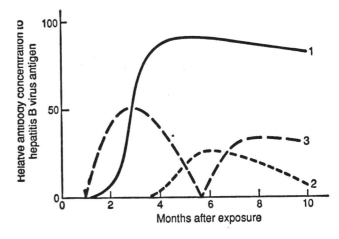

Figure 8–1

784. Figure 8–1 shows the antibody response to clinical acute hepatitis B virus infection. Curve 1 most likely represents which antibody formed against antigen?

(A) HBs
(B) HBe
(C) HBc
(D) HBn
(E) HBr

785. Which one of the following structural features is NOT true of retroviruses?

(A) double-stranded RNA genome

(B) virus-associated reverse transcriptase

(C) lipid envelope

(D) genome in a protein core

786. A brick-shaped 400-nm × 230-nm double-stranded DNA virus that multiplies in the cytoplasm of host cells and causes a skin rash is

(A) herpesvirus

(B) adenovirus

(C) papovavirus

(D) poxvirus

(E) paramyxovirus

787. Development of a vaccine for the "common cold" is difficult because

(A) coronaviruses have a low recombination rate

(B) rhinoviruses have more than 100 serotypes

(C) influenza viruses have a low mutation rate

(D) respiratory syncytial virus induces life-long immunity

788. All normal cells contain genes that can cause transformation of cells if these genes are altered in some way. These genes are called proto-oncogenes. Proto-oncogenes are

(A) virally encoded

(B) altered versions of normal genes

(C) always transduced by retroviruses

(D) activated by viral and nonviral mechanisms

(E) associated with the suppression of cell growth

789. A 10-year-old healthy boy suddenly developed a fever of 100°F, sore throat, and swelling at the parotid, maxillary, and sublingual glands. Microbiological tests indicated that he had mumps. This disease could best have been prevented by

(A) prophylactic administration of acyclovir

(B) daily doses of zidovudine

(C) prophylactic administration of ribavirin

(D) immunization with the live attenuated mumps virus

790. You infect a cell line with poliovirus at m.o.i. (multiplicity of infection) of 10. Radioactive amino acids are added to the cells. During the *latent period*, you expect to detect

(A) infectious virus particles released from the cells

(B) viral proteins that are being translated

(C) viral messenger RNAs that are being transcribed

(D) viral genomes undergoing replication

791. Herpes simplex virus type 1 most commonly causes cold sores. The site of reactivation for this virus is the

(A) vagus nerve

(B) B lymphocyte

(C) epidermal cell

(D) trigeminal nerve

(E) eighth cranial nerve

792. A rapid method that may be useful for the specific diagnosis of cytomegalovirus (CMV) infections is

(A) Gram stain

(B) acid-fast stain

(C) silver stain to detect capsid antigens

(D) labeled DNA probe and DNA hybridization

(E) agglutination using latex particles tagged with virus

793. A procedure used to detect some of the orthomyxoviruses and paramyxoviruses that produce little or no cytopathic effect in cell culture is the use of

(A) neutralization
(B) hemadsorption
(C) plaque reduction
(D) complement fixation
(E) interference

794. The most generally accepted laboratory method for the diagnosis of most common viral infections is the use of

(A) hen's egg inoculation
(B) mouse inoculation
(C) direct antigen detection
(D) DNA probe analysis
(E) cell culture

795. A 71-year-old woman with chronic leukemia developed slow impairment of memory, as well as deterioration of intellectual power and orientation. Brain autopsy specimens showed demyelination due to viral damage of oligodendroglial cells. Abundant JC virus particles were also found in the brain. The MOST likely diagnosis is

(A) progressive multifocal leucoencephalopathy
(B) rabies
(C) Reye syndrome
(D) papillomatosis

796. Which of the following viruses is MOST resistant to chemical physical agents?

(A) mumps
(B) measles
(C) influenza
(D) serum hepatitis
(E) poliomyelitis

797. All of the following statements about viruses are true EXCEPT

(A) a viral genome is composed of either DNA or RNA, but not both

(B) the protein capsid may be covered by a lipid membrane (envelope)
(C) the protein capsid is taken into the cell and then disassembled, liberating the viral genome
(D) viruses replicate by a gradual increase in size, followed by division
(E) virion components are synthesized and then assembled into progeny within the infected cell

798. For viruses, the burst size is the

(A) average number of progeny viruses released per infected cell
(B) interval between infection and appearance of program viruses
(C) average number of viruses that infect a cell
(D) number of viruses per unit volume of the growth medium

799. The antibody induced by which of the following parts of influence virus is most protective?

(A) envelope
(B) neuraminidase
(C) hemagglutinin
(D) nucleic acid
(E) internal protein

800. A 5-month-old baby had constant nonproductive cough and a temperature of 39.5°C. Radiographs, physical examination, and laboratory tests indicate that the baby has viral pneumonia. Which of the following viruses is LEAST likely to cause this illness?

(A) adenovirus
(B) rotavirus
(C) respiratory syncytial virus
(D) parainfluenza serotype 3 virus

801. All of the following viruses are replicated in the nucleus EXCEPT

(A) poxviruses
(B) papovaviruses
(C) adenoviruses
(D) herpesviruses
(E) parvoviruses

802. A 26-year-old farmer has not been feeling well during the past 4 months. He has taken antifungal, antiprotozoan, and antibacterial drugs without improvement in his health. Laboratory tests show high serum alanine aminotransferase, aspartate transaminase values of 500 to 2,000 units, leucopenia, decreased serum albumin, and increased serum globulin levels. The MOST likely diagnosis is

(A) sandfly fever
(B) poliomyelitis
(C) hepatitis A
(D) West Nile fever
(E) rabies

803. Human papillomaviruses have a

(A) linear, double-stranded DNA genome
(B) circular, double-stranded DNA genome
(C) circular DNA genome that is partially double-stranded and partially single-stranded
(D) linear single-stranded DNA genome
(E) positive strand, single-stranded RNA genome

804. The following figure shows various structures of a virus. According to this figure, which part of the virus is indicated by arrow 2?

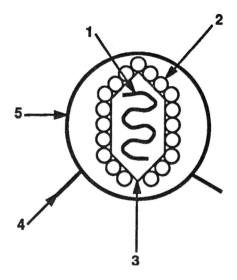

Figure 8-2

(A) spike
(B) envelope
(C) matrix protein
(D) nucleic acid
(E) capsomer

805. Protection from which of the following is NOT provided by a live attenuated virus vaccine?

(A) poliomyelitis
(B) hepatitis B
(C) measles
(D) mumps
(E) rubella

806. Viruses are attractive vectors for gene therapy because

(A) they infect cells with a much lower efficiency as compared to chemical or physical means of gene transfer

(B) the genes inserted into viruses may be expressed in a regulated way

(C) adenovirus vectors cannot be used to target gene transfer into cells of the respiratory tract

(D) retrovirus vectors can be produced in extremely small quantities from producer cell lines

807. The first event following paramyxovirus infection of a cell is

(A) synthesis of individual messenger RNAs by the RNA-dependent RNA polymerase associated with the RNA genome

(B) translation of the incoming RNA genome

(C) degradation of the minus sense RNA

(D) budding of the genome through the plasma membrane

(E) reverse transcription of the negative strand RNA genome

808. When antibody titers are used in the laboratory diagnosis of viral infections, the diagnosis can only be made if

(A) the acute titer is less than 10

(B) the convalescent titer is greater than 20

(C) there is a two-fold rise in titer

(D) there is a four-fold rise in titer

(E) there is no change in titer

809. A child receiving chemotherapy presents with a disseminated varicella-zoster virus (VZV) infection. The MOST likely reason for the severity of the case was

(A) induction of a hypogammaglobulinemia

(B) synergism between the chemotherapy and VZV

(C) induction of a T-cell deficiency

(D) induction of a B-cell deficiency

(E) outgrowth of virus from a VZV IgG immunization

810. A 55-year-old woman has shingles. The MOST likely treatment with antiviral agents is

(A) isatin-6-thiosemicarbazone

(B) rifampin

(C) adenosine vidarabine

(D) azidothymidine

(E) amantadine

811. The replication of Rauscher murine leukemia virus, an RNA virus, is sensitive to actinomycin D. This sensitivity is due to effects occurring on which of the following steps in the viral replication cycle?

(A) the reverse transcriptase

(B) ribonuclease H

(C) transcription of the viral information

(D) integration of the viral genome into the host cell genome

(E) translation of the viral information

812. Messenger RNAs (mRNAs) in mammalian cells are usually monocistronic, whereas many bacterial mRNAs are polycistronic. This difference refers to the fact that

(A) initiation of transcription in mammalian cells occurs at the promoter closest to the 5′ end of the gene, whereas in bacterial cells it can occur at several different locations within the gene

(B) mammalian mRNAs have a polyadenylated tail, but bacterial mRNAs do not

(C) mammalian mRNAs are capped, but bacterial mRNAs are not

(D) initiation of translation in mammalian cells usually occurs at the first start codon from the 5′ end of the mRNA, whereas in bacterial cells it can occur at several different locations on the mRNA

(E) bacterial mRNAs often contain sequences encoding several proteins, whereas mammalian mRNAs do not

813. The effectiveness of azidothymidine (AZT) therapy for the control of HIV infection declines with continued administration. What is the primary reason for this?

   (A) cellular DNA polymerases are 100 times more susceptible to inhibition by this drug that the HIV reverse transcriptase

   (B) the patient responds by increasing production of enzymes capable of inactivating the drug

   (C) cellular kinases mutate for forms unable to recognize the drug

   (D) viral reverse transcriptase mutates to a form resistant to the drug

   (E) the drug precipitates in the kidneys

814. A patient is infected with a paramyxovirus. The cytopathic effect for this virus is

   (A) syncytia formation

   (B) major destruction of the tissue culture monolayer

   (C) intranuclear inclusion formation

   (D) Negri body formation

815. The viral envelopes are

   (A) polysaccharide bilayers

   (B) lipid bilayers

   (C) nucleoprotein bilayers

   (D) glycoprotein bilayers

816. If there are 2,500 amino acids in a virus capsid, the number of purine and pyrimidine base pairs needed to code for this capsid, disregarding any bases that directly do not code for an amino acid, is

   (A) 2,500

   (B) 10,000

   (C) 7,500

   (D) 5,000

817. All of the following are positive-stranded RNA viruses EXCEPT

   (A) St. Louis encephalitis virus

   (B) measles virus

   (C) Rous sarcoma virus

   (D) rhinovirus

   (E) poliovirus

818. The cytopathic effect that is seen when a virus infects a specific cell culture

   (A) will vary with the various types of cells used

   (B) is characteristic of each virus and can be used for presumptive identification

   (C) is so characteristic that it is used for specific identification

   (D) is the same for most viruses

   (E) is not useful in diagnostic virology

819. Which one of the following viruses is LEAST likely to be transmitted by arthropod vectors?

   (A) flaviviruses

   (B) yellow fever virus

   (C) bunyaviruses

   (D) coronaviruses

   (E) togaviruses

820. All of the following statements about negative-stranded RNA viruses are true EXCEPT

   (A) they contain a genome that is of opposite polarity to viral messenger RNAs

   (B) mammalian cells they infect do not contain mammalian RNA-dependent RNA polymerases

   (C) viral nucleic acid itself is not infectious

   (D) positive-stranded RNA viruses do not contain RNA-dependent RNA polymerase

   (E) two groups whose genomes are single-stranded uninterrupted RNA molecules are the rhabdoviruses and the paramyxoviruses

821. Which of the following statement about rhabdoviruses is NOT true?

   (A) rabies virus cannot be transmitted directly to humans by insect vectors

   (B) they are positive-stranded RNA viruses

   (C) they are enveloped

   (D) they have a bullet-shaped morphology

(E) the viral genome must first be transcribed to produce viral messenger RNAs

822. Which one of the following viruses is NOT classified as a paramyxovirus?

(A) mumps virus
(B) measles virus
(C) respiratory syncytial virus
(D) parainfluenza virus
(E) influenza C virus

823. Which of the following viruses does not cause upper respiratory tract infections, including symptoms of the common cold?

(A) orthomyxoviruses
(B) paramyxoviruses
(C) papovaviruses
(D) coronaviruses
(E) rhinoviruses

824. Influenza virus A has all of the following features EXCEPT

(A) a nonsegmented RNA genome
(B) a helical capside
(C) negative-stranded RNA
(D) a lipid envelope of cellular origin
(E) hemagglutinin and neuraminidase spikes embedded on their surfaces

825. Which of the following diseases is NOT associated with herpesviruses?

(A) scrapie
(B) central nervous system diseases
(C) venereal diseases
(D) skin rashes
(E) congenital diseases

826. Which statement regarding viruses is true?

(A) they do not pass through filters that retain bacteria
(B) they are sensitive to antibiotics
(C) they are not sensitive to interferon
(D) they depend on host cells for energy production

(E) they are composed of DNA or RNA capsid proteins and are envelope

827. The etiologic agent of chickenpox is

(A) vaccinia virus
(B) variola virus
(C) varicella-zoster virus
(D) rubella virus
(E) rubeola virus

828. Following infection, complete uncoating of the genome cannot occur until after transcription of some viral genes and synthesis of one or more viral polypeptides in

(A) herpes simplex virus
(B) varicella-zoster virus
(C) vaccinia virus
(D) adenovirus
(E) SV-40

829. In which of the following viruses is the genome a linear double-stranded DNA molecule that can exist in four possible isomeric forms in which the L and S components of the genome can exist in all possible orientations with respect to each other?

(A) herpes simplex virus
(B) adenovirus
(C) hepatitis A virus
(D) variola virus
(E) rotavirus

830. In equatorial eastern Africa, infection with which of the following viruses is closely associated with the development of Burkitt's lymphoma?

(A) HTLV-I
(B) HTLV-II
(C) HTLV-III
(D) Epstein–Barr virus
(E) hepatitis A virus

831. 0.1 mL of a phage suspension was diluted as shown and plated with a sensitive bacterium. The relevant number of plaques are shown below:

Dilution	Plaque Count
10^{-1}	too many to count
10^{-2}	200
10^{-3}	20
10^{-4}	2
10^{-5}	0

Therefore, the number of phages per mL of the original suspension is

(A) 20×10^{-4}

(B) 2×10^{-2}

(C) 2×10^{-5}

(D) 200,000

832. The virus that has been associated with primary hepatocellular carcinoma is

(A) hepatitis A virus (HAV)

(B) hepatitis B virus (HBV)

(C) non-A/non-B hepatitis (NANB)

(D) delta-associated agent

(E) Marburg virus

833. The genome of a given virion is DNA. Following uncoating, the viral DNA is transcribed into plus-stranded RNA, the pregenome. After being translated, the pregenome is encapsidated into immature cores, and subsequently reverse transcribed into DNA within the maturing progeny virions. This replication cycle is characteristic of

(A) hepatitis A virus

(B) retroviruses

(C) hepatitis B virus

(D) polyomavirus

(E) non-A/non-B hepatitis

834. Which of the following diagnostic techniques would be LEAST useful for the detection of a virus infection in tissue culture cells during the eclipse phase of virus replication?

(A) radioimmunoassay (RIA)

(B) enzyme-linked immunosorbent assay (ELISA)

(C) immunofluorescence

(D) electron microscopy

835. The agent of viral disease with prominent liver involvement spread by the fecal–oral route is

(A) hepatitis A virus

(B) hepatitis B virus

(C) agents of non-A/non-B hepatitis

(D) cytomegalovirus

(E) Epstein–Barr virus

836. The drug frequently used in the treatment of influenza virus infections is

(A) vidarabine

(B) amantadine

(C) phosphonoacetic acid

(D) acyclovir

(E) bromodeoxyuridine

837. The function of the nucleocapsid proteins of measles virus is to

(A) give the virion particle a geometric symmetry

(B) protect the DNA from nuclear digestion

(C) allow the virion to assemble in the icosahedral shell

(D) protect the genome RNA from nuclease digestion and recognize the location in the cell membrane for budding

(E) promote virion entry into the susceptible cell

838. Herpesvirus type 2 involves primarily the

(A) mouth

(B) throat

(C) genitalia

(D) respiratory

(E) eyes

839. Spread of herpesvirus type 1 occurs primarily by

(A) breast milk

(B) blood

(C) frozen plasma

(D) direct personal contact

(E) contaminated syringes

840. A Tzanck smear is a diagnostic test that

(A) requires a blood sample

(B) reveals intranuclear inclusions in herpesvirus infections

(C) is used to monitor the efficacy of acyclovir therapy

(D) requires T lymphocytes

(E) is used to distinguish between varicella virus and herpesvirus infections

841. Which of the following statements correctly describes the varicella-zoster virus?

(A) it does not infect the newborn

(B) it affects the trigeminal nerve

(C) it does not cause vesicles

(D) it represents a reactivation of a prior cytomegalovirus infection

(E) it is not troublesome in immunosuppressed patients

842. Which of the following statements is NOT true concerning cytomegalovirus?

(A) the virus may be transmitted sexually

(B) the virus may be acquired via blood transfusion

(C) organ transplant patients may acquire this virus

(D) it is an important cause of morbidity in immunosuppressed patients

(E) vertical transmission does not occur

843. The primary target for the human immunodeficiency virus (HIV), which causes acquired immunodeficiency syndrome (AIDS), is the

(A) T4 cell

(B) B cell

(C) polymorphonuclear cell

(D) eosinophil

(E) basophil

844. The HIV retrovirus is a member of the

(A) oncoviruses

(B) spuma viruses

(C) foamy viruses

(D) lentiviruses

(E) reoviruses

845. Generally, the sarcoma/acute leukemia viruses are known to

(A) be double-stranded RNA viruses

(B) replicate only when a nondefective helper virus infects the same cell

(C) be unable to transform fibroblasts in tissue culture

(D) fail to transform hematopoietic cells in tissue culture

(E) possess naked virions

846. The retroviruses are known to

(A) possess reverse transcriptase

(B) contain a nonsegmented genome

(C) lack glycoproteins in their envelopes

(D) mature in the nuclei of their host cells

(E) have genomic DNA molecules

847. The *env* gene of HIV, which causes AIDS, is known to

(A) encode the viral lipoproteins

(B) encode the viral hemagglutinins

(C) encode the viral glycoproteins of the nucleocapsid

(D) be highly variable

(E) be very stable

848. HIV differs from the RNA tumor viruses in that it

(A) does not require T4 receptor protein for adsorption to host cells

(B) contains two copies of single-stranded RNA in its virion

(C) contains the *gag* gene

(D) contains the *pol* gene

(E) lyses the host cells

849. The *pol* gene of retroviruses codes for

(A) viral RNase

(B) polymeric viral capsomeres

(C) nucleocapsid proteins

(D) reverse transcriptase

(E) polymeric envelope viral proteins

850. Which of the following statements correctly descirbues the *myc* oncogene?

(A) it encodes for guanine nucleotide-binding proteins

(B) it encodes for a cytoplasmic threonine-specific kinase

(C) it can induce cell immortality

(D) it is needed for the synthesis of tyrosine-specific protein kinase

(E) it is required for the synthesis of reverse transcriptase

851. The normal cell gene that may be converted to an oncogene is called a

(A) retrogene

(B) metagene

(C) proto-oncogene

(D) para-oncogene

(E) *cis*-oncogene

852. Viruses with segmented double-stranded genomes are

(A) reoviruses

(B) papovaviruses

(C) influenza viruses

(D) arenaviruses

(E) rhabdoviruses

853. The *Ha-ras* oncogene is correctly described as

(A) found in myelocytomatosis retrovirus

(B) derived from the PDGF gene

(C) associated with bursal lymphomas

(D) encoding for the guanine nucleotide binding proteins

(E) found only in DNA-containing oncogenic viruses

854. A 6-year-old boy is coughing, has nasal congestion, fever, headache, chills, and muscular pains that have definitely been attributed to a viral infection. Electron microscopic examination of throat washings show the virus sketched below. He is most likely suffering from a respiratory illness caused by

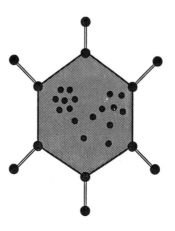

Figure 8–3

(A) influenza virus

(B) parainfluenza virus

(C) adenovirus

(D) mumps virus

(E) measles virus

855. You are faced with the problem of controlling a virus infection in a community and are told that it has already been determined it is a togavirus (arbovirus). You know then that your problem most likely is one of

(A) stopping the spread by respiratory droplets and dust of a virus that enters by the respiratory tract

(B) controlling or eliminating biting animals

(C) improving the treatment of sewage, preventing carriers from working as food handlers, and setting up methods for proper treatment of feces and urine from infected persons

(D) stopping spread by reducing the close contact of children in schools

(E) identifying and controlling an insect vector, and identifying and controlling an animal reservoir

856. An outbreak of hantavirus infection in the southwestern United States was recently described. Transmission of this virus usually occur by

(A) fecal–oral contamination
(B) bites from infected ticks
(C) inhalation of infected rodent excreta
(D) bites from infected mosquitoes

857. Infectious naked viral nucleic acids are produced by

(A) orthomyxoviruses
(B) paramyoviruses
(C) rhabdoviruses
(D) picornaviruses

858. Defective interfering virus particles are known to

(A) occur when there is phenotypic mixing
(B) be induced during repeated viral passage at high multiplicities of infection
(C) generally have excess genetic material compared with the normal virus
(D) generally have the same capsid as the normal virus
(E) be identical to prions

859. A poliovirus type 2 has been isolated from the stool of a 55-year-old patient who has been clinically diagnosed as having poliomyelitis. There have been no previous cases of polio reported; however, an infant grandchild was vaccinated about three weeks prior to onset of the disease. How can the laboratory determine whether the isolated virus is related to the vaccine strain or is a wild-type virus?

(A) inoculate the virus into mice to determine whether it kills mice
(B) inoculate several different kinds of tissue culture to determine the host range
(C) do neutralization studies using the infant's serum

(D) stain the virus with fluorescent antibody
(E) do oligonucleotide mapping of the unknown virus and compare with maps of wild-type and vaccine strains

860. All of the following viruses carry molecules of an RNA-dependent RNA polymerase as structural components of the virion EXCEPT

(A) respiratory syncytial virus
(B) rabies virus
(C) influenza viruses
(D) retroviruses

861. A college freshman has the typical symptoms of infectious mononucleosis. The most sensitive means of confirming this infection is

(A) antibody to hemagglutinin
(B) antibody to neuraminidase
(C) heterophile antibody that reacts with antigens on sheep erythrocytes
(D) antibody that reacts with Epstein–Barr virus nuclear antigen (EBNA)
(E) nucleic acid hybridization assays for the presence of Epstein–Barr viral nucleic acid

862. Which of the following viruses is not inactivated by mild detergents that solubilize phospholipid membranes?

(A) poliovirus
(B) eastern equine encephalitis virus
(C) variola virus
(D) vaccinia virus
(E) cowpox virus

863. A viral genome that does not replicate in the cytoplasm of the infected cell is

(A) poliovirus
(B) rabies virus
(C) mumps virus
(D) cytomegalovirus
(E) rubella virus

864. The viral genome is maintained as a covalently closed circle that is distinct from the cellular chromosomes in cells transformed by

(A) polyomavirus
(B) human papillomaviruses
(C) Rous sarcoma virus
(D) rabies virus

865. Exanthem subitum (roseola infantum) is a common infection of infancy characterized by fever and skin rash of 2 to 4 days' duration. This disease is caused by

(A) cytomegalovirus
(B) rubella virus
(C) varicella-zoster virus
(D) human herpesvirus type 6

866. Viral genetic information is covalently integrated into the cellular chromosomes in cells transformed by

(A) adenoviruses
(B) HTLV-I
(C) SV-40 virus
(D) hepatitis B virus
(E) all of the above

867. A 35-year-old woman, who has not been previously exposed to German measles, is infected with this virus during the third trimester of pregnancy. Laboratory tests indicate that the baby has also been infected with the German measles virus. All of the following features of congenital German measles syndrome are likely to be encountered EXCEPT

(A) aortic stenosis
(B) lack of IgM antibody
(C) ventricular septal defect
(D) blindness
(E) deafness

867. Transmission of measles is MOST likely to occur by

(A) contact with the rash of an infected person
(B) bite from an infected flea

(C) ingestion of contaminated food or water
(D) bite from an infected mite
(E) inhalation of aerosol droplets from the sneeze of an infected patient

869. Children undergoing chemotherapy are given immunoglobulins for certain common childhood viral diseases such as chickenpox. This procedure is an example of

(A) postexposure vaccination
(B) stimulation of immune response
(C) induction of specific cellular immunity
(D) passive immunization

870. Viruses that encode an RNA-dependent RNA polymerase that is a physical component of the virion include

(A) rubella virus
(B) mumps virus
(C) HTLV-III
(D) variola virus
(E) herpesvirus

871. Which of the following herpesviruses regularly causes manifestations of recurrent infection in otherwise healthy people?

(A) Epstein–Barr virus (EBV)
(B) varicella-zoster virus (VZV)
(C) cytomegalovirus (CMV)
(D) herpes simplex virus (HSV)

872. Primary infection with herpes simplex virus (HSV) is characterized by all of the following EXCEPT

(A) vesicle formation
(B) systemic signs and symptoms (fever, chills, malaise)
(C) widespread local lesions
(D) average course of 14 to 21 days
(E) a few lesions on the lips or genitals that resolve over 8 to 10 days

873. Viroids or prions are correctly described as

(A) naked RNA molecules of 30 to 400 nucleotides
(B) viruses that cause hemorrhoids

(C) virus shells without the nucleic acid core

(D) animal pathogens responsible for slow viral diseases

(E) virus-like particles that confer antibiotic resistance to susceptible bacteria

874. A disease that is thought to be caused by a slow-developing viral agent is

(A) Creutzfeldt–Jakob disease

(B) St. Louis encephalitis

(C) Eastern encephalitis

(D) Western encephalitis

(E) Lassa fever

875. The route of transmission is gastrointestinal in

(A) non-A/non-B hepatitis

(B) hepatitis B

(C) delta-associated agent

(D) hepatitis A

876. The use of acyclovir to treat human herpesvirus infections results in the emergence of mutant viruses. These mutants typically

(A) exhibit enhanced virulence for the central nervous system than the parent strain

(B) can experience permissive growth in neurons but not neuroglia

(C) have lost the capacity to express viral thymidine kinase

(D) retain their sensitivity to acyclovir

877. Replication is inhibited by alpha-amanitin, a drug that inhibits the cellular enzyme RNA polymerase II, in which of the following viruses?

(A) SV-40

(B) retroviruses

(C) adenoviruses

(D) influenza viruses

(E) all of the above

878. The effectiveness of acyclovir as an antiherpes drug lies in the fact that it is utilized by or inhibits which of the following viral en-

zymes much more readily than the corresponding cellular enzyme?

(A) threonine kinase

(B) RNA polymerase

(C) protein kinase

(D) thymidine kinase

879. Vidarabine (ara-A) effectively inhibits replication of herpes simplex virus at concentrations at which it is relatively nontoxic to uninfected cells. The basis for this selectivity involves the enzyme

(A) ribonucleotide reductase

(B) Enolase

(C) protein kinase

(D) DNA polymerase

880. Viral disease for which passive immunization is commercially available

(A) yellow fever

(B) Lassa fever

(C) cytomegalovirus infection

(D) hepatitis A

881. Carcinogenic viruses are known to

(A) include DNA but not RNA retroviruses

(B) transform cells by integrating new genes into the DNA of infected cells

(C) do not induce permanent cell transformation when virus multiplication is impossible

(D) lack genes in the DNA-containing papovaviruses that can cause cell transformation

882. For retroviruses, the transforming genes are

(A) not normal cellular genes

(B) slightly modified cellular genes

(C) not hyperactivated in the host cell

(D) integral parts of the virus genome

(E) none of the above

883. Characteristics of virus-transformed cells include

(A) alterations in glycoproteins and glycolipids of the cell surface

(B) enhanced agglutination by lectins

(C) loss of actin microfilaments

(D) reduction or absence of surface fibronectin

(E) all of the above

DIRECTIONS (Questions 884 through 923): Each group of items in this section consists of lettered headings followed by a set of numbered words or phrases. For each numbered word or phrase, select the ONE lettered heading that is most closely associated with it. Each lettered heading may be selected once, more than once, or not at all.

Questions 884 and 885

(A) enteroviruses

(B) papovaviruses

(C) poxviruses

(D) herpesviruses

(E) arenaviruses

884. Common feature is their zoonotic reservoir (small rodents)

885. Viral particles have a "sandy" appearance

Question 886

(A) adsorption

(B) penetration

(C) loss of infectivity

(D) translation

(E) synthesis of nucleocapsid

886. Viral eclipse period

Question 887

(A) rickettsia

(B) *Chlamydia*

(C) viruses

(D) L forms

(E) *Mycoplasma*

887. Contain either DNA or RNA

Questions 888 and 889

(A) nonsegmented, positive-stranded RNA

(B) segmented, negative-stranded RNA

(C) nonsegmented, negative-stranded RNA

(D) nonsegmented, double-stranded RNA

(E) segmented, double-stranded RNA

888. Rhinoviruses

889. Influenza viruses

Questions 890 and 891

(A) one

(B) two

(C) three

(D) four

(E) seven

890. Number of clinically important dengue serotypes

891. Number of clinically important poliovirus serotypes

Questions 892 and 893

(A) herpes

(B) chickenpox

(C) poliomyelitis

(D) measles

(E) hepatitis B

892. Oral live trivalent virus used for active immunization in the United States

893. Purified surface viral protein used for active immunization

Questions 894 and 895

(A) measles vaccine

(B) influenza killed viral vaccine

(C) hepatitis B vaccine

(D) diphtheria vaccine

(E) pneumococcal vaccine

894. Should not be given to immunosuppressed individuals

895. Guillain–Barré syndrome occurs on rare occasions

Questions 896 and 897

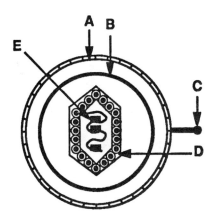

Figure 8–4

896. Essential protein for the budding of retrovirus from the host cells

897. Required for adsorption and entry of retrovirus into the host cells

Questions 898 and 899

 (A) herpes simplex virus
 (B) papovavirus BKV
 (C) Lassa fever virus
 (D) poliomyelitis virus
 (E) smallpox virus

898. Latent infection

899. Inapparent infection

Questions 900 and 901

 (A) neuraminidase
 (B) association with single plus stranded RNA
 (C) prion
 (D) hemagglutinating glycoprotein
 (E) β-lactamase

900. Poliovirus

901. Scrapie

Questions 902 and 903

 (A) coronaviruses
 (B) polioviruses
 (C) myxoviruses
 (D) paramyxoviruses
 (E) poxviruses

902. Do not grow well in cell culture

903. Envelope with petal-shaped spikes

Questions 904 and 905

 (A) rabies virus
 (B) poliovirus
 (C) German measles virus
 (D) measles virus
 (E) influenza virus

904. Purified genome is infectious

905. Virion does not contain RNA polymerase

Questions 906 through 908

The following figure represents one-step growth of a virus. From this figure, select the letter that most closely approximates the relationship described in questions 906 through 908.

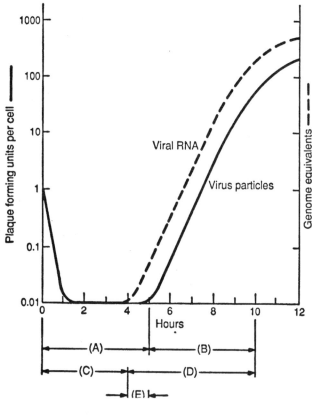

Figure 8–5

906. Eclipse period

907. Rise period

908. Period necessary to encapsidate viral genome

Questions 909 and 910

    (A) hepatitis virus A
    (B) hepatitis virus B
    (C) hepatitis virus C
    (D) hepatitis virus D

909. Principal vaccine used for prevention of disease in humans

910. Short incubation period (15 days)

Questions 911 and 912

    (A) dengue fever virus
    (B) Rous sarcoma virus
    (C) St. Louis encephalitis virus
    (D) eastern equine encephalitis virus
    (E) Russian spring–summer encephalitis virus

911. Tick is the usual vector

912. Possession of the *src* gene

Questions 913 and 914

    (A) normal fibroblast cells
    (B) transformed cells
    (C) normal fibroblast cells containing muramic acid
    (D) transformed cells containing diaminopimelic acid
    (E) both normal fibroblast cells and transformed cells

913. Loss of contact inhibition of growth

914. Anchorage dependence

Questions 915 and 916

    (A) adenoviruses
    (B) Epstein–Barr virus
    (C) adenoviruses and Epstein–Barr viruses
    (D) orthomyxoviruses
    (E) coronaviruses

915. Implication in Burkitt's lymphoma

916. Transformation of cells in culture

Questions 917 and 918

    (A) herpesvirus type 2
    (B) hepatitis B virus
    (C) Rous sarcoma virus
    (D) herpesvirus type 2 and hepatitis B virus
    (E) papillomavirus

917. Definitive causal relationship between virus and malignancy is lacking

918. Dane particles

Questions 919 through 921

Establish the most likely association between these viruses with the clinical symptoms described in questions 919 through 921.

 (A) rabies virus

 (B) coronavirus

 (C) poxvirus

 (D) parvovirus

 (E) rotavirus

 (F) adenovirus

 (G) Lassa virus

919. An 11-month-old child has severe diarrhea and vomiting that has resulted in dehydration. The illness has been attributed to a wheel-shaped, nonenveloped, double-stranded RNA virus which has a genome that contains 11 segments.

920. A zoological gardenkeeper who has been bitten by a dog complains of headache, excitation, nervousness, great difficulty swallowing, and even the sight of liquid induces painful contractions of the throat muscles (hydrophobia). Then he develops convulsions, lethargy, and coma. Laboratory tests show a bullet-shaped, linear, single-stranded, negative-sense RNA virus in the saliva of the gardenkeeper.

921. A Nigerian villager becomes infected with a virus by contact with contaminated rodent urine. The villager develops high fever, mouth ulcers, skin rashes with hemorrhages, severe muscle aches, and pneumonia, and died from heart and kidney failure. It was found that the infection was due to a spheri-

cal, enveloped virus that had a sandy appearance and contained single-stranded, double-segmented, negative-sense RNA, as well as ribosome-like particles.

Questions 922 and 923

For each structure, select the function in the diagram.

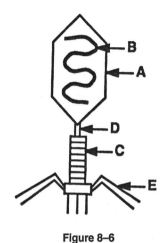

Figure 8–6

922. Recognition of specific binding sites on host cells

923. Collapses to drive a hollow tube through the envelopes of the bacterial cell

Medical Virology
Answers and Explanations

782. **(D)** The most noticeable symptom of mumps is the painful swelling of the parotid glands, accompanied by pain during eating, mild pharyngitis, headache, and general malaise. In adult males the genital organs are commonly involved and about 30% develop orchitis with painful swelling of the testicles. These are precisely the symptoms of the 20-year-old man who is suffering from a viral infection that does not respond to nonviral antimicrobial agents. Measles, German measles, chickenpox, and shingles viruses produce erythematous vesicular infections. (*Joklik et al, pp 959–961,1004–1018*)

783. **(D)** Interferons suppress the intracellular growth of many viruses, and have little if any action on the host cells of viruses. They act by inducing the synthesis of three proteins that inhibit the translation of viral mRNA. The proteins involved in the inhibition of viral mRNA are a 2,5 oligonucleotide synthetase that forms an adenine trinucleotide, an endonuclease that is degrades viral but not cellular mRNA, and a protein kinase that phosphorylates and thus inactivates the eIF-2 initiation factor for protein synthesis. Interferons do not prevent viral host cell entry, or cell host uncoating of virions, and they do not neutralize extracellular virions or destroy the host cell DNA polymerase. (*Levinson and Jawetz, p 160*)

784. **(C)** Hepatitis B virus (HBV) is the causative agent. Serum hepatitis is usually transmitted to humans by HBV infected blood or blood products. HBV is a polymorphic hepadnavirus containing circular, double-stranded DNA. The virus has a nucleocapsid core protein called hepatitis B virus core antigen (HBcAg). It also has a form of HBcAg, known as ABeAg, that may be present in serum during HBV infection, and, finally, this virus contains an envelope or surface protein known as HBsAg. Antibody to HBcAg usually is detected when clinical disease occurs 2 to 4 weeks after HBsAg reactivity appears. Since HBcAg antibody response is against the internal capsid of the hepatitis B virus, this antibody response signals viral replication. In typical acute cases of HBV infections, high levels of IgM anti-HBc are found. HBV does not have HBn, or HBm antigens, and thus antibody responses to these antigens cannot be expected. Curve 2 represents antibody formed against HBe, while curve 3 represents antibody formed against HBs. (*Brooks et al, pp 458–460*)

785. **(A)** Retroviruses are single-stranded, linear, positive polarity RNA viruses 90 to 120 nm in diameter. The RNA is surrounded by an inner protein envelope and an outer envelope that contains lipid and glycoprotein spikes, which serve to attach the virus to the host cells. Retroviruses have been associated with leukemia, sarcoma, mammary tumors, and especially with AIDS. The word retro refers to the possession of the enzyme reverse transcriptase, which transcribes RNA into DNA during the process of viral nucleic acid synthesis. (*Joklik et al, pp 878–879*)

786. **(D)** The poxviruses are very large, brick-shaped 400-nm × 230-nm double-stranded DNA viruses, which multiply in the cytoplasm of the host cells and are usually associated with skin rashes. The most important human poxvirus is smallpox (variola). Herpesviruses, adenoviruses, and papovaviruses are spherical or ovoid viruses, 100, 75, 55, and 100 nm, respectively, and have a double-stranded genome. Paramyxoviruses contain single-stranded RNA. Herpesviruses, adenoviruses, and papovaviruses multiply in the nucleus of the host cells. Adenoviruses and papovaviruses do not ordinarily produce skin rashes. The varicella-zoster viruses are members of the herpesviruses and produce skin rashes. Similarly, the measles viruses, which are members of the paramyxoviruses, also produce skin rashes. (*Joklik et al, pp 949, 959,968,975,1011*)

787. **(B)** The "common cold" is caused by a variety of viruses that include the coronaviruses, the rhinoviruses, the influenza viruses, and the respiratory syncytial virus. Development of a vaccine against the common cold requires inclusion of the viruses indicated above and all of their antigenic varieties. This is an extremely difficult, if not impossible, task because coronaviruses have a high recombination rate that can lead to numerous antigenic types; rhinoviruses have more than 100 serotypes that will have to be included in the vaccine; influenza viruses exhibit a high rate of mutation of their H and N key antigens; and finally, the human immune response to respiratory syncytial virus is incomplete and of short duration. (*Joklik et al, pp 989,994,999–1001*)

788. **(D)** An oncogene is an altered version of a normal gene. A proto-oncogene is a normal gene that can be converted to an oncogene. Proto-oncogenes have been maintained in the mammalian cell genome, and they may play some role in the normal cellular metabolism. At this time, approximately 24 proto-oncogenes have been discovered using retroviruses, which can infect mammalian cells containing proto-oncogenes and transfer the proto-oncogenes to other cells that can infect.

The majority of the proto-oncogenes may be activated via retroviruses. However, it has been shown that a nonvirally induced single-base pair mutation was sufficient to convert the benign proto-oncogene *ras* into an oncogene. Thus, proto-oncogenes may be activated either by association with retroviruses or they may be altered via mutational nonviral events. (*Joklik et al, pp 887–895*)

789. **(D)** The best way to prevent and reduce mumps infection and possible death is immunization with the live, attenuated strain of mumps virus. The vaccine provides protection against mumps for at least 10 years. It has induced 95% protection to persons exposed to mumps, and it may be administered in combination with the measles and rubella vaccine at 15 months of age and again before entering school. Vaccinated individuals have a subclinical, noncommunicable infection. Immunization against mumps is not recommended for individuals allergic to vaccine components, persons receiving immunosuppressive therapy or with defective immune systems, and pregnant women. Administration of acyclovir, zidovudine, or ribavirin has not been shown to prevent mumps. (*Ryan et al, pp 212–213,467,476*)

790. **(B)** The synthesis of the viruses involves the uncoating of the viral genome, the replication of the viral genome, the synthesis of the viral proteins, and the assembly of the progeny virus particles. The late period of the viral synthetic phase is the period during which structural, nonstructural, and enzymes of the viral particles are formed. Since amino acids are the building blocks of proteins, detection of radioactive amino acids, following addition to a cell line infected with poliovirus, will most likely be made when viral proteins are translated during the late period. (*Joklik et al, pp 792–795*)

791. **(D)** Upon contact with the mucous membranes or broken skin of a susceptible individual, herpesvirus type 1 multiplies in the parabasal and intermediate epithelial cells, the lysis of which results in the formation of vesicles. Following this initial multiplication in epithelial skin cells, herpesvirus type 1 invades local nerves and then moves to the dorsal root ganglia, including the trigeminal ganglia. Herpesvirus type 1 infections lead to latent infections in the trigeminal ganglia. Epidermal cells are the sites of initial multiplication of herpesvirus type 1 and not the sites of reactivation for this virus. There is no evidence that the vagus nerve, the eighth cranial nerve, or the B lymphocyte is the site of reactivation of herpesvirus type I. (*Brooks, pp 421–426*)

792. **(D)** DNA homology (in the case of DNA viruses such as CMV) is most accurately determined by the DNA–DNA hybridization technique using labeled DNA probe. DNA from a suspected viral strain is denatured by heating or treatment with alkali so as to separate the two strands. These are then adsorbed on some supporting matrix. To them are added small, broken, radioactively labeled denatured DNA oligonucleotide strands derived from a known strain of CMV. The mixture is then heated and allowed to anneal by cooling slowly. If the two DNA samples are entirely homologous, radioactively labeled DNA is hybridized and converted to the DNAse-resistant form. If they are completely dissimilar, all radioactive DNA remains DNAse sensitive. Retention of radioactivity with the supporting matrix after DNAse treatment and washing becomes a measure ofhybridization and DNA homology. (*Joklik et al, pp 945–948*)

793. **(B)** When guinea pig erythrocytes are added to monkey kidney cell cultures of influenza virus, the red cells are aggregated about and adsorbed by the cells in which viral proliferation is occurring. Viruses that demonstrate this phenomenon are called hemadsorption viruses. (*Joklik et al, pp 766,995–996*)

794. **(E)** Cell culture techniques are the most widely used for isolating viruses from clinical specimens. When viruses multiply in cell culture, they produce biologic effects (cytopathic changes, viral interference, or the production of a hemagglutinin) that permit detection and isolation of the agent. The identity of an isolated virus is established with type-specific antiserum, which inhibits virus growth or reacts with the viral antigen. Other techniques such as inoculation DNA probe analysis and direct antigen detection using immunological techniques are also useful for the diagnosis of certain viruses. (*Joklik et al, pp 942–947*)

795. **(A)** JC virus is a member of the polyomaviruses, which include the JC virus (JCV) and the BK virus (BKV) of humans and simian 40 virus (SV-40). These are double-stranded DNA nonenveloped viruses that are widely distributed in various animal species, which usually do not produce disease. Progressive and multifocal leukoencephalopathy is a rare illness that may be encountered in individuals with chronic diseases such as AIDS and reticuloendothelial cancer. This disease causes progressive deterioration of mental and neuromuscular function. At autopsy, foci of demyelination are found, surrounded by giant bizarre astrocytes containing intranuclear inclusions. Demyelination is due to viral damage of oligodendroglial cells which synthesize myelin. Abundant JC virus particles can be found in the brain when brain tissue is examined by electron microscopy. Rabies virus induces the formation of Negri bodies in the brain; is associated with bites of rabid dogs, bats, or other animals; foaming of the mouth; and hydrophobia. Reye syndrome is an acute, noninflammatory illness usually encountered in childhood and is characterized by cerebral edema, hepatic dysfunction, and hyperammonemia. Influenza A and B as well as varicella-zoster viruses have been implicated in Reye syndrome. Concomitant aspirin (salicylate) therapy has been proposed as a contributing factor. Papillomatosis is a viral infection that causes human warts. (*Ryan et al, pp 537–540,557–560,785–786*)

796. **(D)** Hepatitis B virus is practically indestructible; hence, the need for the use of disposable syringes, needles, and other equipment that may carry the virus. This agent has been of special importance in the dental profession, where cold sterilization with disinfec-

tant solutions is commonly practiced. This virus is not inactivated by most disinfectants used. It is now recommended that dentists be vaccinated against hepatitis B. The increased use of self-injected drugs has greatly increased the occurrence of hepatitis B. *(Brooks et al, p 454)*

797. (D) Viruses do *not* replicate by a gradual increase in size followed by division. During the replicative cycle, in general, numerous copies of viral nucleic acid and coat proteins are synthesized. The coat proteins assemble to form the capsid, which surrounds the viral nucleic acid, stabilizing it against the extracellular environment. The capsid may play a role in the attachment and, perhaps, penetration of the new host cell. *(Joklik et al, pp 741–747)*

798. (A) The term "burst size" is defined as the average number of progeny viruses released per infected host cell. *(Joklik et al, pp 790–795)*

799. (C) The attachment of influenza virus to host cells occurs through a reaction of the hemagglutinin membrane. Thus, antibody that blocks this reaction will prevent the disease. Antineuraminidase antibodies reduce viral spread and can diminish the severity of the disease. *(Joklik et al, pp 824–827)*

800. (B) Infections with rotaviruses are especially common in children 1 to 24 months of age. However, these viruses cause diarrhea, not viral pneumonia. Adenoviruses can cause pneumonia with cough and fever, particularly among children less than 3 years old. Parainfluenza serotype 3 virus frequently causes pneumonia in children less than 1 year old. In older individuals, parainfluenza serotype 3 is the etiologic agent of upper respiratory tract infections or tracheobronchitis. Respiratory syncytial virus is the major cause of bronchiolitis and pneumonia in infants less than 1 year old. *(Ryan et al, pp 458–459,463,522)*

801. (A) Of the viruses listed in the question, only the genomes of poxviruses are replicated in the cytoplasm; the others are replicated in the nucleus. *(Brooks et al, p 375)*

802. (C) Alanine aminotransferase (ALT) assays are conducted to assess the function of liver. In hepatitis A, laboratory tests show high serum alanine transaminase and aspartate transaminase values of 500 to 2,000 units. There is also leukopenia in the preicteric phase of the disease. Additional evidence of liver damage is indicated by decreased serum albumin and increased gamma globulin levels. West Nile Fever is a viral disease characterized by lymphadenopathy and rash. Sandfly fever features papules on the skin, fever, nausea, and stiffness of the back and neck. Rabies is characterized by excitement, hydrophobia, paralysis, convulsive seizures, coma, and death. Poliomyelitis is an acute viral illness which in its severe form damages the central nervous system leading to motor neuron damage and paralysis. *(Brooks et al, pp 458,471,496,500,540)*

803. (B) Both papillomaviruses and polyomaviruses are members of the papovavirus group, which includes viruses that possess circular, double-stranded DNA. The outstanding characteristic of these viruses is that they stimulate cell DNA synthesis; thus, they are members of the tumor-associated viruses. The papillomaviruses cause different kinds of warts, such as genital condylomas, skin warts, and pharyngeal papillomas. *(Joklik et al, pp 975–979)*

804. (E) The viral particles, or virions, contain either DNA or RNA (arrow 1), which is protected by a surrounding protein layer known as capsid (arrow 3). The capsid consists of polypeptide units called capsomers (arrow 2). Six viral families—Parvoviridae, Papovaviridae, Adenoviridae, Picornaviridae, Calciviridae, and Reoviridae—do not have envelopes. The remaining 12 viral families (Herpesviridae, Poxviridae, Hepadnaviridae, Togaviridae, Flaviviridae, Arenaviridae, Coronaviridae, Retroviridae, Bunyaviridae, Orthomyxoviridae, Paramyxoviridae, Rhabdoviridae) have a lipid-containing envelope (arrow 5). On the surface of the viral envelope some viruses, such as the orthomyxoviruses and the paramyxoviruses, form glycoproteinaceous projections known as spikes (arrow 4). Matrix proteins are found as a myristylated protein layer below the envelope of most retroviruses. *(Brooks et al, pp 366, 367; Joklik et al, p 880)*

805. (B) Hepatitis B virus (HBV) licensed vaccines (Heptavax B, Recombivax HB) consist of the purified surface antigen of the hepatitis B virus. Immunization with surface antigen of HBV has been shown to confer excellent immunity against HBV. Prevention of measles and rubella (German measles) rests upon use of an attenuated, live virus vaccine, which is recommended for all healthy, susceptible children after 15 months of age. This vaccine has reduced measles and rubella by at least 90%. The live virus attenuated Jaryl–Lynn strain of mumps virus is 95% effective in preventing mumps. This vaccine can induce immunity, which can last up to 20 years. It is administered in combination with the rubella and measles vaccines, and it is recommended for all susceptible, healthy children, adolescents, and adults. Prevention and control against poliomyelitis is attained by use of both live virus (Sabin vaccine) and formalin killed virus (Salk vaccine). Both vaccines contain the three serotypes (1, 2, and 3) of poliomyelitis viruses and both reduce drastically the incidence of paralytic poliomyelitis. However, the live virus vaccine is transmissible and thus increases the number of immune individuals. Furthermore, live virus vaccine is less expensive to produce than the formalin killed virus vaccine. *(Joklik et al, pp 985,1008,1013,1045)*

806. (B) The concept of gene therapy is based on the assumption that definitive treatment for any genetic disease should be possible by directing treatment to the site of the defect itself, the mutant gene, and not to the secondary effects of that mutant gene. Since there are many hereditary diseases that are caused by defects in a single gene, there are many potential applications of this type of therapy to the treatment of human diseases. In addition, gene therapy may be useful for acquired diseases such as cancer or infectious diseases. One of the problems encountered in gene therapy is the need of introducing the desired gene into the host cells. Viruses with weak pathogenic potential, capable of entering into host cells, have been found to be useful gene carriers. They are attractive vectors in gene therapy for the following reasons: They infect cells with a much higher efficiency as compared to chemical or physical means of gene transfer. The genes inserted into viruses may be expressed in a regulated way. Adenovirus vectors may be used to target gene transfer into cells of the respiratory tract. Retrovirus vectors can be produced in large quantities from producer cell lines. *(Brooks et al, pp 95–104)*

807. (A) Paramyxoviruses have an unsegmented single-stranded RNA genome. This RNA genome is a negative strand, single molecule surrounded by a nucleocapsid. One of the proteins of the nucleocapsid is an RNA polymerase. Viral multiplication proceeds as follows:

First, virions fuse to specific sites on the cell surface. As with orthomyxoviruses, the nucleocapsid enters the cytoplasm where the RNA is uncoated, probably by host enzymes.

Second, since the genome RNA is a negative strand, it first is transcribed into mRNAs. Although not confirmed, the RNA probably contains a single promoter site for transcription. This would imply that the genome is copied into one mRNA, which could be subsequently cleaved into shorter mRNAs corresponding to the virion proteins that are found in infected cells.

Third, as viral proteins are made, they begin to form nucleocapsids, HN protein, F protein, and M protein. Progeny viral RNA is made from + strand templates and begins to complex with the nucleocapsids.

Fourth, the budding process follows a similar specificity as that of the orthomyxoviruses. HN- and F glycoproteins are embedded in the plasma membrane, M protein aligns itself to that location, and then the RNA-nucleocapsids begin budding through these structures. *(Brooks et al, pp 520–521; Joklik et al, p 819)*

808. (D) Serologic diagnosis of a microbial disease, be it viral, bacterial, fungal, or protozoan, demands analysis of the serum antibody concentration (antibody titer) at both the acute and convalescent stage of the disease. Serologic diagnosis of a particular disease is usually made when there is a fourfold rise or higher in antibody titer between the acute and the convalescent phase of a given illness. That is, assuming the acute stage antibody concentration was 20, an antibody titer of 80 will be required to establish the serologic diagnosis for a specified viral or other microbiological agent. *(Brooks et al, pp 612–613)*

809. **(C)** Varicella-zoster virus (VZV) is an obligate intracellular parasite. In general, protection against intracellular parasites rests, to a large extent, on the presence of an adequate number of properly functioning T lymphocytes that have the CD4 and CD8 proteins. KD8 T lymphocytes are cytotoxic for virus-infected cells as well as tumor cells. CD4 T lymphocytes are involved in the alteration of B cells to the antibody-producing plasma cells. CD4 T lymphocytes also assist CD8 T lymphocytes to become cytotoxic for virus-infected and tumor cells. Induction of T-cell deficiency usually leads to disseminated infections caused by VZV or other intracellular parasites. *(Joklik et al, p 337)*

810. **(C)** Shingles, or herpes zoster, is a disease of the nerves of the skin and other tissues they supply. Shingles is also called adult chickenpox. Immunocompromised individuals have an increased risk of developing skin and visceral disseminated herpes zoster infections. A chronic form of herpes zoster with wart-like skin lesions has been described in AIDS patients. Adenosine arabinoside (vidarabine) suppresses the synthesis of varicella-zoster and herpes simplex viruses, and it tends to diminish new lesion formation and the duration of fever and to prevent the spread of virus through the viscera. Isatin——thiosemicarbazone inhibits the multiplication of poxviruses in cell cultures, but is has little value in the treatment of established cases of smallpox or other diseases caused by poxviruses. Rifampin is basically an antibacterial agent that binds to RNA polymerase and thus inhibits transcription. Azidothymidine inhibits the reverse transcriptases of retroviruses, and thus it is used for the treatment of AIDS. Amantadine interferes with the penetration and uncoating of the influenza virus, and it has been used for prophylaxis and treatment of influenza A virus. *(Joklik et al, pp 856–860,960)*

811. **(C)** Actinomycin D is an antibiotic composed of few amino acids that inhibits eukaryotic and prokaryotic cells. Inhibition of these cells occurs at the level of the DNA-dependent RNA synthesis (transcription). During transcription, the genetic information contained in DNA is copied to a complementary sequence of mRNA nucleotides by RNA polymerase. Antibiotics that either modify DNA or interfere with the action of RNA polymerase usually block the synthesis of RNA and thus interfere with the transcription of the viral information. Actinomycin D alters the structure of the DNA template and in doing so blocks the transcription of the viral information. Translation of viral information refers to the RNA-dependent protein synthesis. Chloramphenicol, erythromycin, lincomycin, and puromycin are inhibitors of translation of prokaryotic cells. Reverse transcriptase is found in retroviruses and makes a DNA copy of the virus RNA; it subsequently synthesizes double-stranded DNA molecules. After the DNA is liberated from the RNA–DNA hybrid by ribonuclease H, double-stranded DNA circularizes. *(Joklik et al, pp 167–168)*

812. **(D)** Only statement D is correct. All the other statements are incorrect. *(Joklik et al, pp 104–114)*

813. **(D)** The reason azidothymidine (AZT) is therapeutically useful against HIV is that cellular DNA polymerases are 100 times less susceptible to inhibition by AZT than the HIV reverse transcriptase. However, the effectiveness of AZT therapy for the control of HIV infection declines with continued administration. The primary reason for this is that the viral reverse transcriptase mutates to a form that is resistant to AZT. *(Ryan et al, pp 554–555)*

814. **(A)** Viruses can induce cells to fuse and form multinucleated cells called syncytia. A number of viruses, such as paramyxoviruses, herpesviruses, and respiratory syncytial virus, are well known for their ability to form giant syncytia. Cell fusion by paramyxoviruses is induced by alteration in host cell membranes by the F spike glycoproteins. Enteroviruses grow quickly in cell culture and they can completely destroy a monolayer. Herpes simplex or the varicella-zoster virus can cause the formation of intranuclear inclusions. The rabies virus forms intracytoplasmic inclusions known as Negri bodies. *(Joklik et al, pp 838–839,943,1029)*

815. **(B)** The viral envelopes are lipid bilayers. The envelopes contain glycoproteins but are not glycoprotein, nucleoprotein, or polysaccharide bilayers. The outer surface of the viral envelope may contain virus-encoded glycoproteins, while the inner surface of the envelope tends to be associated with membrane or matrix proteins. The matrix proteins traverse the lipid bilayer and seem to bond with the internal areas of the glycoproteins and with the nucleocapsid proteins. *(Joklik et al, pp 750–751)*

816. **(C)** Elaborate molecular biology experiments have now clearly established that successive groups of three purine and pyrimidine pairs (nucleotide base pairs) code for each amino acids. Therefore, since the viral capsid in this question is composed of 2,500 amino acids, 7,500 nucleotide base pairs will be needed to code for the amino acids of the viral capsid. *(Brooks et al, pp 90–94)*

817. **(B)** Measles is not a positive-stranded virus, as are all of the other viruses listed in the question. Measles (rubeola) virus is a member of the genus *Morbillivirus*, in the Paramyxoviridae family, which includes negative-stranded, single-stranded RNA viruses. *(Joklik et al, pp 773–775)*

818. **(B)** On microscopic examination, virus-infected cells may appear unaltered, or they may show damage known as the cytopathic effect. The cytopathic reactions include necrosis, hypertrophy, giant cell formation, hypoplasia, metaplasia, syncytia, destruction of the host cell monolayer, and inclusion body formation in the nucleus or the cytoplasm of the host cells. For example, enteroviruses destroy the host cell monolayer in 48 to 72 hours. Intranuclear inclusion bodies are found in the lesions induced by the yellow fever, herpes, and varicella viruses. Intracytoplasmic inclusion bodies are found associated with vaccinia, variola, rabies, and certain other viral diseases. These cytologic changes provide useful presumptive evidence for the diagnosis of the viruses that induce the cytopathic effects. *(Joklik et al, p 943)*

819. **(D)** Coronaviruses can cause respiratory disease in adults and gastroenteritis in infants. Transmission to humans occurs via respiratory and gastrointestinal tract excretions and expectorations. Flaviviruses and togaviruses are the etiologic agents of viral encephalitis. St. Louis encephalitis is the most important arthropod-borne human infection. Mosquitoes, especially *Culex tarsalis,* act as vectors of encephalitis. Bunyaviruses were initially found in California but now have spread to other states. They are transmitted to humans by *Aedes triseriatus* mosquitoes and cause the typical signs of encephalitis, that is, severe bifrontal headache, fever, vomiting, lethargy, and possible convulsions. Yellow fever is caused by a flavivirus that is transmitted to humans by *Aedes* mosquitoes and is characterized by high fever, jaundice, hemorrhages, and neurologic symptoms. *(Brooks et al, pp 489–505,536–538)*

820. **(D)** Since mammalian cells do not contain the necessary enzyme, negative-stranded RNA viruses, which cannot serve directly as messenger RNA (mRNA), must carry the RNA-dependent RNA polymerase as a structural component of the infecting virion. However, the positive-stranded RNA viruses, whose RNA can serve as mRNA, synthesize the viral RNA-dependent RNA polymerase following infection, and enzyme molecules are not incorporated into progeny virions. *(Joklik et al, pp 819–829)*

821. (B) Rhabdoviruses are negative-stranded viruses, not positive-stranded viruses. *(Joklik et al, pp 820–822,1028–1030)*

822. (E) Influenza virus, such as influenza C virus, is classified as an orthomyxovirus rather than a paramyxovirus, as are all the other viruses listed in the question. *(Joklik et al, pp 777–779)*

823. (C) Papovaviruses produce latent and chronic infections in their hosts and can induce tumors in some animal species. All the other viruses listed in the question cause upper respiratory tract infections, including symptoms of the common cold. *(Joklik et al, pp 975–979,989–1014,1057–1059)*

824. (A) Influenza viruses (orthomyxoviruses) are enveloped viruses with segmented, single-stranded, negative-stranded RNA genomes, exhibiting helical symmetry. Thus, statement A is wrong; it is segmented, and all the other statements are correct *(Joklik et al, pp 779,824–827)*

825. (A) Scrapie is a degenerative central nervous system disease of sheep. The etiologic agent has been associated with a proteinaceous material devoid of any detectable amounts of nucleic acid and is called a prion instead of a virus. A severe form of encephalitis may be produced by herpesvirus type 1. Herpesvirus type 2 may be transmitted to the newborn during passage through an infected birth canal. Severely infected infants may have permanent brain damage. Genital herpes caused by herpesvirus type 2 is characterized by vesiculo-ulcerative lesions of the penis, cervix, vulva, vagina, or perineum and may be transmitted venereally. Vesicles and skin rashes are also caused by the varicella-zoster virus. *(Joklik et al, pp 957,1065–1067)*

826. (D) The size of viruses ranges between 0.025 μm and 0.2 μm. Most bacterial filters have a pore size a little larger than 0.2 μm and thus with a few exceptions will pass through filters that retain bacteria. Since they lack any independent biosynthetic capabilities and depend on host cells for energy production, viruses are not sensitive to antibiotics. Their replication is inhibited by interferon, which blocks translation of viral mRNA. Viruses may contain either RNA or DNA, but not both, and they may or may not contain an envelope. *(Brooks et al, pp 366–388)*

827. (C) A double-stranded DNA virus causes chickenpox in the human host. Recurrent infection of adults with this virus results in shingles. *(Joklik et al, pp 769–770)*

828. (C) Although most viruses contain proteins (enzymes) required for starting the initial process of replication within the host cells, vaccinia virus is one of those viruses that require a newly synthesized protein (polypeptide) for complete uncoating. This required protein is encoded in the viral DNA and transcribed by the DNA-dependent RNA polymerase that is present within the virus. *(Joklik et al, pp 795–812)*

829. (A) Although adenoviruses and variola viruses are double-stranded DNA viruses, their genomes have a uniform structure and cannot exist in four possible isomeric forms. Rotavirus is a double-stranded RNA virus, and hepatitis A virus is a single-stranded RNA virus. *(Joklik et al, pp 804–805)*

830. (D) Epstein–Barr virus (EBV) is linked to the development of Burkitt's lymphoma. It is not possible to state with certainty whether the relationship between EBV and nasopharyngeal carcinoma is unequivocal or not. The cells of most of the Burkitt's tumors that arise contain EBV DNA. EBV has an etiologic role in Burkitt's lymphoma and nasopharyngeal carcinoma, but other cofactors must also be involved. *(Joklik et al, pp 876–877,963–964)*

831. (D) The number of phages per mL in the original suspension is 200,000. Dilutions 1:100 (10^{-2}), 1:1000 (10^{-3}) and 1:10000 (10^{-4}) all indicate that there are 20,000 phages per 0.1 mL, or 200,000/mL of the original suspension. That is, the 200 plaque count obtained with a 1:100 dilution must be multiplied by 100 to account for the dilution and then multiplied again by 10 to convert the number of phages to 1 mL instead of the 0.1 mL that was used to obtain the plaques that resulted as a result of the lysis of bacteria by the phage particles: 200 × 100 × 10 equals 200,000. *(Brooks et al, pp 84–87)*

832. **(B)** Among the viruses listed in the question, HBV is the only virus that has cirrhosis and primary hepatocellular carcinoma as sequelae. The HBV genome (DNA) is known to be integrated into the DNA of tumor cells. Marburg virus is an RNA virus similar to rhabdovirus and is not related to hepatitis viruses. Marburg virus causes African hemorrhagic fever. *(Joklik et al, pp 1031–1032, 1039–1049)*

833. **(C)** Hepatitis A virus (HAV) and retroviruses are RNA viruses. The nature of the genome of non-A/non-B hepatitis virus is not known. Polyomavirus is a double-stranded DNA virus. The genome of polyomavirus is replicated bidirectionally using the DNA polymerase of the host cell. *(Joklik et al, pp 796–798,810–812,829,878–884)*

834. **(D)** During the eclipse phase of viral replication, uncoating of the virion occurs; the viral nucleic acid is separated from its capsid as well as other envelopes that may surround the capsid; the virus no longer can be distinguished by electron microscopy. Thus, electron microscopy becomes useless at this point of viral replication. Radioimmunoassay (RIA) is an assay used to quantitate antigens that can be radioactively labeled. Enzyme-linked immunosorbent assay (ELISA) depends on the conjugation of an enzyme to an antibody or antigen, and this enzyme can be detected by the addition of its substrate. The sensitivity of ELISA approaches that of RIA. Immunofluorescence depends on the conjugation of the fluorescent dye fluorescein, or auramine, to antibody, which may be made detectable by ultraviolet light with a fluorescence microscope. The three immunological assays described above can be used to detect viral antigens during the eclipse phase of viral replication. *(Joklik et al, pp 790–795; Brooks et al, p 121)*

835. **(A)** The major source of infection of hepatitis A virus is feces. Hepatitis B virus and agents causing non-A/non-B are transmitted through blood and other body fluids. Cytomegalovirus is transmitted by several different routes, including the intrauterine route, sexual route, and via blood and other body fluids. Liver involvement is minimal in Epstein–Barr virus infections. *(Joklik et al, pp 1039–1046)*

836. **(B)** Amantadine (Symmetrel) inhibits an early event in the multiplication cycle of influenza virus as well as arenaviruses. It blocks the uncoating process. Mutations in the M protein genes result in the development of drug-resistant mutants. The drug is not used extensively in the United States because it seems impractical to control this type of infectious disease that is not fatal. To protect individuals at high risk and those in whom infection is of potential danger, there is a choice between this drug and the influenza vaccine. In most cases, the vaccine seems to be preferred. *(Joklik et al, pp 858, 996–997)*

837. **(D)** Measles virus is an RNA-containing human virus that is membrane bound. The nucleocapsid proteins are arranged in an helical symmetry inside the viral membrane. Therefore answers B, C, and E are not correct. D becomes the Best answer since A does not provide a function for the nucleocapsid protein. *(Joklik et al, pp 823,1011–1024)*

838. **(C)** Two types of herpes simplex virus have been identified: herpes simplex virus type 1, which usually infects the oral cavity, lips, respiratory tract, eyes, or the central nervous system; and herpes simplex virus type 2, which involves mainly the genitalia and is known as the genital strain. *(Joklik et al, pp 956–957)*

839. **(D)** Transmission of herpes simplex virus type 1 occurs primarily by direct personal contact. Breast milk, blood, frozen plasma, and contaminated syringes have been implicated in the transmission of human immu-

nodeficiency virus and are not considered the primary vehicles of herpes simplex virus type 1. *(Joklik et al, pp 955–959)*

840. (B) In a Tzanck smear, fixed stained scrapings from the vesicle base reveal multinucleated giant cells and intranuclear inclusions in herpesvirus infections. Because similar intranuclear inclusions may be caused by the varicella-zoster virus, the Tzanck smear cannot be employed to distinguish between varicella-zoster virus and herpes simplex virus infections. To perform a Tzanck smear, an intact vesicle is located and ruptured with a razor blade. The base of the vesicle is scraped with the blade, and the blade is wiped off a clean slide that is stained with Wright's stain. The smear is finally examined to locate multinucleated giant cells with intranuclear inclusions. These are seen in herpes simplex and in varicella-zoster virus lesions. *(Joklik et al, p 958)*

841. (B) The varicella-zoster virus (VZV) remains latent in the nerve root cells of the posterior root ganglia or cranial nerve roots. The most frequently affected cranial nerve is the trigeminal. Infections due to VZV are thought to represent a reactivation of a prior varicella infection. This frequently occurs when humans become immunosuppressed. Zoster may appear in a newborn after maternal chickenpox. Following a prodromal symptom of pain, vesicles appear along the course of the affected cranial or sensory nerves. *(Joklik et al, pp 959–961)*

842. (E) At the beginning of the twentieth century, pathologists observed the presence of large swollen cells in the lungs, liver, and kidneys of infants dying of congenital (vertical) cytomegalovirus (CMV) infection. Infants who survive CMV congenital infections may become mentally retarded. The CMV is transmitted venerally, by blood transfusion, congenitally, or via organ transplantation. Thus, heart, bone, and renal transplant patients may acquire CMV. Since these patients are receiving immunosuppressive drugs to suppress organ rejection, CMV in-

fections in organ transplant patients are an important cause of morbidity for them. *(Joklik et al, pp 961–963)*

843. (A) The human T-cell lymphotrophic/lymphadenoma-associated virus (HTLV-III/LAV), now known as HIV, has been identified as the cause of AIDS. This virus has been shown to replicate and destroy the T4 cells, which constitute the primary targets for this virus. *(Joklik et al, pp 1051–1054)*

844. (D) The HIV retrovirus is an important member of the lentiviruses. The virus replicates in and kills helper T cells of the T4 class, a finding that explains much of the pathology of AIDS. The oncoviruses produce leukemias, lymphomas, breast carcinomas, and sarcomas. The spuma or foamy viruses produce cytopathic effect in tissue culture cells, but no known disease. The lentiviruses, oncoviruses, and spuma viruses constitute the three groups into which the retroviruses are divided. *(Joklik et al, pp 779–780,1051–1054)*

845. (B) The sarcoma/acute leukemia viruses are single-stranded RNA viruses. The RNA is segmented, and the viruses possess ether-sensitive envelopes. They are able to transform fibroblasts and hematopoietic cells in tissue culture. With the exception of the Rous sarcoma virus, they are defective viruses and can replicate only when a nondefective helper virus infects the same cell. They are defective because they have picked up pieces of genetic information from their host cells and in the process have deleted information encoding essential viral proteins. *(Joklik et al, pp 779–780,886–887)*

846. (A) Each genomic RNA molecule of the retroviruses has the same polarity as the viral messenger RNA (mRNA). However, unlike the positive-stranded RNA viruses, genomic RNA does not serve as mRNA immediately following penetration of the virus into the cell. Instead, genomic RNAs are copied to produce linear double-stranded DNA copies of the viral RNA retrovirus genome. This step is catalyzed by the retroviral enzyme reverse transcriptase. The RNA genome of retroviruses is segmented. The viruses mature in the cytoplasm of their host cells and contain glycoproteins in their envelopes. *(Joklik et al, pp 880–884)*

847. **(D)** The *env* gene of HIV (AIDS retrovirus) is extremely variable. Marked mutation of the *env* gene was recently discovered even during the course of AIDS in the same patient. Because the *env* gene encodes the highly variable envelope glycoproteins of HIV, this situation has been offered as an explanation for the progressive course of AIDS within each patient and for the way HIV evades the host immune response. *(Joklik et al, pp 880–884)*

848. **(E)** An important difference between HIV and the RNA tumor viruses is that it lyses the host cells while RNA tumor viruses transform the cells that they invade but do not possess cytolytic activity. The tropism of HIV for the T4 lymphocytes depends on the presence of the T4 protein on the surface of the T4 lymphocyte. This protein serves as the receptor for the adsorption of HIV to T4 lymphocytes. HIV is a member of the retroviruses. Retroviruses contain two copies of the genome's RNA molecule. The genomic RNA molecule contains the *gag*, *pol*, and *env* genes. Therefore, HIV cannot be expected to differ from the RNA tumor retroviruses. *(Joklik et al, pp 880–887)*

849. **(D)** The genomic RNA molecule of retroviruses contains three important genes: the *pol* gene, which codes for the reverse transcriptase (DNA polymerase) that transcribes the retroviral RNA genome into DNA; the *gag* gene, which codes for a protein that is the precursor to four structural proteins of the nucleoid; and the *env* gene, which codes for the retroviral envelope proteins. *(Joklik et al, pp 880–890)*

850. **(C)** The *myc* gene, found in the animal retrovirus avian MC20 myelocytomatosis, is capable of inducing immortality of the transformed cells. It encodes for nuclear matrix proteins that are possibly involved in regulating transcription. The guanine nucleotide

binding proteins are encoded by the *Ha-ras*, *Ki-ras*, or the *N-ras* oncogenes. Protein kinases specific for serine or threonine are encoded by the *fms*, *mos*, or the *raf* oncogenes. Finally, oncogenes *skc*, *yes*, *fps*, *abl*, *ros*, *fgr*, and *erbB* are needed for the synthesis of tyrosine specific kinases. *(Joklik et al, pp 887–892)*

851. **(C)** By definition, the normal cell gene that can be transformed to an oncogene is called a proto-oncogene. *(Joklik et al, pp 887–888)*

852. **(A)** The genome of reoviruses is segmented double stranded. It has a cubic symmetry and it is resistant to ether. Rotaviruses are members of the reoviruses. They have a wheel-shaped morphology and are the causative agents of infantile gastroenteritis. Papovaviruses are ether-resistant, circular double-stranded DNA viruses. They cause human warts and they can be tumorigenic. Influenza viruses are members of the orthomyxoviruses, containing a segmented, single-stranded RNA genome. Orthomyxoviruses have hemagglutinin, or neuraminidase, on their surface, and they are sensitive to ether. The genome of arenaviruses is segmented and single-stranded. The Lassa fever virus is a member of the arenaviruses, which are prominent in tropical America. Lassa fever is characterized by ulcers, skin rashes, higher fever, hemorrhages, pneumonia, and kidney and heart lesions. The mortality rate ranges between 36 and 37%. Rhabdoviruses have a single-stranded, nonsegmented RNA genome. The rabies virus is an example of a rhabdovirus. It has a bullet-shaped morphology, and it is ether sensitive. *(Brooks et al, pp 368–370)*

853. **(D)** The *Ha-ras* oncogene is found in the Harvey murine sarcoma retrovirus, which contains single-stranded RNA. The *Ha-ras* oncogene encodes for guanine nucleotide-binding proteins with guanine triphosphate activity. The oncogene that is derived from the PDGF gene is the *sis* oncogene of the simian sarcoma retrovirus. The nonviral tumor avian bursal lymphomas have been associated with the *Blym* oncogene. *(Levinson and Jawetz, pp 559–561)*

854. (C) The disease syndromes that adenoviruses are associated with include acute respiratory track infections, conjunctivitis, and epidemic keratoconjunctivitis. The fact that the majority of tonsils and adenoids will yield adenoviruses following surgical removal exemplifies the common nature of their infections. Therefore, coughing, nasal congestion, fever, headache, chills, and muscular pains will be expected in respiratory tract infections caused by adenoviruses. Some, or all, of these symptoms are found in infections caused by influenza, parainfluenza, mumps, or measles viruses; however, these viruses are all enveloped viruses, without projecting fibers from their nucleocapsids. In contrast to these viruses, adenoviruses do not have envelopes and they can be readily separated from other icosahedral viruses, because they possess characteristic projections known as fibers from each of their vertices, or penton bases. *(Brooks et al, pp 408–409)*

855. (E) Togaviruses contain viral species which cause encephalitis. They are transmitted via mosquito vectors with birds serving as reservoirs of infection. Western and Eastern encephalitis viruses cause infections that have high mortality in children and in aged individuals. These viruses enter the bloodstream from insect inoculation. The virus is removed by the reticuloendothelial cells and multiplies in the spleen and lymph nodes. From these tissues a secondary viremia is established spreading the virus to the CNS by passage through the blood–brain junction (virus grows through the vascular endothelium or in some way is passively transported across the blood–brain barrier). The brain and spinal cord become edematous and show vascular congestion and small hemorrhages. There are no human vaccines, and control is limited to controlling the insect vectors and identifying and controlling the animal reservoirs of infection. *(Brooks et al, pp 492–495)*

856. (C) The chief reservoirs of hantavirus are small rodents such as mice and voles. The virus is believed to be transmitted to humans most frequently by inhalation of infected rodent excreta, by the conjunctival route, or by direct contact with skin lesions. Transmission from one individual to another has not been documented. The disease is diagnosed serologically. *(Ryan et al, pp 534–535)*

857. (D) The nucleic acids of several groups of animal viruses (eg, those of togaviruses, papovaviruses, adenoviruses, and herpesviruses) are not infectious. These all are nucleic acids that either can act as messenger RNA (mRNA) themselves or that are transcribed into mRNA by host-coded RNA polymerases. Of the viruses listed in the question, only nucleic acids of picornaviruses are infectious. *(Brooks et al, pp 408,418,469 489,562)*

858. (C) Defective interfering (DI) viruses lack one or more functional genes for virus replication. They do not have excess genetic material. They arise spontaneously when passaged at high multiplicity of infection but not when there is phenotypic mixing. DI virus particles have normal capsid proteins. Prions are unconventional viruses. *(Levinson and Jawetz, pp 379–380,384; Joklik et al, p 1064)*

859. (E) To determine whether the poliovirus is a wild-type virus or related to that used for vaccination, it will be necessary to prepare oligonucleotide maps of the isolated virus and compare them with the oligonucleotide maps of the wild type and vaccine strains. Many viruses may kill mice; thus, one cannot determine by mouse lethality studies that he is dealing with related or unrelated poliovirus strains. Similarly, cytopathology cannot be used for definitive diagnosis of poliovirus strains or other types of viruses. Viral neutralization assays using the grandchild's serum will only indicate if the grandchild has been exposed and vaccinated to the polioviruses in question, but will not establish whether the poliovirus isolated from the stool of the 55-year-old grandfather is related to the poliovirus used to vaccinate his grandchild. *(Joklik et al, p 768)*

860. (D) The negative-stranded, single-stranded RNA viruses (the first three viruses listed in the question) must all carry RNA-dependent RNA polymerase as a structural component because their negative-stranded RNA cannot serve directly as messenger RNA (mRNA). The retroviruses carry a reverse transcriptase, an RNA-directed DNA polymerase. *(Levinson and Jawetz, pp 510,517,539,553)*

861. **(E)** Infectious mononucleosis is caused by Epstein–Barr virus (EBV), which is a member of the herpesviruses. Nucleic acid hybridization assays for EBV DNA is the most sensitive means of diagnosing infectious mononucleosis. Important antigens that also may be used, but which are less sensitive for diagnostic purposes, include the viral capsid protein (VCA), the early proteins (EA), and the Epstein–Barr virus nuclear antigen (EBNA). Infectious mononucleosis patients develop antibody titers exceeding 1:320 and 1:20 against VCA and EA, respectively, during the acute phase of infectious mononucleosis. Antibodies to EBNA develop 1 to 2 months after acute infection. The majority of infectious mononucleosis patients develop what is known as heterophile antibody: that is, antibodies which cross react with unrelated antigens, such as those found on sheep and horse erythrocytes. Hemagglutinins and neuraminidases are associated with ortho- and paramyxoviruses. *(Brooks et al, pp 436–437; Joklik et al, pp 963–964)*

862. **(A)** Poliovirus is not enveloped and therefore is not inactivated by mild detergents that solubilize the phospholipid cytoplasmic membranes derived by budding through the host cell. *(Brooks et al, p 468)*

863. **(D)** All of the viral genomes listed in the question, except that of cytomegalovirus, a herpesvirus, replicate in the nucleus. *(Brooks et al, p 375)*

864. **(D)** Polyomavirus DNA becomes stably integrated into multiple sites of the DNA of the host. As a result, it *cannot* multiply except as a cellular gene, and no progeny of virus is produced. Rous sarcoma virus and avian leukemia virus belong to RNA tumor viruses containing transforming genes. Its genome is

integrated into the host chromosome, from which the genome of its progeny is transcribed. *(Joklik et al, pp 803,870–887)*

865. **(D)** Roseola infantum is a disease that is encountered frequently in infants and children 6 months to 4 years old. The term "exanthem subitum" means sudden rash. The etiologic agent most commonly associated with roseola infantum is the human herpesvirus type 6. The key clinical features of this disease include fever and rash of 2 to 4 days' duration. Leukopenia and some brief convulsions may be also encountered. *(Ryan et al, p 477)*

866. **(E)** Viral genomes are stably integrated into the host cell chromosomes in adenoviruses, HTLV-I, SV-40 virus, and hepatitis B virus. *(Joklik et al, pp 796–803;810–812)*

867. **(B)** The communicability of German measles (rubella) is much lower than that of measles (rubeola). Thus, 15 to 20% of women may reach adult age and still remain susceptible to German measles. Usually, uneventful recovery occurs following infection in many women. However, if a woman is infected during the third trimester of her pregnancy, the German measles virus following viremia can cause congenital infection. Intrauterine infection has been shown to lead to such severe complications of an infected fetus as aortic stenosis, ventricular septal defect, blindness, deafness, mental retardation, and death. Immunization of women early in life with a live, attenuated rubella vaccine protects mother and fetus against rubella. *(Joklik et al, pp 1016–1018)*

868. **(E)** The measles virus is usually transmitted by inhalation of aerosol droplets produced by sneezing and coughing during the prodromal phase of the disease and for several days after the appearance of the rash. Most nonimmunized children contract measles upon exposure to the measle virus. In the last few years a marked increase in the number of measle cases has been reported in the United States. This increase has been attributed to failure to immunize many preschool children, insufficient immunity in children im-

munized before 15 months of age, and declining immunity in individuals who received only one dose of the vaccine. *(Levinson and Jawetz, p 188)*

869. **(D)** By definition, passive immunity is immunity obtained following the administration of antibodies preformed in another host. The injection of immunoglobulins against such common viral diseases as chickenpox, or such bacterial diseases as diptheria, tetanus, and botulism provides immediately available antibodies which neutralize the specific virus or toxin that causes the disease under consideration. Induction of specific cellular or immune response involves the injection of a specific microorganism or the antigens to a given host, which in turn produces antibodies specific for the antigen or microorganism injected. *(Brooks et al, pp 105–108)*

870. **(B)** Mumps virus is single negative-stranded RNA virus. The RNA polymerase in the nucleocapsid transcribes the minus-stranded RNA into plus-stranded RNA of two types. The one type is the faithful transcription of the minus strands into plus strands, which in turn serve as templates for the synthesis of numerous progeny minus-strands (minus-strand replication). The second type is the transcription of the minus-stranded RNA into plus-stranded RNA molecules that can serve as the messenger RNA through which the viral RNA expresses itself. *(Joklik et al, pp 819–824)*

871. **(D)** Regular recurrent infections occur following primary infection with either herpes simplex virus 1 or herpes simplex virus 2. Recurrent disease is not usually as severe as primary disease, and most recurrences are due to reactivation of endogenous virus rather than to reinfection. Varicella-zoster virus causes varicella (chickenpox), which most people contract before reaching adulthood. Recurrent infection of adults results in zoster (shingles). Regular recurrent infections are not outstanding features of Epstein–Barr virus, varicella-zoster virus, or cytomegalovirus infections. *(Joklik et al, pp 955–965)*

872. **(A)** Because of the viremia that accompanies primary infection with herpes simplex virus, systemic manifestations usually accompany more severe local disease. Some primary infections go unrecognized or are subclinical. A few labial or genital lesions that resolve in a week to 10 days are the manifestation of reactivation of latent virus in sacral, trigeminal, and vaginal ganglia. *(Joklik et al, pp 956–957)*

873. **(A)** Viroids or prions, which produce diseases in plants, are small molecules of circular single-stranded RNA (ssRNA) with no proteinaceous capsid coat. They have extensive internal base pairing, which presumably protects them from extracellular nucleases. It is suspected that they may cause diseases in animals, perhaps being involved in some of the slow viral diseases such as kuru and scrapie, but this theory is only speculative. *(Ryan et al, pp 72,565; Brooks et al, p 370)*

874. **(A)** Creutzfeldt–Jakob disease is a progressive fatal disease of the central nervous system occurring in middle life. Vague prodromal symptoms are followed by dementia, with subsequent rapid progression to coma and death, usually within 2 years after development of the initial symptoms. Scrapie is a chronic, related disease that affects the central nervous system of sheep. The disease may be transmissible, indicating a causative role by infectious agents (collectively called slow viruses or prions). One of the unique features of this group of illnesses is the lack of an inflammatory reaction in involved tissues. *(Joklik et al, pp 1064–1068)*

875. **(D)** Except for hepatitis A virus, which is transmitted via the mouth, all the hepatitis-causing viruses are transmitted parenterally, mainly via contaminated blood. *(Joklik et al, pp 1041–1045)*

876. **(C)** Acyclovir is a relatively inert compound, but herpes simplex virus (HSV) thymidine kinase present in infected cells preferentially phosphorylates acyclovir to its monophosphate form. Cellular thymidine kinase has a significantly lower affinity for the drug, so phosphorylation by the host enzyme is un-

likely to occur. Further phosphorylation to the triphosphate form is mediated by cellular enzymes. Acyclovir triphosphate then can act as an inhibitor of, and substrate for, the HSV DNA polymerase, effectively blocking viral replication. (Joklik et al, p 857)

877. (E) The multiplication of all of the viruses listed in the question is inhibited by alpha-amanitin, an inhibitor of cellular RNA polymerase. This compound is a toxic component of the poisonous mushroom *Amanita phalloides*, and ingestion of this mushroom is often fatal. (Joklik et al, p 1082)

878. (D) Initially, acyclovir is preferentially phosphorylated by viral enzyme (thymidine kinase) to become acyclovir monophosphate, which is further phosphorylated by cellular enzymes. Acyclovir triphosphate inhibits herpes simplex virus DNA polymerase, thus inhibiting viral replication. (Joklik et al, p 857)

879. (D) Vidarabine (adenosine arabinoside, or ara-A) and similar compounds (cytosine arabinoside and ara-AMP) are inhibitors of DNA polymerase, which is more sensitive to the drugs than are host cell DNA polymerases. (Joklik et al, pp 856–857)

880. (D) Immune gamma globulin that is obtained from pools of healthy adult individuals has been shown to confer passive immunity to approximately 90 to 95% of those exposed to hepatitis A virus when it was administered 1 to 2 weeks after exposure to this virus. (Brooks et al, p 465)

881. (B) Two kinds of carcinogenic viruses have been identified: DNA viruses and the RNA-containing retroviruses. These viruses transform cells by permanently incorporating new genes into the DNA of the infected cells. The DNA-containing papovaviruses have genes that transform cells by creating in cells a growing state that promotes viral multiplication. Permanent cell transformation occurs when viral multiplication is not feasible. (Joklik et al, pp 370–371,870–893)

882. (B) For DNA viruses, the known transforming genes are integral parts of the virus genome. For the RNA-containing retroviruses, the transforming genes are thought to be normal or slightly altered cellular genes that are either appropriated from or hyperactivated in the host cell. (Joklik et al, pp 370–371, 870–893)

883. (E) The glycoproteins and glycolipids that are found in large amounts on the surface of normal cells are modified in transformed cells. For example, the protein-linked *N*-acetylneuraminic acid is decreased, as well as the ganglioside content of lipids. Transformed cells are agglutinated by lectins at a much lower level than are the normal cells. Also, transformed cells either lack fibronectin or contain significantly diminished levels. Finally, transformed cells show loss of actin microfilaments. (Joklik et al, pp 870–873)

884. (E) A common feature of arenaviruses is their zoonotic reservoir of infection. Small rodents such as mice or hamsters are the principal sources of infection for lymphocytic choriomeningitis, or hemorrhagic fevers, such as Argentinean hemorrhagic fever, Bolivian hemorrhagic fever, and Lassa fever. Small rodents do not play a major role in the transmission of enteroviruses, papovaviruses, poxviruses, or herpesviruses. (Ryan et al, pp 532–533)

885. (E) The virions of arenaviruses incorporate host cell ribosomes during their maturation and the incorporation of these ribosomes into the viral particles gives them a "sandy" appearance. This viral morphologic event usually does not occur during the maturation of enteroviruses, papovaviruses, poxviruses, or the herpesviruses. (Brooks et al, pp 369–371)

886. (C) The period when the infectivity of the virus particles is destroyed, or eclipsed, following uncoating is called the viral eclipse period. (Joklik et al, pp 790–795)

887. **(C)** Viruses contain only a single type of nucleic acid, either RNA or DNA, but not both. *(Brooks et al, p 374)*

888. **(A)** Rhinoviruses, which are picornaviruses, have a nonsegmented, positive-stranded RNA genome. *(Brooks et al, p 369)*

889. **(B)** Influenza viruses, which are orthomyxoviruses, have a segmented negative-stranded RNA genome. *(Brooks et al, p 370)*

890. **(D)** Dengue viruses have four clinically important serotypes. *(Brooks et al, pp 499–500)*

891. **(C)** There are three important polio serotypes. *(Brooks et al, p 471)*

892. **(C)** Two vaccines are currently used for active immunization against poliomyelitis, the inactivated polio vaccine (IPV) and a trivalent oral live virus vaccine (OPV). Both vaccines produce immunity in more than 90% of the recipients. However, the OPV has a higher benefit-to-risk ratio. In contrast to IPV, the OPV does not require booster injections. It is simple to administer, establishes intestinal immunity to reinfection, and is well received by patients. *(Brooks et al, pp 473–475)*

893. **(E)** The hepatitis B vaccine consists of purified hepatitis B virus surface antigen (HBsAg) obtained from the blood of high-titered carriers of HBsAg. Field trials have demonstrated that the vaccine provides excellent protection (80 to 95% efficacy) to high-risk groups, and commercially prepared vaccine is now available. *(Brooks et al, pp 128,464)*

894. **(A)** Measles virus vaccine is composed of live, attenuated measles virus and as such it is contraindicated for immunosuppressed individuals who might become infected or fail to respond. *(Brooks et al, pp 531–535)*

895. **(B)** The vast majority of the side effects from the influenza vaccine administration have been encountered in children. These include hypersensitivity, fever, and the Guillain–Barré syndrome. This condition manifests itself in approximately 2 months in ten of every million vaccinations. The syndrome is a self-limiting paralysis. Five to ten percent of individuals afflicted with Guillain–Barré syndrome show muscle weakness, and roughly 5% die. *(Brooks et al, pp 514–516)*

896. **(B)** Retroviruses contain a core where the two similar plus-stranded RNA molecules with the enzyme reverse transcriptase (E) are localized. The retrovirus core is enclosed in two shells. The inner nucleocapsid shell (D) that is encoded by the *gag* gene and an outer lipid bilayer shell (A). Below the lipid bilayer shell there is another myristilated protein layer known as the matrix protein (B), which is encoded by the *gag* gene and is essential for the budding of retrovirus from the host cells. *(Joklik et al, pp 878–884)*

897. **(C)** The initial events during retroviral or any other viral multiplication cycle are the adsorption and entry of the virus into the host cell. Each virus has specific structures on its surface layer that allows the virus to be adsorbed and enter into the host cell. In the case of retrovirus, it is the surface protein (C) that is required for the adsorption and entrance of viral particles into the host cells. The surface protein of retrovirus is encoded by the *env* gene and contains the major antigen against which neutralizing antibodies are formed. *(Joklik et al, p 880)*

898. **(A)** Some viruses such as the herpesviruses can exist for a long time in infected cells without producing overt disease. Apparently, synthesis of infectious virus has been arrested at a certain stage of the viral multiplication cycle. For reasons that have not been clarified, the arrest in the production of infectious virus can be either permanent or temporary. This phenomenon is known as latency, and the infections produced by herpesvirus types 1 and 2, varicella-zoster virus, Epstein–Barr virus, and cytomegalovirus are called latent infections. *(Joklik et al, p 840)*

899. **(B)** Inapparent infections are those in which viral multiplication and gene expression proceeds at such a low pace that their presence can be manifested only when the host immune response has been suppressed. For example, papovavirus BKV initiates inapparent urinary tract infections in most persons by the time they become adolescents, yet the infection becomes evident when the normal host defense mechanisms are overcome by chemotherapy, radiation, corticosteroids, or other immunosuppressive drugs. (*Joklik et al, p 840*)

900. **(B)** Poliovirus is a single, plus-stranded RNA virus. It lacks neuramidase and hemagglutinating glycoproteins that are components of the ortho- and paramyxoviruses. Poliovirus contains the VP1 surface protein that can induce virus neutralizing antibodies that remain for many years. Once the poliovirus reaches the brain and spinal cord, it is not affected by blood virus neutralizing antibodies. (*Brooks et al, p 473*)

901. **(C)** Scrapie is a central nervous system disease of sheep. Infected animals fail to grow, become excitable, and develop itching, ataxia, and spastic tremors, or they die. The itching causes sheep to scratch constantly against trees. It is from this scratching that the term scrapie is given to this disease. Normal sheep can be infected by grazing on pastures previously used by animals with scrapie. Thus, scrapie is transmissible. A unique 27- to 30-kd protein called prion protein 27-30 has been isolated from the brains of infected sheep. This protein is resistant to proteinase K digestion, as well as to physical and chemical treatments that modify nucleic acids. Agents or substances that cause transmissible diseases and have the characteristics described above are called prions. (*Joklik et al, pp 1064–1067*)

902. **(A)** Coronaviruses are spherical, 80 to 160 nm in diameter, and possess a helical nucleocapsid. Their genome is a linear, nonsegmented, positive single-stranded RNA. Another outstanding characteristic of coronaviruses is that they do not grow well in cell culture. Polioviruses, ortho- and paramyxoviruses, as well as poxviruses do not present difficult problems with regard to their cultivation in cell cultures. (*Brooks et al, pp 536–538*)

903. **(A)** The name coronaviruses is derived from the fact that these viruses possess envelopes with unique petal-shaped spikes resembling a solar corona. These petal or club-shaped envelope projections consist of a 180 to 200-kd glycoprotein. (*Brooks et al, pp 536–538*)

904. **(B)** For the purified viral genome to be infectious it must be able to serve directly as messenger RNA. Therefore, it must be positive-stranded. Poliovirus is a positive-stranded RNA virus. Rabies, measles, German measles, and influenza viruses are negative-stranded RNA viruses. Also see answer to question 812. (*Joklik et al, p 765*)

905. **(B)** The germane step during viral multiplication, following attachment, penetration, and uncoating of the viral particle, is the transcription of the viral genome into messenger RNAs (mRNAs). Once this is accomplished, the viral particle uses host cell components to translate the mRNAs, and new viral particles are synthesized. Depending on the nature of the viral nucleic acid, viruses employ diverse pathways to form their mRNAs. Rabies, measles, German measles, and influenza viruses are negative-stranded RNA viruses and must have in their virions RNA polymerases to form their mRNAs. They are called negative-stranded RNA viruses because their RNA has a nucleotide base sequence that is complementary to mRNA. Poliovirus is a positive-stranded RNA virus and does not need to carry RNA polymerase in its virion because the RNA in this case can serve directly as mRNA. (*Brooks et al, pp 380–381*)

906. **(A)** The time interval 0 to 5 hours (A) is called the eclipse period. During this period of the viral growth cycle, the virus is adsorbed to the host cell via ionic interactions and specific viral receptors on the host cell. Once the virus becomes adsorbed on the surface of the host cell, penetration of the virus into the cytoplasm of the host cell occurs and can be observed by electron microscopy. Finally, during the eclipse period, uncoating of the viral particle is observed. Now the viral nucleic acid is separated from its capsid as well as other envelopes that may surround the capsid. These events lead to loss of viral infectivity, so that the infectivity is eclipsed. The time interval 0 to 4 hours is known as the early period (C). It differs from the eclipse period in that it is slightly shorter than the eclipse period and in that no encapsidation of the viral genome has taken place. The appearance of the first progeny of viral nucleic acid signifies the start of the late period (D), and it is also shown by the curve drawn with a broken line. *(Joklik et al, pp 790–795)*

907. (B) The time interval 5 to 10 hours is known as the rise period (B). It indicates the complete synthesis of mature virus, the first appearance of progeny viral particles, and their increase as shown by the curve drawn with a solid line. This period is part of the late period (D) which according to the figure begins at the fourth hour and ends at the tenth hour. The duration of all periods during viral multiplication is dependant upon the nature of the virus and its host cell. *(Joklik et al, pp 790–795)*

908. (E) According to the figure, the late period (D) in the one-step growth cycle of a virus begins at the fourth hour and ends on the tenth hour of the growth cycle. The time period between the fourth and fifth hours (E) is the period necessary to encapsidate the viral genome. It is essentially the time required to assemble the proper sequences of amino acids into capsid proteins. That is, the proteins form a shell or a coat that encloses and protects the nucleic acid of the viral genome. *(Joklik et al, pp 790–795)*

909. (B) Hepatitis B virus (HBV) is the etiological agent of serum hepatitis, which is transmitted to humans by HBV infected blood or blood products. The virus contains an envelope or surface protein known as hepatitis B virus surface antigen (HBsAg). Purified HBsAg is now available for active immunization and prevention against HBV infection. The licensed vaccine is called Heptavax-B, or

Recombivax by the vaccine manufacturers. Since the mechanism of resistance against HBV is based on an antibody response to HBsAg it is understandable that the vaccine has been found to be effective against HBV infection in 85 to 95% of vaccinated individuals. There are no vaccines available against hepatitis A, C, D, or E. *(Joklik et al, pp 1042–1046)*

910. (A) Patients with short-incubation hepatitis A virus remain asymptomatic for as little as 15 days following exposure. Then fever, vomiting, and abdominal pain develop for about 1 week. At this time, jaundice with other symptoms may occur. Hepatitis B, C, and D viruses have a longer incubation period (45 to 160 days) than hepatitis A. *(Brooks et al, p 457)*

911. (E) The usual vector of Russian spring–summer encephalitis virus is the *Ixodes* or *Dermacentor* tick. The invertebrate vectors of dengue fever, St. Louis encephalitis, and Eastern equine encephalitis viruses are the *Aedes* or *Culex* mosquitoes. Development of Rous sarcoma depends on the conversion of proto-oncogenes such as the *src* gene to oncogene. *(Joklik et al, pp 887–888,1023–1024)*

912. (B) The Rous sarcoma virus possesses the *src* proto-oncogene. Dengue, St. Louis encephalitis, Eastern equine encephalitis, and the Russian spring–summer viruses lack oncogenic properties because they lack the *src* gene, which is required for cell transformation to oncogenic state. *(Joklik et al, pp 887–891)*

913. (B) When an untransformed cell comes into contact with another similar cell, this untransformed cell can no longer divide to produce a progeny of new cells. This phenomenon is called contact inhibition of growth. Cells transformed by tumor viruses lose this property and thus pile up on the top of each other and form tumors. Normal fibroblast cells or transformed cells do not contain muramic or diaminopimelic acid. These acids are components of the procaryotic bacterial cells. *(Joklik et al, pp 870–873)*

914. (A) Untransformed fibroblast cells require attachment to a solid surface in order to divide. This need of the untransformed cells is called anchorage dependence of multiplication. By comparison, transformed cells can multiply in suspension. *(Joklik et al, pp 870–873)*

915. (B) The Epstein–Barr virus has been implicated in Burkitt's lymphoma and nasopharyngeal carcinoma. The evidence for this is that sera from patients with Burkitt's lymphoma and nasopharyngeal carcinoma contain antibodies to Epstein–Barr virus. Also, many Burkitt's lymphoma patients exhibit a characteristic chromosomal translocation, the result of which is to place the cellular proto-oncogene *c-myc* near elements in the cell that activate it. *(Joklik et al, pp 963–964)*

916. (C) Both the adenoviruses and the Burkitt's lymphoma virus transform cells in culture. Adenoviruses induce tumors in laboratory animals but have not been implicated in any human tumors. The Epstein–Barr virus has been associated with Burkitt's lymphoma and nasopharyngeal carcinoma in humans. The E1A region of the adenoviral genome is involved in cell transformation. Cells transformed by adenoviruses contain the integrated viral DNA. Similarly, tumor cells obtained from Burkitt's lymphoma patients contain the entire Epstein–Barr genome and express the Epstein–Barr nuclear antigen, or EBNA. *(Joklik et al, pp 876,964)*

917. (D) There is some evidence that suggests that infection with herpes simplex virus type 2 is associated with carcinoma of the cervix. Similarly, hepatitis B virus has been associated with primary hepatocellular carcinoma in humans. However, although suggestive, this evidence is not sufficient to establish a definitive etiologic association between herpes simplex virus type 2 or the hepatitis B virus and malignancy in humans. *(Joklik et al, pp 855,878,957,959)*

918. (B) Large 45-nm spherical bodies called Dane particles have been demonstrated in the sera of patients with hepatitis B viral infections. They are composed of an envelope that contains the hepatitis B surface antigen and an inner core that contains the hepatitis B virus core antigen. DNA polymerase, as well as DNA, has been found in the inner core of the Dane particle. *(Joklik et al, p 811)*

919. (E) Children under 2 years of age appear particularly susceptible to rotaviral infections. Fever and severe diarrhea, followed by vomiting, are the main symptoms. The principal site of viral multiplication appears to be the duodenal mucosa with secretion of virus on the feces most prominently during the first several days of infection. Viral isolation may be difficult, but virions can be detected in fecal material using electron microscopy of concentrated samples. The viral particles are nonenveloped, wheel-shaped, 60 to 80 nm, and contain double-stranded RNA in 11 segments. Coronaviruses (B) are spherical, 80 to 160 nm. Their genome is a linear, nonsegmented, positive-sense, single-stranded RNA. The viral particles are enveloped and contain unique petal-shaped projections resembling a solar corona. The human coronaviruses cause common colds and have been implicated in gastroenteritis in infants. Poxviruses (C) are the largest and most complex enveloped brick-shaped virions measuring approximately 400 nm. Poxviruses contain a double-stranded DNA, linear genome. They produce such diseases as smallpox and vaccinia that are basically exanthematous skin infections in which macules, papules, vesicles, and pustules develop. Parvoviruses (D) are the smallest viruses, measuring about 20 nm. They lack envelopes and contain linear, single-stranded DNA and have an icosahedral capsid. A typical member of the parvoviruses is the human adeno-associated virus that depends upon adenovirus for coinfection, growth, and spread in the human population. Parvoviruses have not been associated with any known human disease. Adenoviruses (F) lack envelopes and have a linear, continuous piece of double-stranded DNA. Thirty-five serotypes have been described. The antigenic characteristics of these viruses are determined by the protein polypeptides, which comprise their icosahedral capsid with unique fiber projections from each vertex.

Adenoviruses are associated with acute respiratory infections, conjunctivitis, and keratoconjunctivitis. (*Brooks et al, pp 369–370,408, 441,482,537,583*)

920. **(A)** Rabies is a 75-nm bullet-shaped virion that contains a single molecule of single-stranded RNA with negative-sense polarity. The RNA genome is surrounded by several proteins that form the nucleocapsid. One of these proteins is an RNA polymerase. Bites or scratches that break the skin are required for virus transmission from an infected dog, bat, or other animal's saliva. Initial signs of infection include headache, fever, vomiting, and sore throat. A tingling sensation at the site of the wound, nervousness, apprehension, and anxiety follow as symptoms. Then throat spasms leading to hydrophobia, increased perspiration, convulsions, seizures, and coma precede death. Human antiserum for the rabies virus is available for passive protection, and an attenuated vaccine appears promising. See the previous answer for reasons why the other choices are incorrect. (*Brooks et al, pp 539–544*)

921. **(G)** The initial cases of Lassa fever were reported in the Nigerian village of Lassa. The causative agent was an arenavirus. This is an enveloped virus, which possesses a single-stranded negative-polarity RNA genome in two segments and enclosed in a helical capsid. The viral particles incorporate host cell ribosomes, which gives the virions a sandy appearance. Arenaviruses pathogenic for humans cause chronic infections in rodents. Thus, Lassa fever transmission to individuals can occur by contact with infected rodents or their excretions. Transmission can also occur by human-to-human contact. Arenavirus can attack any organ of the body. However, patients with Lassa fever usually develop high fever, mouth ulcers, skin rashes with hemorrhages, and muscular pain, as well as kidney and heart damage. This kidney and cardiac damage can cause death in 36 to 67% of Lassa fever patients. See answers 924 and 925 for reasons why the other choices are not correct. (*Brooks et al, pp 470,488–489,504*)

922. **(E)** Bacteriophages (phages) are viruses that infect bacteria. A number of medically important diseases, such as diphtheria, scarlet fever, and botulism, are caused by bacteriophage products. For example, diphtheria toxin is the product of a lysogenic phage that resides in *Corybacterium diphtheriae*. Likewise, toxin production by *Streptococcus pyogenes* and *Clostridium botulinum* depends upon the presence of phages. Many bacteriophages have proteinaceous structures on their tails known as tail fibers (E), which serve to recognize specific binding sites on the bacterial host cells. See answer 928 for reasons why the other choices are incorrect. (*Brooks et al, pp 84–85*)

923. **(C)** Basically, phages consist of a head (A) and a tail. The tail functions both as an attachment organ and as a tube through which the phage genome (B) is injected into the bacterial cell. The tail has a hollow core (D), most of which is covered by a sheath (C) that collapses to drive the hollow tube of the tail through the envelopes of the bacterial cell. The head (A) consists of a protein coat that surrounds and protects the phage genome. This head coat usually contains two to three major structural proteins and some other minor components. Phages may have DNA or RNA as their genome (B). RNA is always linear and usually single-stranded. DNA may be either linear or circular and double- or single-stranded. (*Brooks et al, pp 84–85*)

REFERENCES

Brooks GF, Butel JS, Ornston LN, et al. *Medical Microbiology*, 19th ed. Norwalk, CT: Appleton & Lange; 1991.

Joklik WK, Willett HP, Amos BD, Wilfert CM. *Zinsser Microbiology*, 20th ed. Norwalk, CT: Appleton & Lange; 1992.

Levinson WE, Jawetz E. *Medical Microbiology and Immunology*, 2nd ed. Norwalk, CT: Appleton & Lange; 1992.

Ryan KJ, Champoux JJ, Drew WL, et al. *Sherris Medical Microbiology*, 3rd ed. Norwalk, CT: Appleton & Lange; 1994.

CHAPTER 9

Practice Test

READ THE FOLLOWING INSTRUCTIONS CAREFULLY BEFORE TAKING THE PRACTICE TEST

---

1. This examination consists of 100 questions, covering the subject areas listed in the table of contents.
2. The practice test simulates an actual examination in question types and integration of subject areas.
3. You should set aside 1 hour and 25 minutes of *uninterrupted*, distraction-free time to take the practice test. This averages out to 50 seconds per question.
4. Be sure you have a clock (to time and pace yourself) and an adequate number of No. 2 pencils and erasers.
5. You should tear out and use the answer sheet that is provided on pages 287 to 288.
6. Be sure to answer all of the questions, and be sure the number on the answer sheet corresponds to the question number in the practice test.
7. Use any remaining time to review your answers.
8. After completing the practice test, you can check all of your answers on pages 270 to 284. A score of 75% or higher should be considered as a passing score (75 correct answers).
9. After checking your answers and your score, you can analyze your strengths and weaknesses using the Practice Test Subspecialty List on page 285. To do this, you should check off your incorrect practice test answers on the subspecialty list. You may find a pattern developing. For example, you may find you do well on medical bacteriology but poorly on immunology. In such an instance, you can go back and review the immunology section of this book and supplement your review with your texts and with the references cited in that section.

Questions

which part of the virus is indicated by arrow 2?

DIRECTIONS (Questions 1 through 79): Each of the numbered items or incomplete statements in this section is followed by answers or by completions of the statement. Select the ONE lettered answer or completion that is BEST in each case.

1. Which of the following statements is true concerning blood groups and blood typing?

   (A) type AB individuals can always receive blood from a donor of any other ABO blood group
   (B) antibodies to the ABO blood group antigens are "natural" antibodies
   (C) the blood types A, B, O, and Rh are adequate information in determining compatibility for crossmatch purposes
   (D) antibodies to the Rh blood group antigens are "natural" antibodies

2. Skin may be BEST disinfected by washing with

   (A) isopropyl alcohol
   (B) soap
   (C) mercurochrome
   (D) 1% hydrogen peroxide
   (E) 1% solution of iodine in 70% ethanol

3. The following figure shows various structures of a virus. According to this figure,

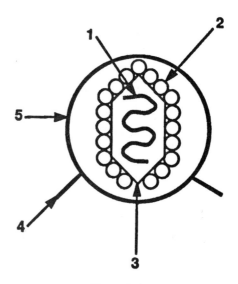

Figure 9–1

   (A) spike
   (B) envelope
   (C) matrix protein
   (D) nucleic acid
   (E) capsomer

4. The periplasmic space

   (A) is within the lysosome
   (B) is within the cytoplasm
   (C) contains biosynthetic enzymes
   (D) contains mesosomal enzymes
   (E) is between the cell wall and the cytoplasmic membrane

5. A mixed lymphocyte reaction that results in marked cellular differentiation and a very good induction of cytotoxic T lymphocytes is a result of

   (A) similarity at major histocompatibility complex (MHC) class I and MHC class II loci
   (B) disparity at MHC class I and MHC class II loci
   (C) disparity at MHC class I loci and similarity at MHC class II loci
   (D) disparity at MHC class II loci and similarity at MHC class I loci

6. One difference that distinguishes the genetics of heavy chains from that of light chains is the

   (A) presence of V genes
   (B) presence of J genes
   (C) presence of C genes
   (D) processing of nuclear messenger RNA by splicing out intervening sequences
   (E) ability to translocate variable-region gene clusters to different C genes

7. The tolerance of facultative anaerobic bacteria to superoxide is due to

   (A) the lack of cytochrome C oxidase
   (B) the presence of cytochrome C oxidase
   (C) the lack of peroxidase
   (D) the presence of superoxide dismutase and catalase
   (E) the inability to form the superoxide radical

8. The process in which any bacterial gene can be packaged inside a phage particle and then introduced into another bacterium by infec-

tion of that cell with the phage, leading to a change in the phenotype of the recipient cell, is called

   (A) generalized transformation
   (B) specialized transduction
   (C) generalized transfection
   (D) sexduction
   (E) generalized transduction

9. A procedure used to detect some of the orthomyxoviruses and paramyxoviruses that produce little or no cytopathic effect in cell culture is the use of

   (A) neutralization
   (B) hemadsorption
   (C) plaque reduction
   (D) complement fixation
   (E) interference

10. A lymphoma patient starts to complain of frequent cough and mild chest pain. A chest x-ray examination reveals a coin-sized round shadow that resembles cavitary tuberculosis. The tuberculin reaction of the patient is, however, negative. Microscopic examination of fresh sputum reveals the presence of wide (4 to 7 µm) septate filamentous elements of relatively uniform width. Cultures of patient's sputa yield colonies with abundant aerial mycelia. The MOST likely diagnosis of this patient is

   (A) candidiasis
   (B) cryptococcosis
   (C) aspergillosis
   (D) histoplasmosis
   (E) zygomycosis

11. Mice depleted of T cells by neonatal thymectomy failed to produce antibody to most antigens tested. The capacity of these animals to form antibody will be restored if

    (A) mature B cells are injected into the mice
    (B) normal bone marrow cells are transplanted
    (C) thymus cells are injected into the mice
    (D) interleukin-2 is injected into the mice
    (E) the mice are irradiated

12. The demonstration of spherules in infected tissues is useful for the diagnosis of

    (A) histoplasmosis
    (B) sporotrichosis
    (C) blastomycosis
    (D) coccidioidomycosis
    (E) dermatophytosis

13. Benzylpenicillin is still the antibiotic of choice during the initial treatment of

    (A) erysipelas
    (B) staphylococcal pyoderma
    (C) intra-abdominal abscess
    (D) shigellosis
    (E) typhoid fever

14. Gram-negative anaerobes such as *Bacteroides*

    (A) are common normal inhabitants of the colon, where they outnumber coliform bacilli
    (B) produce an exotoxin that is responsible for intestinal epithelial cell necrosis
    (C) are mostly insensitive to clindamycin
    (D) do not require anaerobic conditions for growth
    (E) are rarely involved in mixed infections

15. The leukocytes from a potential kidney transplant recipient (R) were tested in five separate mixed leukocyte reaction cultures with irradiated leukocytes from five potential donors (1, 2, 3, 4, and 5). The results of the test (counts per minutes of ^{3}H-thymidine incorporated into each culture) are summarized below:

Donor + Recipient	Count per Minutes
1 + R	16,750
2 + R	28,830
3 + R	85,000
4 + R	2,500
5 + R	42,000

The best kidney donor would be

(A) donor 1
(B) donor 2
(C) donor 3
(D) donor 4
(E) donor 5

16. Antibody diversity is generated primarily by

(A) somatic mutation
(B) gene rearrangements that affect a cluster of heavy-chain genes
(C) post-translational modification
(D) gene rearrangements that affect a cluster of light-chain genes
(E) random splicing of messenger RNA

17. A 2-year-old girl comes to your office with a 3-day history of fever to 102°F, running nose, conjunctivitis, cough, and diffuse erythematous macular rash over her face, chest, and back. Her rash appears confluent. When you examine her mouth, you would expect to find

(A) pseudomembrane
(B) large ulcerative lesions
(C) Koplik spots
(D) a large number of vesicles on her tongue
(E) strawberry tongue

18. In a patient with a consistently reactive Venereal Disease Research Laboratory test but lacking clinical evidence of syphilis, the physician should

(A) start treatment immediately
(B) conclude that the patient has latent syphilis
(C) order a Wassermann test
(D) order a fluorescent treponemal antibody absorption test
(E) instruct the patient to come back for reexamination in 3 months

19. The following figure shows the ultraviolet light (UV) death curve of a bacterial culture:

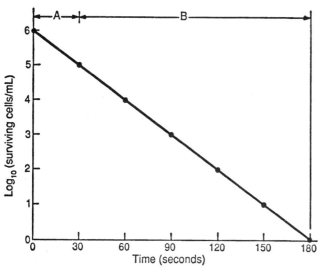

Figure 9–2

If during B, 10% of the cells survive any 30-second dose

(A) the number of viable cells remaining after an additional 30-second dose is 1% of the original

(B) the number of viable cells remaining at 1 minute is 0.1% of the original

(C) 90% of the cells are killed with each additional 60-second dose of UV

(D) the killing curve cannot be modified markedly by irradiating the cells with white light following UV irradiation

(E) the killing curve can be modified markedly by irradiating the same number of cells in a larger volume of liquid

20. A 4 year-old child with a history of recurrent pulmonary infections has been brought to the emergency room in obvious respiratory distress. Gram stain of the sputum reveals numerous polymorphonuclear leukocytes and gram-positive cocci in grape-like clusters. The drug of choice to be employed until the antibiotic susceptibility report is received from the laboratory is

(A) penicillin

(B) methicillin

(C) streptomycin

(D) gentamicin

(E) chloramphenicol

21. Which of the following structural features is NOT true of retroviruses?

(A) lipid envelope

(B) double-stranded RNA genome

(C) virus-associated reverse transcriptase

(D) genome is in a protein core

(E) replication via a DNA intermediate

22. Infection of a single cell by influenza A_2 virus can be blocked by

(A) specific IgG

(B) amantadine hydrochloride

(C) specific IgM

(D) all of the above

23. Diphtheria toxin mediates

(A) dissociation of eukaryotic ribosomal subunits

(B) inhibition of peptide bond formation

(C) hydrolysis of messenger RNA

(D) adenosine diphosphate ribosylation of eukaryotic elongation factor 2

(E) destruction of the endoplasmic reticulum

24. Staphylococcal scalded skin syndrome is related to the organism's ability to produce

(A) α-toxin

(B) lipase

(C) exfoliatin

(D) hyaluronidase

(E) coagulase

25. An extrachromosomal element that can replicate either autonomously in the cell cytoplasm or as an integral part of the cell chromosome is a(n)

    (A) plasmid
    (B) transposon
    (C) episome
    (D) competence factor
    (E) Hfr

26. Which of the following parasitic organisms is acquired by ingestion of poorly cooked freshwater crabs or crayfish?

    (A) *Opisthorchis viverrini*
    (B) *Paragonimus westermani*
    (C) *Schistosoma japonicum*
    (D) *Schistosoma mansoni*
    (E) *Diphyllobothrium latum*

27. The biosynthesis of fungal ergosterol is inhibited by

    (A) amphotericin B
    (B) griseofulvin
    (C) flucytosine
    (D) nystatin
    (E) ketoconazole

28. Humans are the only natural reservoir of the causative agents of all of the following infections EXCEPT

    (A) syphilis
    (B) typhoid fever
    (C) gonorrhea
    (D) listeriosis
    (E) influenza

29. One of your patients is found to have a pancreatic disorder in which her immune system is producing antibodies against her pancreatic islet cells. Tests have revealed an increased T4:T8 ratio. You may conclude that

    (A) the patient has acquired immunodeficiency syndrome (AIDS)
    (B) the patient has lost tolerance to the islet cell antigens as a result of a loss of T-suppressor cells

    (C) the patient has hypersensitivity to insulin
    (D) T-cytotoxic cells have been abnormally activated by pancreatic enzymes
    (E) the patient has a viral infection

30. A 38-year-old male, who underwent emergency surgery for the gunshot wounds he sustained in the abdomen 2 weeks earlier, complains of fever and abdominal discomfort. Subsequently, he is found to have intra-abdominal abscesses. Cultures of the pus obtained from the abscess is likely to yield

    (A) anaerobic bacteria only
    (B) aerobic bacteria only
    (C) both aerobic and anaerobic bacteria
    (D) gram-positive cocci only
    (E) gram-negative cocci only

31. Lymphocytes leaving fetal liver or bone marrow will be rich in

    (A) sheep cell resetting factors
    (B) idiotype determinants
    (C) OK8 or LEU1 determinants
    (D) cytotoxic potential
    (E) cell surface TdT

32. Human immunodeficiency virus (HIV) causes

    (A) an abnormal increase of cytotoxic natural killer cell function
    (B) an increase of delayed cutaneous hypersensitivity reactions
    (C) polyclonal hypogammaglobulinemia
    (D) severe lymphopenia primarily in the CD4$^+$ T-cell subset
    (E) enhanced monocyte function

33. *Hemophilus influenzae*, *Streptococcus pneumoniae*, and *Neisseria meningitidis* are common bacteria that infect normal children less than 2 years old. This is due to

    (A) the inability of their immune systems to produce antibodies against polysaccharides

(B) the inability of their immune systems to produce antibodies against proteins

(C) their undeveloped cell-mediated immune systems

(D) the transient neutropenia occurring during this stage of development

(E) the lack of certain complement components at this stage of development

34. Lysogenic phage conversion has been implicated in the pathogenesis of

(A) diphtheria

(B) whooping cough

(C) cholera

(D) pneumococcal pneumonia

(E) typhoid fever

35. All of the following organisms cause sexually transmissible diseases EXCEPT

(A) *Treponema pallidum*

(B) herpes simplex

(C) HIV

(D) adenoviruses

(E) *Chlamydia trachomatis*

36. Bence Jones proteins are

(A) immunoglobulin light chains found in the urine of myeloma patients

(B) immunoglobulin heavy chains found in the urine of myeloma patients

(C) monomeric IgA

(D) Fc fragments of myeloma proteins

(E) Fab fragments of myeloma proteins

37. *Escherichia coli* mutants lacking the catabolite activator protein (CAP) will express the *lac* operon if

(A) cyclic adenosine monophosphate (cAMP) is added to the culture

(B) lactose is added to the culture

(C) cAMP and lactose are added to the culture

(D) a reverse mutation occurs and lactose is present as a sole carbon source

(E) genetically engineered CAP protein is added to the culture

38. The anaphylactic reaction involves

(A) IgA antibody as a mediator of the response

(B) interaction of antibody with the eosinophilic leucocyte

(C) mediation by IgE

(D) attraction of eosinophils by antibody

39. A feature of the DiGeorge syndrome is

(A) developmental failure of the second and third pharyngeal pouches

(B) decrease in the serum immunoglobulin levels

(C) strong T-lymphocyte mediated immune responses

(D) deficiency in B-lymphocytes

40. Aflatoxins

(A) are carcinogenic bacterial toxins

(B) may cause hepatic carcinoma

(C) are of no significance in America

(D) are equally toxic to all animal species

41. An icosahedral RNA and DNA virus that is sensitive to ether is

(A) picornavirus

(B) respiratory syncytial virus

(C) varicella virus

(D) herpesvirus

(E) poxvirus

42. The Fc moiety of an IgG molecule is

(A) involved in passage of the IgG through the placenta

(B) localized in light chain

(C) involved in the idiotypic identification of the IgG molecule

(D) involved in secretion of the IgG molecule

(E) involved in the specificity of the IgG molecule

43. The drug of choice for infections caused by *Pseudomonas aeruginosa* is

(A) clindamycin

(B) penicillin G

(C) rifampin

(D) tetracycline

(E) tobramycin or gentamicin

44. Sabin poliovirus vaccine can be described as a

(A) heat-killed virus preparation

(B) monovalent attenuated virus preparation

(C) trivalent, attenuated virus preparation, which establishes an active infection in the respiratory tract

(D) genetically engineered viral coat protein preparation

(E) trivalent, attenuated virus preparation, which establishes an active but subclinical infection in the intestine

45. Adenine arabinoside is effective as a treatment for viral encephalitis because it

(A) inhibits viral DNA synthesis

(B) blocks virus-uncoating protein

(C) augments the host immune response

(D) prevents the formation of double-stranded replicative intermediates

(E) binds double-stranded replicative intermediates

46. A bacterial cell wall component susceptible to lysozyme is

(A) lipopolysaccharide

(B) teichoic acid

(C) peptidoglycan

(D) lipoprotein

(E) outer membrane

47. *Escherichia coli* is a

(A) gram-negative facultative anaerobe

(B) gram-negative aerobe

(C) gram-negative anaerobe

(D) gram-positive facultative anaerobe

(E) gram-positive aerobe

48. The toxic effects of the endotoxin molecule appears to reside in the

(A) common core polysaccharide

(B) O-specific polysaccharide

(C) polypeptide side chain

(D) lipid A

(E) 2-keto-3-deoxyoctonate

49. An adult patient with a history of severe penicillin allergy has a sore throat and low-grade fever. Results of a throat culture show a large number of beta-hemolytic streptococcal colonies. Of the following, the most likely antibiotic selected would be

(A) ampicillin

(B) oxacillin

(C) cephalothin

(D) tetracycline

(E) phenoxymethylpenicillin

50. The lactose operon is correctly described as

(A) containing five genes

(B) constitutive

(C) controlled at the transcriptional level

(D) an example of a positive control mechanism

(E) independent of the *lacI* gene product

51. Each of the following mechanisms relates to modes of regulation of messenger RNA synthesis EXCEPT

(A) attenuation

(B) feedback inhibition

(C) feedback repression

(D) catabolite repression

(E) autoregulation

52. Lymphocyte "capping" can be induced by

(A) surface immunoglobulin–anti-immunoglobulin reactions

(B) phytohemagglutinin

(C) pokeweed mitogen

(D) complement

(E) fructose

53. Which of the following applies to transformation by *Streptococcus pneumoniae?*

(A) donor cells remain intact

(B) competence factor is not required

(C) transformation is inhibited by DNAse

(D) transformation has not conducted with *Hemophilus influenzae*

54. A disease in which activated macrophages play a key role is

(A) diphtheria

(B) pneumococcal pneumonia

(C) furunculosis

(D) tuberculosis

(E) botulism

55. Pili of *Neisseria gonorrhoeae* are known to

(A) be responsible for the absence of secretory IgA in urethral exudates

(B) impart resistance to intracellular killing on piliated strains

(C) have endotoxic properties

(D) be organelles of attachment

(E) be composed of lipopolysaccharides

56. In clusters of infections caused by *Salmonella* species, the best method used to define the epidemic is

(A) phage typing

(B) serotyping

(C) antibiotic susceptibility

(D) pyocin typing

(E) plasmid profile

57. The most common site of recognized extraintestinal amebiasis is

(A) skin

(B) liver

(C) lung

(D) pericardium

(E) brain

58. Hyperacute graft rejection is primarily mediated by

(A) activated macrophages

(B) high-titer antibodies to major histocompatibility complex determinants

(C) IgE

(D) B lymphocytes

(E) basophils

59. Causative agents of mild and acute respiratory tract infections, conjunctivitis, and pharyngitis in humans are

(A) arenaviruses

(B) rotaviruses

(C) arboviruses

(D) herpesviruses

(E) adenoviruses

60. Cervicofacial actinomycosis is caused by *Actinomyces* that is commonly found

(A) in the soil

(B) in drinking water

(C) on mucous membranes

(D) in prepared foods

(E) on inanimate objects

61. It can usually be determined in the laboratory whether a proper sputum specimen has been collected for the diagnosis of bacterial pneumonia by determining the

(A) viscosity of the material

(B) ratio of white blood cells to epithelial cells in a Gram stain

(C) ratio of gram-positive to gram-negative cocci

(D) ratio of aerobic to anaerobic bacteria

(E) presence of *Streptococcus pneumoniae* on culture

62 A 55-year-old Caucasian male was hospitalized with pneumonitis after 5 days of unremitting fever (104°F) and recurrent rigors. He is suspected of having legionellosis. All of the following statements about such cases are true EXCEPT

(A) for fastest diagnosis, a monoclonal antibody test for *Legionella* species should be requested

(B) there is no good antibiotic treatment for legionellosis

(C) a request should be made for culture of the suspected *Legionella*

(D) misdiagnosis is common unless *Legionella* is suspected

63. A single-stranded DNA virus family is the

(A) Papovaviridae

(B) Parvoviridae

(C) Adenoviridae

(D) Herpesviridae

(E) Poxviridae

64. The antibody that develops after an episode of pneumococcal pneumonia may not protect against subsequent pneumococcal disease because

(A) the antibody is only against the pneumococcal C substance (phosphocholine-containing teichoic acid)

(B) antibody levels are present for only a few weeks

(C) the polysaccharide is not immunogenic

(D) the 84 different pneumococcal polysaccharides and their antibodies do not cross- protect

(E) anticapsular antibody is not protective

65. A 20-year-old pregnant woman (third trimester) developed pyuria, dysuria, and flank pain. She had no previous history of urinary or genital infections. The organism that is most likely to be isolated from urine culture is

(A) *Candida albicans*

(B) *Neisseria gonorrhoeae*

(C) alpha-hemolytic streptococci

(D) *Staphylococcus aureus*

(E) *Escherichia coli*

66. The phosphoenol pyruvate–phosphotransferase system

(A) is independent of the heat-stable protein

(B) requires adenosine triphosphate as an energy source

(C) is inhibited by enzymes I and II

(D) changes the molecular nature of the substance that is being transported

(E) is utilized for the transport of amino acids

67. CO_2 is required for primary isolation of

(A) *Yersinia pestis*

(B) *Mycobacterium tuberculosis*

(C) *Treponema pallidum*

(D) *Neisseria gonorrhoeae* and *Brucella abortus*

(E) *Mycobacterium leprae*

68. The virus that has been implicated in nasopharyngeal carcinoma is

(A) Epstein–Barr virus

(B) rotavirus

(C) rhabdovirus

(D) reovirus

(E) cytomegalovirus

69. The virulence of *Streptococcus pyogenes* is directly related to

(A) possession of streptolysin O

(B) possession of streptolysin S

(C) presence of M protein in its cell wall

(D) presence of the Vi antigen

(E) presence of V/W antigen

70. Lyme disease is transmitted through the bite of a

(A) louse

(B) flea

(C) dog

(D) tick

(E) human

71. Interferon

    (A) may be induced by synthetic double-stranded polyribonucleotides

    (B) is composed of DNA

    (C) is a lipoidal substance

    (D) activates the C3 component of complement

    (E) is produced in large quantities (grams per liter of tissue culture medium)

72. Echoviruses

    (A) contain double-stranded DNA

    (B) can cause aseptic meningitis

    (C) can cause variola

    (D) multiply primarily in the central nervous system

    (E) are not excreted by humans

73. *Neisseria gonorrhoeae*

    (A) types 2 and 4 are pathogenic

    (B) lacks indophenol oxidase

    (C) grows best anaerobically (80% CO_2 tension)

    (D) may cause blindness in the newborn

    (E) produces a protease that cannot degrade IgA

74. Antibiotics A and B are added alone or combined to cultures of *Streptococcus pyogenes*.

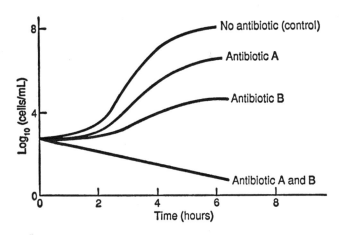

Figure 9–3

The results presented in Figure 9–3 illustrate

    (A) antagonism

    (B) indifference

    (C) addition

    (D) synergism

75. Pending the results of cultures, meningitis in children 8 to 10 months of age should be treated with

    (A) cefotaxime

    (B) ampicillin

    (C) penicillin G

    (D) tetracycline

    (E) gentamicin

76. Natural resistance to malaria caused by *Plasmodium vivax* has been demonstrated in populations who are

    (A) Duffy blood group antigen-positive

    (B) glycophorin A-positive

    (C) glucose-6-phosphate dehydrogenase-deficient

    (D) Duffy blood group antigen-negative

77. A 20-year-old homosexual man complains of dysphagia, malaise, and loss of body weight. Physical examination shows oral thrush and bilateral swelling of neck lymph nodes. There are no records showing that the patient has been under antibiotic medication or other drug treatment. Appropriate measures that you should take immediately do NOT include

    (A) amphotericin B treatment

    (B) anti-human immunodeficiency virus antibody titer

    (C) T4:T8 ratio

    (D) microscopic examination and culture of oral plaque

    (E) routine blood cell counts and differential

78. A 26-year-old farmer has not been feeling well during the past 4 months. He has taken antifungal, antiprotozoan, and antibacterial drugs without improvement in his health. Laboratory tests show high serum alanine aminotransferase, and aspartate transaminase values of 500 to 2,000 units, leukopenia, decreased serum albumin, and increased serum globulin levels. The MOST likely diagnosis is

(A) sandfly fever
(B) poliomyelitis
(C) hepatitis A
(D) West Nile fever
(E) rabies

79. All normal cells contain genes that can cause transformation of cells if these genes are altered in some way. These genes are called proto-oncogenes. Proto-oncogenes are

(A) virally encoded
(B) altered versions of normal genes
(C) always transduced by retroviruses
(D) activated by viral and nonviral mechanisms
(E) associated with the suppression of cell growth

DIRECTIONS (Questions 80 through 100): Each group of items in this section consists of lettered headings followed by a set of words or phrases. For each numbered word or phrase, select the ONE heading that is most closely associated with it. Each lettered heading may be selected once, more than once, or not at all.

Question 80

(A) herpesviruses
(B) adenoviruses
(C) poxviruses
(D) togaviruses
(E) paramyxoviruses

80. Viruses that do not have an envelope

Question 81

(A) interleukin-10
(B) interleukin-3
(C) interferon-gamma
(D) interleukin-2
(E) tumor necrosis factor

81. Induces fever

Question 82

(A) poxviruses
(B) reoviruses
(C) picornaviruses
(D) herpesviruses
(E) paramyxoviruses

82. The genomes of these viruses are replicated in the nucleus of the host cell

Question 83

(A) ethylene oxide
(B) ultraviolet light
(C) ethyl alcohol
(D) mercurochrome
(E) phenol

83. Causes the formation of thymine dimers

Question 84

(A) dogs
(B) cats
(C) turtles
(D) pigs
(E) humans

84. The reservoir of *Salmonella typhi* is

Question 85

    (A) repressor

    (B) enhancer

    (C) operator

    (D) promoter

    (E) inducer

85. Nucleotide sequence in DNA that binds RNA polymerase

Question 86

    (A) chloramphenicol

    (B) piperacillin

    (C) sulfamethoxazole

    (D) tetracycline

    (E) erythromycin

86. Causes bacterial lysis and death

Question 87

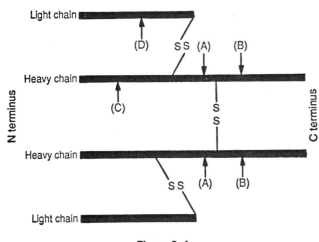

Figure 9–4

87. Cleavage of the molecule at this point produces two Fab fragments

Question 88

    (A) toxoid

    (B) toxin

    (C) living, attenuated microorganisms

    (D) killed, virulent microorganisms

    (E) endotoxin

88. Vaccine component for rubeola (measles)

Question 89

    (A) conjugation

    (B) lysogenic conversion

    (C) generalized transduction

    (D) transversion

    (E) transformation

89. A process that is not useful for gene transfer

Question 90

Kinetics of a primary humoral immune response to a foreign antigen is illustrated in Figure 9–5:

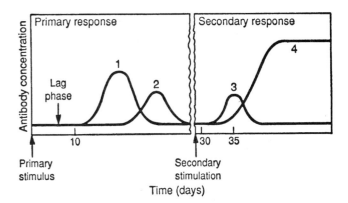

Figure 9–5

    (A) IgM

    (B) IgG

    (C) IgD

    (D) IgM and IgG

    (E) none of the above

90. The class of immunoglobulin predominant in peak 2

Question 91

    (A) IgE

    (B) antigen-sensitized T cells and lymphokines

    (C) secretory IgA

    (D) endotoxin

    (E) IgD

91. Mediation in contact dermatitis

Questions 92 and 93

You performed a double-immunodiffusion plate (Ouchterlony) in which the center well contained anti-bovine serum albumin (anti-BSA). Bovine serum albumin (BSA) and human serum albumin (HSA) were placed in wells 1 and 2, respectively. The precipitation pattern that developed after 24 hours of incubation was as follows:

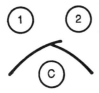

Figure 9–6

(A) immunologically identical
(B) immunologically partially identical
(C) immunologically unrelated
(D) none of the above

92. BSA and HSA

93. If you replaced HSA in well 2 with bovine gamma globulin (BGG), which shares no antigenicity with BSA, and added BGG to the central well (the central well would now contain anti-BSA and anti-BGG), this is the precipitation you would expect:

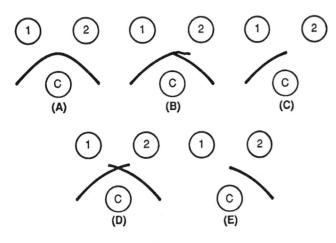

Figure 9–7

Question 94

(A) failure to enter cells
(B) decreased uptake
(C) active efflux
(D) enzymatic inactivation of drug
(E) alteration of target

94. Resistance of *Pseudomonas aeruginosa* to β-lactam antibiotics

Questions 95 through 97

(A) botulinum toxin
(B) tetanus toxin
(C) diphtheria toxin
(D) cholera toxin
(E) pertussis toxin
(F) staphylococcal enterotoxin
(G) amatoxin
(H) aflatoxin
(I) vero toxin
(J) *Shigella* toxin
(K) anaphylotoxin
(L) anthrax toxin

95. Inhibits acetylcholine release at myoneural junction

96. Superantigen

97. Responsible for whooping cough symptoms

Question 98

(A) Tsutsugamushi disease
(B) Rocky Mountain spotted fever
(C) murine typhus
(D) epidemic typhus
(E) bubonic plague

98. Tick is the arthropod vector

Question 99

    (A) an unsubstituted protein

    (B) a glycolipid

    (C) a glycoprotein

    (D) a mucopolysaccharide

    (E) a nucleic acid

99. Composition of the plasma membrane receptor for influenza virus

Question 100

    (A) myeloperoxidase–hydrogen peroxide–halide system

    (B) oxygen metabolites

    (C) lysozyme and other hydrolytic enzymes

    (D) iron chelating proteins, such as lactoferrin

    (E) catalase

100. Direct contribution to the intracellular killing of microbes by neutrophiles has not been shown

Practice Test
Answers and Explanations

1. **(B)** In addition to ABO and Rh antigens on the red blood cell, there are many other antigens that can induce antibody production and cause problems in the crossmatch. An important purpose of the crossmatch is to check for problems that may be caused by these other antibodies and/or antigens. Thus, an AB individual cannot always receive blood from a donor of any other ABO group, and the ABO Rh types are not adequate information in determining compatibility. ABO antibodies are termed "natural" antibodies because they appear soon after birth and their stimulus is not known for sure. Rh antibodies are not "natural." They are present after antigenic stimulation from pregnancy or incompatible blood transfusion. (*Brooks et al, p 123*)

2. **(E)** Disinfection is defined as the destruction of pathogenic microorganisms. Isopropyl alcohol at 70% concentration has been used for skin disinfection because it denatures microbial proteins and enzymes that the microbes need to function. At unspecified concentrations, its action cannot be predicted. The most effective skin disinfectant currently in use is a solution of 1% iodine in 70% ethanol. Iodine oxidizes the free sulfhydryl groups of enzymes. This leads to enzyme inactivation. Seventy percent ethanol acts as a protein denaturant. Mercurochrome easily loses its disinfective properties by extraneous organic material or unclean skin surfaces. Soap removes mechanically pathogenic and nonpathogenic bacteria, but it does not kill necessarily pathogenic bacteria. Three percent hydrogen peroxide has a modest disinfective action. However, it is not as effective as 1% solution of iodine in 70% ethanol. (*Brooks et al, pp 46–47*)

3. **(E)** The viral particles, or virions, contain either DNA or RNA (arrow 1), which is protected by a surrounding protein layer known as capsid (arrow 5). The capsid consists of polypeptide units called capsomers (arrow 2). Six viral families—Parvoviridae, Papovaviridae, Adenoviridae, Picornaviridae, Calciviridae, and Reoviridae—do not have envelopes. The remaining 12 viral families (Herpesviridae, Poxviridae, Hepadnaviridae, Togaviridae, Flaviviridae, Arenaviridae, Coronaviridae, Retroviridae, Bunyaviridae, Orthomyxoviridae, Paramyxoviridae, and Rhabdoviridae) have a lipid-containing envelope (arrow 3). On the surface of the viral envelope, some viruses, such as the orthomyxoviruses and the paramyxoviruses, form glycoproteinaceous projections known as spikes (arrow 4). Matrix proteins are found as a myristylated protein layer below the envelope of most retroviruses. (*Brooks et al, pp 366, 367; Joklik et al, p 880*)

4. **(E)** The periplasmic space constitutes the area between the cytoplasmic cell membrane and the outer membrane of the cell wall of gramnegative bacteria. It contains proteins that bind amino acids, sugars, vitamins, and ions. In addition to these binding proteins, the periplasmic space contains various phosphatases, proteases, endonuclease I, and such antibiotic-inactivating enzymes as β-lac-

tamases, as well as aminoglycoside-phosphorylating enzymes. *(Joklik et al, pp 25–26)*

5. **(B)** In a mixed lymphocyte culture, leukocytes from two unrelated (allogeneic) individuals are mixes in vitro. After 5 to 7 days, substantial proliferation (primarily T helper and some cytotoxic cells) can be measured because of the recognition of foreign major histocompatibility antigens on the leukocytes. Antigens of class I regions react preferentially with precursors of cytotoxic T effector cells (CD8) and antigens of class II regions react preferentially with helper T cells (CD4). Thus, for a maximum response, disparity at both class I and II loci is needed. No proliferation occurs if class I and II loci are similar. A fair cytotoxic T-lymphocyte response can be seen when disparity is only at class I determinants and a strong (but not maximum) cell proliferation is seen when disparity is only at class II determinants. *(Joklik et al, pp 259, 266–268,274–275)*

6. **(E)** *V, J,* and *C* genes are present in both heavy and light-chain genes. Processing of nuclear messenger RNA (mRNA) (primary RNA transcript) by splicing out intervening sequences (introns) to produce mRNA takes place during gene recombination of both heavy and light chains. In both mouse and man, the kappa light-chain locus has a single C gene, and the genes for heavy-chain constant regions (C_H) of different isotypes are arranged in a tandem array. The newly assembled heavy-chain V-D-J gene set can be translocated to a position immediately 5′ to any of the heavy-chain C-region genes. However, in a given light chain (kappa or lambda), the newly assembled V-J gene set (light chain lacks D segment) is always combined with the same C-region gene (C kappa or C lambda). *(Joklik et al, pp 23–235; Roitt et al, pp 6.2–6.6)*

7. **(D)** The facultative anaerobic bacteria tend to have cytochrome C oxidase and peroxidase. However, their tolerance to superoxide radical (O_2^-) is not due to cytochrome C oxidase. Their tolerance to O_2^- is thought to be primarily due to the possession of superoxide dismutase and catalase. Obligate anaerobic bacteria do not possess these enzymes. Superoxide dismutase converts the potentially lethal O_2^- to hydrogen peroxide, which also possesses antibacterial properties in appropriate concentrations, while catalase breaks down H_2O_2 to H_2O and O_2. *(Joklik et al, p 46)*

8. **(E)** Generalized transduction is a mechanism that alters the phenotype of the host by transfer of *any* bacterial genes from one bacterial cell to another via bacteriophage. Bacteria infected with a lytic virus or a lysogenic cell is induced to produce lytic virus. During the maturation process, fragmented bacterial DNA may be packaged into the phage. Upon lysis of the cell, one or more of the phage particles will carry bacterial DNA (transducing phage) instead of phage DNA. The incorporation of bacterial DNA into the phage head is a random event, and any bacterial genes could be transduced by these phages. There is no generalized transformation or generalized transfection. *(Brooks et al, pp 87–89; Joklik et al, p 138)*

9. **(B)** When guinea pig erythrocytes are added to monkey kidney cell cultures of influenza virus, the red cells are aggregated about and adsorbed by the cells in which viral proliferation is occurring. Viruses that demonstrate this phenomenon are called hemadsorption viruses. *(Joklik et al, pp 766,995–996)*

10. **(C)** Both the clinical and mycologic findings are consistent with the diagnosis that this patient has pulmonary aspergillosis. The most common species that causes pulmonary aspergillosis in humans is *Aspergillus fumigatus*. Infections in compromised hosts occur through the inhalation of air-borne conidia. Causative fungi and zygomycosis (*Mucor* and *Rhizopus*) are nonseptate. *Candida albicans*, which causes candidiasis, forms cream colonies. *Cryptococcus neoformans*, causative fungus for cryptococcosis, and *Histoplasma capsulatum*, causative fungus for histoplasmosis, proliferate in the yeast form in infected tissues. *(Joklik et al, pp 1148–1152)*

11. **(C)** B cells generally require the presence of T cells for stimulation by antigen toward antibody formation. In animals, the thymus is regarded as a central lymphoid organ and plays a critical role in the differentiation process from bone marrow stem cells to T lymphocytes. In thymectomized mice, transplantation of normal bone marrow, mature B cells, injection of interleukin-2, or other treatments such as irradiation cannot restore the ability to form antibody. *(Joklik et al, pp 208,256)*

12. **(D)** In infected tissues, *Coccidioides immitis* forms spherules in which numerous endospores are produced. A definitive diagnosis of coccidioidomycosis requires the finding of spherules of *C. immitis* in sputum, draining sinuses, or tissue specimens. *(Joklik et al, p 1095)*

13. **(A)** Erysipelas is caused by group A *Streptococcus pyogenes*, for which benzylpenicillin (penicillin G) is still the antibiotic of choice. This antibiotic is not recommended for infections caused by penicillinase-producing bacteria. Most strains of *Staphylococcus aureus* now isolated from clinical specimens including staphylococcal pyoderma are penicillinase producers and are resistant to penicillin G. Ampicillin, not penicillin G, is the drug of choice for the treatment of shigellosis. Intraabdominal abscess is best treated with clindamycin. Ampicillin or chloramphenicol is the drug of choice for the treatment of typhoid fever. *(Joklik et al, pp 159–160,424–425)*

14. **(A)** *Bacteroides* are gram-negative anaerobic bacteria commonly inhabiting the large colon, where they outnumber coliform bacilli by 100 to 1. *Bacteroides fragilis* is especially important because it is implicated in abdominal abscesses occurring postoperatively. This type of infection is usually a mixed infection in which more than one species of bacteria are involved. Other species of *Bacteroides* (*B. melaninogenicus*) are found in the oral cavity. No exotoxins are produced by *Bacteroides fragilis,* are susceptible to clindamycin. Anaerobic conditions are essential for culturing *Bacteroides.* *(Joklik et al, pp 145,175,628)*

15. **(D)** The results of the mixed lymphocyte reaction correlate with the degree of dissimilarity of histocompatibility. High counts indicate more stimulation, suggesting immunologic unrelatedness of tissues tested. Human leukocyte–antigen-identical sibs do not stimulate mixed leukocyte reaction, indicating their tissues are mutually transplantable. *(Joklik et al, p 269)*

16. **(B)** Although somatic mutation and gene rearrangement that affect light-chain genes contribute to the diversity of antibody, the major cause for generation of antibody diversity is gene rearrangements that affect a cluster of heavy-chain genes. The light-chain genes lack D segments; thus, the number of combinations is much smaller. Post-translational modification does not significantly contribute to antibody diversity. Transcripts of immunoglobulin genes are not spliced randomly. *(Joklik et al, pp 206–207)*

17. **(C)** All clinical symptoms indicate that this patient has measles. Diagnosis is ascertained on the basis of the typical history and clinical findings. A prodromal stage marked by catarrhal symptoms of cough, coryza, and conjunctivitis is accompanied by fever, which rises steadily until the appearance of rash 2 to 4 days after onset. Preceding the rash, the pathognomotic Koplik spots appear. They are pinpoint and grayish white surrounded by bright red inflammation and found over the lateral buccal mucosa and inner lips, occasionally involving the entire inner mouth cavity. Koplik spots do not develop on the tongue. Pseudomembranes develop, in certain infections, diseases such as diphtheria. Strawberry tongue is a characteristic symptom of scarlet fever, which is caused by a group A *Streptococcus.* *(Joklik et al, pp 423,1012)*

18. **(D)** Under this situation, it is important for the physician to establish that this patient has syphilis. For this purpose, a more specific test (ie, fluorescent treponemal antibody-absorption test) should be employed. This test is relatively specific for disease with virulent trep-

onemal species, usually *Treponema pallidum*. This test is expensive and time consuming. It is therefore recommended not for general screening, but for confirmation of positive nontreponemal tests such as the Venereal Disease Research Laboratory test. Other treatments or tests are inappropriate. *(Joklik et al, pp 663–665)*

19. **(A)** An examination of the death curve shown in the figure given indicates that there is a 90% reduction in the surviving cells for each 30-second exposure to ultraviolet (UV) light. That is, there is one log reduction of the cell population for every 30 seconds. That is, in 30 seconds the surviving cells were reduced from 1,000,000 cells (10^6) to 100,000 cells (10^5). Then the number of viable cells remaining after an additional 30 seconds (1-minute total exposure) were reduced to 10,000 cells (10^4). Ten thousand cells represent 1% of the original cell population. Ultraviolet (UV) light irradiation of bacterial cells causes them to form pyrimidine dimers that distort the shape of the DNA and leads to inhibition of DNA synthesis. If, following UV light irradiation, the bacterial cells are exposed to visible light, the lethal effect of the UV light is significantly reduced. This phenomenon is called photoreactivation and is due to the activation of an enzyme that removes the pyrimidine dimers from the bacterial DNA. *(Brooks et al, pp 43–44; Joklik et al, pp 197–198)*

20. **(B)** The Gram stain of sputum reveals numerous polymorphonuclear leukocytes (suggesting a lung infection) and gram-positive cocci in grape-like clusters. Although staphylococci can't positively be identified by Gram stain (streptococci are also possible), the likelihood is there. Since the vast majority of staphylococci are β-lactamase producers, methicillin is the immediate drug of choice because it is likely to be effective against gram-positive cocci. Penicillin, which is ineffective against β-lactamase producers, would replace methicillin only after the laboratory results showed the absence of a β-lactamase. *(Ryan et al, pp 191–198)*

21. **(B)** Retroviruses are single-stranded, linear, positive-polarity RNA viruses 90 to 120 nm in diameter. The RNA is surrounded by an inner protein envelope with an icosahedral symmetry and an outer envelope that contains lipid and glycoprotein spikes, which serve to attach the virus to the host cells. Retroviruses have been associated with leukemia, sarcoma, mammary tumors, and especially with AIDS. The word retro refers to the possession of the enzyme reverse transcriptase, which transcribes RNA into DNA during the process of the viral nucleic acid synthesis. The virus is produced from a proviral DNA in infected cells. *(Joklik et al, pp 878–879)*

22. **(D)** Amantadine inhibits primary transcription, thus inhibiting uncoating, although it does not block the initial attachment and penetration of the cell membrane by the virus. Both IgG and IgM specific for the virus may neutralize the viral particle, thus blocking its infectivity. *(Joklik et al, pp 854–867, 996–997)*

23. **(D)** Diphtheria toxin is an exotoxin produced by toxigenic strains of *Corynebacterium diphtheriae*. The toxin consists of two subunits, A and B. Subunit A is a toxigenic moiety that enzymatically adenosine diphosphate-ribosylates the elongation factor 2 (EF-2) of the eucaryotic cell. The modification of EF-2 results in the inhibition of protein synthesis and eventual death of the host cell. Subunit B is a receptor-binding component of the toxin. Mg deficiency causes dissociation of ribosomal subunits. Certain antibiotics such as chloramphenicol and puromycin inhibit peptide bond formation. *(Joklik et al, pp 488–495)*

24. **(C)** Staphylococcal scalded skin syndrome is an intoxication in which exfoliation, produced by phage group II organisms growing somewhere in the body (usually the gut), obtain access to the bloodstream. The resultant toxemia is evidenced by changes in the integrity of the integument: The skin separates at the stratum granulosum because of the ef-

fect of the toxin on the desmosomes located there. This causes the skin to appear to float. It has no resilience and will stay wrinkled if pushed in one direction (Nikolsky's sign). (*Joklik et al, pp 406–411*)

25. **(A)** Plasmids are extrachromosomal double-stranded DNA circles that exist in bacterial cytoplasm independently of the host chromosome. They are of tremendous importance to medicine because they play a major role in the development of antibiotic-resistant bacterial strains. Plasmids replicate independently in the bacterial cytoplasm. Occasionally, plasmids will integrate into the bacterial chromosome. Usually, integration is a rare event. These plasmids that can replicate either autonomously in the cell cytoplasm, or as an integral part of the bacterial chromosome, are called *episomes*. Transposons are genetic elements that are highly mobile and that can be transposed from one piece of DNA to another at high frequency. Unlike plasmids, they do not contain genetic information for their synthesis. Competence factor is a special set of proteins required for bacterial transformation. Hfr refers to high frequency recombination donors from which chromosomal DNA is transferred to the donor cells. (*Levinson and Jawetz, pp 85–89*)

26. **(B)** *Opisthorchis viverrini* and *Diphyllobothrium latum* are acquired by ingestion of uncooked fish. Both *Schistosoma japonicum* and *Schistosoma mansoni* are acquired by skin penetration of cercariae (larvae). (*Joklik et al, pp 1187–1215*)

27. **(E)** Ketoconazole inhibits the biosynthesis of ergosterol by blocking demethylation at the C-14 site of the ergosterol precursor, lanosterol. This results in the accumulation of lanosterol-like sterols in the cell, altered properties of the cell membrane, the leakage of potassium ions and small phosphorus-containing compounds. Amphotericin B and nystatin disturb the permeability of the cell membrane by directly complexing with the membrane sterols. The target of griseofulvin is microtubules. Flucytosine (5′-fluorocytosine) is incorporated into RNA after being deaminated and then phosphorylated. It also interferes with DNA synthesis because it is a noncompetitive inhibitor of thymidylate synthetase. (*Joklik et al, pp 165–166,181*)

28. **(D)** Listeriosis is caused by *Listeria monocytogenes*, a facultative intracellular gram-positive bacterium. This bacterium can be isolated from a wide range of animals, birds, fish, ticks, and crustacea. There is a high incidence of plant and soil samples and animal feces. The organism is contracted by humans and animals from many sources. (*Joklik et al, p 283*)

29. **(B)** The disorder is immunologic because the patient's immune system is producing antibodies against her own pancreatic islet cells. An increased T4:T8 ratio suggests, among other possibilities, decreased suppressor T cells. Three CD8 suppressor cell subpopulations have been defined: suppressor precursor T cells, suppressor activator T cells, and suppressor effector T cells. AIDS patients usually show a decreased T4:T8 ratio. Destruction of islet cells (beta cells) by viral infection may cause diabetes, but antibodies against islet cells are not produced. (*Joklik et al, pp 211,259–262,363; Roitt et al, p 20,10*)

30. **(C)** This type of infection is caused by spilling of the contents of the gut during or after the operation. Thus, infection is often a mixed infection in which multiple organisms, including aerobic, facultative anaerobic, and strict anaerobic bacteria, are involved. Usually both gram-positive and gram-negative bacteria can be isolated from intra-abdominal abscesses. Typically, *Bacterioides fragilis* and *Escherichia coli* are the most common organisms isolated from this type of pus. Treatment should be directed to both aerobic and anaerobic bacteria. (*Joklik et al, pp 159,628*)

31. **(E)** Lymphocytes existing in fetal liver, or bone marrow, will be rich in cell surface TdT. This transferase is an indicator of a rather primitive cell state and is found only in very young cells that have not undergone extensive membrane differentiation or developed cell receptors. Sheep cell rosetting factors,

subpopulation determinants, and cytotoxic potential appear after thymic migration. An abundance of idiotype determinants will appear after specific antigen stimulation and an appearance of the final heavy class chain on the cell surface. (*Joklik et al, pp 208,221, 235,250–253*)

32. (D) Human immunodeficiency virus causes decrease of cytotoxic natural killer cell function, lowered delayed cutaneous hypersensitivity reactions, and decreased monocyte function. The virus also causes polyclonal hypergammaglobulinemia. (*Joklik et al, p 1052*)

33. (A) A major deficit in children less than 2 years old is their inability to make antibodies against polysaccharide antigens. There is a period of 2 to 3 months after birth when the transferred maternal antibodies are protective, followed by 2 years of relatively high danger from infection as passively transferred antibody declines. When exposed to a polysaccharide antigen, children in this age range can transiently make IgM antibodies, but IgG antibodies do not develop, and no memory B cells are established. (*Joklik et al, p 362*)

34. (A) *Corynebacterium diphtheriae* becomes toxigenic as the consequence of infection with bacteriophages (beta phage). The toxin gene (*tax* gene) introduced by the phage is integrated into the chromosome of *C. diphtheriae*, enabling the bacteria to produce diphtheria toxin. Similar mechanisms (lysogenic phage conversion) are also responsible for the development of toxin production in *Clostridium botulinum* (botulinum toxin) and group A *Streptococcus pyogenes* (erythrogenic toxin). Lysogenic phage conversion is not involved in either the toxin production or the pathogenicity of bacteria responsible for the other diseases listed in the question. (*Joklik et al, pp 422–423,488–490,927–928*)

35. (D) Adenoviruses are capable of establishing productive infections of the respiratory, conjunctival, and gastrointestinal mucosal lining cells. The major means of transmission is the fecal–oral route. It can be also transmitted through direct contact of contaminated swimming pool water or other infected materials with nose or eyes. Sexual transmission is not a normal mode of transmission of adenovirus infections. (*Joklik et al, pp 969–972*)

36. (A) Plasma cell tumors are known as myeloma or plasmacytoma. In such myeloma cells, an abnormal rise in single molecular type of immunoglobulin occurs. In a certain type of myeloma (light-chain disease), light chains alone are produced greatly in excess of the production of heavy chains. These light chains excreted in urine precipitate when heated at 60°C but redissolve as the temperature is raised to 80°C. Proteins having this unusual property are known as Bence Jones proteins, and their presence in urine is indicative of a myeloma. (*Joklik et al, pp 226–227*)

37. (D) The catabolite activator protein (CAP) in the 3′,5′-cyclic adenosine monophosphate (cAMP)-liganded form is required for the maximum expression of the *lac* operon. The *las* operon would not be expressed in CAP-defective *E. coli* mutants even in the presence of cAMP, lactose, or both. The *lac* operon in such mutants would be expressed only when a reverse mutation restores the CAP and an appropriate substrate such as lactose is provided. Since the *lac* operon requires activation by CAP for efficient transcription, *E. coli* mutants lacking the CAP will not express the *lac* operon even if an inducer (lactose) or a chemical signal (cAMP) is provided. Externally added CAP is unlikely to enter the cytoplasm of *E. coli* because of the permeability barrier. (*Joklik et al, pp 116–117*)

38. (C) The anaphylactic reaction is a rapidly evolving immunologic reaction that occurs within minutes after re-exposure to an antigen to which an individual has already been sensitized. The response is mediated by IgE antibody (reaginic antibody), which interacts with or is bound to basophils and mast cells. IgE-sensitized mast cells release various mediators or vasoactive amines on exposure to the specific antigen. The activation of mast cells and basophils depends on the cross-linkage of adjacent antibody molecules on the cell surface by multivalent antigens. The release of these mediators then occurs in response to a number of hormonal influences, including a decrease in intracellular cyclic AMP levels. The mediators include histamine, eosinophilic chemotactic factor of anaphylaxis, slow-reacting substance of anaphylaxis, and platelet-activating factor. It is the eosinophilic chemotactic factor of anaphylaxis, not antibody, that attracts the eosinophil to the reaction site. *(Ryan et al, pp 127–128)*

39. **(A)** DiGeorge syndrome is a deficiency of T lymphocytes due to thymic hypoplasia. Developmental failure of the third and fourth pharyngeal pouches is responsible for total or partial thymic, parathyroid, thyroid, and ultimobranchial pouch abnormalities. These structural anomalies lead to the absence of the cell-mediated T-lymphocyte immune response, tetany, and congenital heart and great vessel abnormalities. B-lymphocyte and plasma cell populations tend to be normal, as do serum immunoglobulin levels. The syndrome appears to be the result of an intrauterine insult to the fetus sometime before the eighth week of gestation. The syndrome is not genetically determined. As the affected children grow older, T-cell function improves so that by age 5 years many affected children fail to demonstrate a T-cell deficit. Some patients have been successfully treated by transplantation of fetal thymic tissue. *(Levinson and Jawetz, pp 338–339)*

40. **(B)** Aflatoxins are carcinogenic substances produced by the fungi *Aspergillus flavus* and *Aspergillus parasiticus*. Of the 17 aflatoxins identified, B_1 is considered to be one of the most potent of all known carcinogens. The adverse effects of aflatoxins vary with the species of animal on which the toxin is tested, the dose and route of administration, and the duration of exposure. In Thailand, where large amounts of aflatoxins (especially B_1) are found in peanuts, aflatoxicosis frequently occurs as encephalopathy and fatty degeneration of the viscera. In the United States it is estimated that aflatoxins are a problem in the south, where 6% of America's corn is grown.

Aflatoxins have been proved to cause primary liver cancer in laboratory animals, including monkeys. Humans appear to be less susceptible to the carcinogenic effects. However, data show a highly significant correlation between aflatoxin intake and carcinoma in humans. *(Joklik et al, pp 1082–1083)*

41. **(D)** Picornaviruses (RNA viruses) are ether-resistant, but have icosahedral capsid symmetry. Respiratory syncytial viruses (RNA viruses) have *helical* capsid symmetry and are ether-sensitive; varicella viruses (DNA viruses) are ether-resistant and have complex symmetry, but are not icosahedral. Poxvirus is a DNA virus that has no envelope. The only correct answer is herpesviruses (DNA viruses) that have both icosahedral symmetry and are sensitive to ether (enveloped). *(Joklik et al, p 761)*

42. **(A)** Fc fragment is a portion of heavy chain obtained by papain digestion of immunoglobulin molecules. When papain cleaves IgG, it yields two identical Fab fragments concerned with binding to antigen, and one Fc fragment. Fab fragment contains a univalent binding site for hapten or antigen. The Fc region is involved with effector functions, such as complement fixation and placental transmission. It is not involved in secretion of the IgG molecule. Fab fragments are involved in IgG specificity or idiotypic identification of the IgG molecule. *(Joklik et al, pp 225–227)*

43. **(E)** Some aminoglycosides are active against a broad spectrum of gram-negative bacteria including *Pseudomonas aeruginosa*. With the exception of *Staphylococcus aureus*, gram-positive bacteria are generally resistant to all of the aminoglycosides. Gentamicin is widely used for serious gram-negative bacterial infections, but its use is increasingly limited because of an increase in gentamicin-resistant organisms in the hospital environment. Tobramycin has superior activity against *P. aeruginosa* and is the drug of choice for the treatment of bacteremia, pneumonia, and osteomyelitis caused by this organism. Clindamycin is the drug of choice for *Bacteroides*

fragilis infections. Penicillin G is still used for streptococcal and many other bacterial infections, but it is ineffective on *P. aeruginosa*. For rickettsial infections and cholera, tetracycline is the drug of choice. Isoniazid, rifampin, and pyrazinamide are the drugs exclusively used for the treatment of mycobacterial infections including tuberculosis. *(Joklik et al, pp 159–160, 580)*

44. **(E)** The Sabin poliovirus vaccine is a trivalent vaccine consisting of attenuated poliovirus types 1, 2, and 3. It is not a genetically engineered vaccine. This vaccine is given orally in three doses. The first two are given not less than 6 weeks apart and the third dose follows in 8 to 12 months. The viruses multiply in the intestine leading to an active but subclinical infection. The vaccine establishes intestinal immunity to reinfection by breaking the chain of transmission, does not require periodic boosters, and is believed to have eliminated poliomyelitis. In contrast to this, trivalent polio vaccine was developed by Salk in inactivated viruses and is no longer used. *(Joklik et al, pp 365,981)*

45. **(A)** Adenine arabinoside, known as vidarabine, is effective for the treatment of viral (herpes simplex) encephalitis because it inhibits viral DNA synthesis. It has not been shown to block virus uncoating, to prevent the formation of double-stranded replicative intermediates, to bind double-stranded replicative intermediates, or to augment the immune response. *(Joklik et al, p 856)*

46. **(C)** The enzyme lysozyme is found in human tears, saliva, and serum. It has an antibacterial activity because one component of the bacterial cell wall is susceptible to this enzyme. That component is peptidoglycan, which is a polymer of N-acetylmuramyl-N-acetylglucosamine. Lysozyme cleaves the glycosidic bond between N-acetylmuramic acid and N-acetylglucosamine. This enzyme is also used to produce protoplasts of certain bacteria. All other bacterial cell wall components are not susceptible to lysozyme. *(Joklik et al, pp 24–25,76–77,348)*

47. **(A)** *Escherichia coli* is a member of the normal flora of human intestine. Certain strains of *E. coli* are invasive and produce enterotoxins. This is a gram-negative, rod-shaped, motile bacterium and can be isolated from many sources of our surrounding environment. *E. coli* is a facultative anaerobe, which can grown under aerobic as well as anaerobic conditions. *(Joklik et al, pp 55,539)*

48. **(D)** The toxic effects of the endotoxin molecule seem to reside in lipid A, because deacylation of lipid A results in loss of major biologic activities of the lipopolysaccharide (endotoxin), including lethality, toxicity, pyrogenicity, and complement activation. *(Joklik et al, pp 83–87,90–91,391)*

49. **(D)** Individuals who are allergic to penicillin usually tend to show allergy to other beta-lactam antibiotics, such as ampicillin, oxacillin, cephalothin, or phenoxymethyl-penicillin. The responsible antigens appear to be degradation moieties of the penicillin molecule. Skin test with undegraded and degraded penicillin-containing solutions identify individuals allergic to penicillin. Persons hypersensitive to penicillin usually are treated with tetracycline. *(Brooks et al, pp 161–169)*

50. **(C)** The lactose operon contains three genes: the genes for β-galactosidase (*lacZ*), the galactoside permease (*lacY*), and the galactoside acetylase gene (*lacA*). The enzymes are only present when lactose is present. Thus, the lactose operon is *inducible* and not constitutive. It is an example of a *negative control* mechanism in that a controlling element, that is, a repressor protein, binds tightly to a site in the DNA in front of the *lacZ* gene. This site is called an operator. The presence of the bound repressor protein interferes with the initiation of DNA transcription by RNA polymerase. The addition of lactose combines with the repressor protein and thus allows RNA polymerase to function. The operon is influenced by the *lacI* gene product allolactose. *(Brooks et al, pp 92–93; Joklik et al, pp 49,115)*

51. (B) It was observed that even without repression (in mutants) the level of tryptophane (*trp*) operon messenger RNA (mRNA) and the biosynthetic enzymes increased. Feedback inhibition refers to the situation in which the end product of a metabolic pathway directly inhibits the first enzyme of the pathway. Therefore, it has not been shown to play any meaningful role in the regulation of mRNA synthesis. However, high levels of mRNA have been show to inhibit the synthesis of the enzymes responsible for mRNA production (*feedback repression*). Similarly, high levels of frequently utilized substrates such as glucose have been shown to reduce the level of cyclic adenosine monophosphate (cAMP) (*catabolite repression*). cAMP is required for the binding of the mRNA polymerase to the operon and the subsequent synthesis of mRNA. Finally, autoregulation of the mRNA synthesis has been known to occur. Attenuation is a unique mechanism that regulates the transcription of amino acid biosynthetic operons in bacteria. (*Joklik et al, pp 99–107,114–119*)

52. (A) "Capping" is a coordinated movement of membrane molecules to one region of the cell surface after binding by a multivalent ligand such as an antibody or antigen. Human B lymphocytes stained in the cold with fluorescent anti-human immunoglobulin show a patchy surface fluorescence when examined under ultraviolet light. This phenomenon is called lymphocyte capping and is induced by surface immunoglobulin–anti-immunoglobulin reactions. Phytohemagglutinin, pokeweed mitogen, complement, or fructose have not been shown to induce lymphocyte capping. (*Joklik et al, p 213*)

53. (C) There are different ways by which transfer of genes can occur in bacteria. One of these mechanisms of bacterial gene transfer is transformation, which involves passage of DNA from the donor to the recipient cell without the aid of a bacteriophage, cell donor–cell recipient contact, or a bacterial pilus. During transformation in *Streptococcus pneumoniae*, donor cells autolyse, releasing DNA fragments and competence factor. The competence factor induces recipient cells to synthesize a special set of proteins required for transformation. Transformation is inhibited by DNase because this enzyme digests DNA and thus destroys its biological function. Transformation is an important mechanism of gene transfer in *Streptococcus pneumoniae, Streptococcus sanguis, Neisseria gonorrhoeae, Hemophilus influenzae,* and *Bacillus subtilis*. (*Joklik et al, pp 136–137*)

54. (D) Immunity to tuberculosis requires such key players as activated macrophages and T lymphocytes, which had a previous interaction with the antigens of *Mycobacterium tuberculosis* or related mycobacteria that are classified as facultative intracellular parasites. Activation of macrophages occurs via lymphokinins released by immunocompetent T lymphocytes. Now the macrophages, within which the causative agent of tuberculosis was able to multiply, have acquired the ability to suppress the growth of *M. tuberculosis*. Tuberculosis represents the best example of cell-mediated immunity in which activated macrophages play a key role. Diphtheria, pneumococcal pneumonia, furunculosis, and botulism are caused by extracellular parasites for which activated macrophages do not play a key role for their destruction. For these, extracellular parasites, normal macrophages, and/or specific antibody to their main virulence factor(s) will suffice. (*Joklik et al, pp 506–508*)

55. (D) The pili of *Neisseria gonorrhoeae* confer on the cells an enhanced ability to adhere to each other and to host cells. This has been demonstrated in vitro, where piliated organisms of colony types 1 and 2 adhere to cultured human cells better that do nonpiliated organisms of colony type 4. The pili are composed of proteins; therefore, they do not have endotoxin activity. Secretory IgA can be detected early in the urethral secretions of infected males. Thus, pili do not inhibit IgA secretion. Although the piliated strains are relatively resistant to phagocytosis, inside the phagocytic cell they are as readily destroyed as nonpiliated cells. (*Joklik et al, pp 450–456*)

56. **(E)** The best method used to define a cluster of infections caused by *Salmonella* species is a determination of the plasmid profile of *Salmonella* species associated with a given infection. However, these tests are not as reliable as the plasmid profile when used to define the source of and the etiology of and epidemic. *(Joklik et al, pp 146,556–563)*

57. **(B)** Amebiasis is usually an intestinal disease. However, extraintestinal infection can occur by direct extension from the bowel. By far the most common form of extraintestinal amebiasis is amebic hepatitis or liver abscess. Rarely, abscesses may occur in skin, pericardium, lung, brain, and spleen. *(Joklik et al, pp 1164–1168)*

58. **(B)** Hyperacute graft rejection is primarily mediated by high-titer antibodies to major histocompatibility complex antigens of the graft. Neutrophils and platelets play an important role in graft rejection, but macrophages, B lymphocytes, basophils, and IgE are not considered important in this reaction. *(Joklik et al, pp 265–283; Roitt et al, p 246)*

59. **(E)** Adenoviruses cause conjunctivitis, mild or acute respiratory tract infections, and pharyngitis. Arenaviruses cause such deadly diseases as Lassa fever. Rotaviruses cause sporadic diarrhea in infants and young children. Arboviruses are involved in such infections as dengue, yellow fever, and encephalitis. Herpesviruses are the causative agents of cold sores, genital lesions, shingles, chickenpox, infectious mononucleosis, and other diseases. *(Joklik et al, pp 769–781,968,971,1012–1027,1035–1036)*

60. **(C)** Cervicofacial actinomycosis is caused by *Actinomyces israelii*, *Actinomyces bovis*, or *Actinomyces naeslundii*. These organisms are *commonly* found on healthy mucous membranes and in tonsils. Tooth extractions, oral surgery, trauma, pyogenic or necrotizing infection, or aspiration leads to cervicofacial actinomycosis. Although *Actinomyces* may exist in soil, foods, and water, it is not a common source of cervicofacial actinomycosis. *(Joklik et al, pp 528–535)*

61. **(B)** Microscopic examination of gram-stained expectorated sputum is more useful than culture in establishing the rapid diagnosis of pneumococcal pneumonia. The cellular content of the smear should be examined first, since specimens that contain numerous squamous epithelial cells are more representative of "spit" than of the lower respiratory tract flora. The finding of typical lancet-shaped gram-positive diplococci in association with macrophages of polymorphonuclear neutrophils (PMNs) (and in the absence of other bacteria) strongly supports the diagnosis. As a generalization, in a good sample there should be more than 20 PMNs and fewer that 10 squamous cells per low-power microscopic field. *(Brooks et al, pp 588–589)*

62. **(B)** Intravenous erythromycin is the antibiotic of choice for legionellosis treatment. The newest approved test for rapid diagnosis is a specific monoclonal antibody for all *Legionella* species. This test does not depend on a specific antibody increase in the host, which often takes many weeks, but uses monoclonal antibodies to fix to the legionellae in the serum. Patients with legionellosis need not be kept in isolation since they cannot infect others. *(Brooks et al, p 265; Joklik et al, pp 160,695–696)*

63. **(B)** Parvoviridae are very small viruses. They contain single-stranded DNA, have cubic symmetry, and lack envelopes. The Papovaviridae, Adenoviridae, Herpesviridae, and Poxviridae all contain double-stranded DNA. *(Joklik et al, pp 761–762)*

64. **(D)** There are 84 different pneumococcal capsular serotypes, and their antibodies do not cross-react. If the second infection is not of the same capsular serotype as the first infection, the antibodies will not be protective. Type-specific immunity to pneumococcal infection is long-lasting. Recurrent pneumococcal infections are usually caused by pneumococci of a different serologic type. *(Joklik et al, pp 436–439)*

65. **(E)** It is fairly common that *Escherichia coli* causes urinary tract infections in pregnant

women. In the United States, *E. coli* is the leading cause of nosocomial and community-acquired urinary tract infections. The spectrum of infection ranges from cystitis to pyelonephritis. Females are more likely to have urinary tract infections at a younger age because of difference in anatomic structure and sexual maturation, and the changes that occur during pregnancy and childbirth. Urinary tract infections due to other organisms listed in the question do not occur often in pregnant women. *(Joklik et al, p 547)*

66. **(D)** A key feature that distinguishes the phosphoenol pyruvate–phosphotransferase system from the other active transport systems is that the sugar that is being transported becomes phosphorylated prior to its transport. The phosphate group as well as the energy required for the transport are derived from phosphoenol pyruvate, which transfers the phosphate group to the heat stable protein (HPr). Enzyme I participates in this reaction. Enzyme II transfers the phosphate group from HPr to the sugar, which is thus phosphorylated. *(Joklik et al, pp 58–59)*

67. **(D)** *Neisseria gonorrhoeae* and *Brucella abortus* usually require CO_2 for primary isolation from clinical specimens. *Treponema pallidum* and *Mycobacterium leprae* cannot be cultured on artificial laboratory media. *Yersinia pestis* and *Mycobacterium tuberculosis* do not require CO_2 for primary isolation. *(Joklik et al, pp 444–449)*

68. **(A)** The Epstein–Barr virus (EBV) is the causative agent of infectious mononucleosis. Recently, this virus has been implicated in nasopharyngeal carcinoma. This implication stems from the detection of the EBV genome in nasopharyngeal tumors that express EBV antigens. Patients with nasopharyngeal carcinoma also have high titers of antibodies to EBV. Other viruses listed in the question have not been implicated in nasopharyngeal carcinoma. *(Joklik et al, pp 876–877)*

69. **(C)** The main virulence factor of *Streptococcus pyogenes* is the M protein, which inhibits phagocytosis. Immunization with M protein

provides solid immunity against the strain of *S. pyogens* from which the M protein was extracted and used for immunization. This is not the case when the streptolysin O or S is used for immunization. The Vi antigen is found in the capsule of *Salmonella typhi*. The V/W antigen is the main virulence factor for *Yersinia pestis*. *(Joklik et al, pp 421–422)*

70. **(D)** Lyme disease (erythema chronicum migrans) is caused by *Borrelia burgdorferi* (spirochete), which is transmitted through the bite of a tick. In the United States there are three major foci of recognized cases of Lyme disease: the midsection of the west coast, Minnesota and Wisconsin, and the northeast. Usually, a papule developed at the site of the tick bite has sharply demarcated borders, and its appearance is often accompanied by malaise, fever, headache, and stiff neck. Unless the disease is treated properly at this stage, neurologic and cardiac complications may occur, and, in the advanced stage, migrating episodes of arthritis may develop. *(Joklik et al, pp 670–671)*

71. **(A)** Interferons may be induced by a variety of viruses and other compounds, such as double-stranded RNA, synthetic double-stranded polyribonucleotide, bacterial endotoxin, and other polyanions. They are proteinaceous in nature. Interferon is produced in small amounts, typically about 1 mg of interferon per 10 liters of tissue culture supernatant medium. Interferons inhibit viral protein synthesis. Interferons act as immunoregulators. However, activation of the C3 component of complement is not one of their functions. *(Joklik et al, pp 862–866)*

72. **(B)** The echoviruses are members of the genus *Enterovirus* and of the family Picornaviridae, which includes the polioviruses, echoviruses, and coxsackieviruses. Viruses belonging to this family contain a single-stranded RNA genome. Echoviruses are excreted by humans and have been associated with such clinical manifestations as aseptic meningitis, disseminated neonatal infection, pericarditis, exanthems, respiratory disease, and some other minor infections. Echo-

viruses multiply primarily in the tissues around the oropharynx. Echoviruses may multiply in the central nervous system under certain circumstances, it is not the primary site of multiplication for echoviruses. Variola (smallpox) is caused by viruses belonging to the family of Poxviridae. *(Joklik et al, pp 980–985)*

73 **(D)** *Neisseria gonorrhoeae* may cause blindness of the newborn. This disease is called ophthalmia neonatorum and it is acquired during the passage of neonates through an infected birth canal. *N. gonorrhoeae* types 1 and 2 have pili and are pathogenic; types 3 and 4 do not have pili and are not pathogenic. *N. gonorrhoeae* produces indophenol oxidase, requires 5 to 10% CO_2 for growth, and may produce a protease that degrades the secretory immunoglobulin IgA. *(Joklik et al, pp 450–458)*

74. **(D)** An examination of the bacterial cell population per milliliter indicates that the combination of antibiotic A plus B yields a cell count per milliliter that is smaller than that achieved by either antibiotic A or B used alone. Thus, a synergistic action between antibiotics A and B, or synergism has been obtained. Antagonism between antibiotics A and B would have been indicated if the combination of antibiotics A and B yielded a cell population per milliliter that was higher than that achieved by A alone. Indifference refers to the inability of antibiotic A to alter the antibacterial properties of B and vice versa, while addition refers to an additive antibacterial action between antibiotics A and B. *(Brooks et al, pp 158–159)*

75. **(A)** The most frequent cause of meningitis in 2- to 10-month-old children is *Hemophilus influenzae* type b. Many strains of *H. influenzae* type b tend to be susceptible to ampicillin. However, up to 25% produce β-lactamase due to the possession of a transmissible plasmid. Essentially all strains of *H. influenzae* type b are susceptible to the third generation of cephalosporins such as cefotaxime, ceftriaxone, and ceftizoxime. These antibiotics appear in spinal fluid in sufficient concentra-

tions when given in a sufficient dose (2 g intravenously every 8 hours) and are used to treat meningitis caused by gram-negative rods such as *H. influenzae* type b. *(Brooks et al, pp 167,239)*

76. **(D)** *Plasmodium vivax* requires Duffy group receptors on erythrocytes in order to penetrate the erythrocyte membrane, and these receptors are lacking in many Africans, particularly West Africans. *(Joklik et al, pp 1180–1182)*

77. **(A)** Considering the background of this patient, one must immediately suspect the possibility of human immunodeficiency virus (HIV) infection. This diagnosis can be established by observing increased anti-HIV antibody titer and decreased T4 : T8 ratio (T-helper cells characterized by CD4 marker are preferentially affected by HIV). Oral thrush (oral candidiasis) is one of the most common secondary infections seen in AIDS patients. A routine blood cell count and differential are required for all cases showing these symptoms. Amphotericin B treatment is appropriate once the diagnosis of AIDS and candidiasis is established. *(Joklik et al, pp 337,1136–1144)*

78. **(C)** Alanine aminotransferase assays are conducted to assess the function of liver. In hepatitis A, laboratory tests show high serum alanine transaminase and aspartate transaminase values of 500 to 2,000 units. There is also leukopenia in the preicteric phase of the disease. Additional evidence of liver damage is indicated by decreased serum albumin and increased gamma globulin levels. West Nile fever is a viral disease characterized by lymphadenopathy and rash. Sandfly fever features papules on the skin, fever, nausea, and stiffness of the back and neck. Rabies is characterized by excitement, hydrophobia, paralysis, convulsive seizures, coma, and death. Poliomyelitis is an acute viral illness that in its severe form damages the central nervous system leading to motor neuron damage and paralysis. *(Brooks et al, pp 458,471,496,500,540)*

79. **(D)** An oncogene is an altered version of a normal gene. A proto-oncogene is a normal gene that can be converted to an oncogene.

Proto-oncogenes have been maintained in the mammalian cell genome, and they may play some role in the normal cellular metabolism. At this time approximately 24 proto-oncogenes have been discovered using retroviruses that can infect mammalian cells containing proto-oncogenes and transfer the proto-oncogenes to other cells that can infect. The majority of the proto-oncogenes may be activated via retroviruses. However, it has been shown that a nonvirally induced single base pair mutation was sufficient to convert the benign protooncogene *ras* into an oncogene. Thus, proto-oncogenes may be activated either by association with retroviruses or they may be altered via mutational nonviral events. (*Joklik et al, pp 887–895*)

80. **(B)** The adenoviruses are nonenveloped (naked), whereas all others are enveloped. (*Joklik et al, p 771*)

81. **(E)** Tumor necrosis factor-alpha (TNF-alpha) is a cytokine released by activated macrophages that is structurally related to lymphotoxin released by activated T cells. This cytokine is *cytotoxic* for virally infected cells and induces cachexia and fever. TNF is thought to be a major mediator of the circulatory collapse and widespread tissue necrosis that accompanies bacterial septicemia. TNF-alpha appears to be responsible for most of the tumoricidal activity of human monocytes. (*Joklik et al, p 277; Roitt, pp 9.10–9.11*)

82. **(D)** Of the viruses listed in the question, only herpesvirus genomes are replicated in the nucleus. The others are replicated in the cytoplasm. (*Levinson and Jawetz, p 375*)

83. **(B)** The primary effect of ultraviolet light on DNA is the formation of "thymine" dimers, better described as pyrimidine dimers. Usually, the dimers are formed by linking bonds on adjacent pyrimidines in a single chain. Although other agents kill microorganisms, thymine dimer formation does not occur in the DNA of inactivated organisms. (*Joklik et al, pp 197–198*)

84. **(E)** Household pets such as dogs, cats, and turtles are the reservoirs of gastroenteritis but not of typhoid fever caused by *Salmonella typhi*. The sources of infection for typhoid fever are individuals who are suffering from typhoid fever or who have become carriers of *S. typhi*. (*Salmonella* is a biochemically and serologically diverse bacterial group. Besides humans, *Salmonella* species infect animals, but they cause enteric fevers, the most serious of which is typhoid fever. Since 1983, on the basis of DNA hybridization studies, one species, *Salmonella cholerasuis* has been designated for the *Salmonella–Arizona* group. Reports from reference laboratories that serotype isolates include the serotype name, eg, *Salmonella* serotype *typhimurium* rather than the more taxonomically correct *Salmonella enterica* subspecies *enterica* serotype typhimurium.) (*Brooks et al, pp 218–221; Joklik et al, pp 559–562*)

85. **(D)** The synthesis of all types of RNA present in bacterial cells is mediated by DNA-dependent RNA polymerase. The core form of the enzyme is incapable of using double strand DNA as a template as formed in the chromosome, unless sigma protein is added to the core polymerase. This sigma addition allows the core polymerase to use ds DNA as a template and allows initiation of RNA synthesis at specific regions called promoters, a process that leads to proper initiation of transcription. (*Joklik et al, pp 114–119*)

86. **(B)** Piperacillin is a synthetic penicillin that interferes with cell wall synthesis, resulting in the formation of osmotically sensitive bacterial cells that lyse and cause death. Therefore, piperacillin is a bactericidal chemotherapeutic agent. Chloramphenicol, tetracycline, erythromycin, and sulfamethoxazole are bacteriostatic chemotherapeutic agents. Chloramphenicol, tetracycline, and erythromycin interfere with protein synthesis; sulfamethoxazole acts as a competitive inhibitor or para-amino-benzoic acid utilization. (*Joklik et al, pp 154–163*)

87. (A) When an IgG molecule is treated with papain, it cleaves the molecule at site A (the carboxyl terminal side of the single inter–heavy-chain disulfide bond), producing two Fab fragments and one Fc fragment. *(Joklik et al, pp 225–227)*

88. (C) Measles can be prevented by appropriate use of attenuated, live virus preparations for all healthy children slightly over 1 year of age. *(Joklik et al, pp 365,999,1011)*

89. (D) Transversion refers to the alteration of the nucleotide sequence in the DNA, that is, a change of the nucleic acid bases adenine–thymine to guanine–cytosine (AT → GC) by mutagens. Therefore, there is no gene transfer in transversion. Conjugation, lysogenic conversion, generalized transduction, and transformation involve gene transfer. Conjugation involves transfer of episomes (genetic material) such as the fertility F factor to bacterial cells. Lysogenic conversion has been encountered in *Corynebacterium diphtheriae* and other bacteria, toxigenic strains carry the prophage beta, and nontoxigenic strains can be made toxigenic by infection with beta phage. Generalized transduction refers to the transfer of virtually any gene from one bacterial cell to another by a virus. Transformation involves gene transfer by soluble DNA. *(Joklik et al, pp 133–144)*

90. (B) In the primary response, first IgM antibody is produced after a log period (peak 1); later IgG appears in the serum. *(Joklik et al, pp 248–249)*

91. (B) Contact hypersensitivity is a form of delayed hypersensitivity (type IV hypersensitivity reaction). Antigen-sensitized T cells release lymphokines following a secondary contact with the same antigen. Lymphokines induce inflammatory epidermal reactions by attracting activated macrophages (Langerhans' cells), which release cytotoxic mediators. Unlike other types of hypersensitivity, no antibodies are involved. No endotoxin is involved in this type of hypersensitivity. Neither IgE nor IgA is involved in contact dermatitis. *(Joklik et al, p 323; Roitt, p 22.2)*

92. (B) This double-diffusion precipitin reaction shows a reaction of partial identity (cross-reaction). The spur is caused by the fraction of antibody that is not precipitated by human serum albumin placed in the well 2. *(Joklik et al, p 239; Roitt, pp 25.1–25.2)*

93. (D) Since there is no cross-reaction between bovine serum albumin (BSA) and bovine gamma globulin (BGG), the anti-BSA forms no precipitate with BGG, and anti-BGG and anti-BSA form separate lines of precipitate. *(Golub and Green, p 161; Roitt, pp 25.1–25.2)*

94. (A) *Pseudomonas aeruginosa* is intrinsically resistant to β-lactams because it cannot penetrate the outer surface barrier. *(Joklik et al, p 180)*

95. (A) *Clostridium botulinum* exotoxin causes a lethal food poisoning in humans. Ingested botulinum toxin gains access to the peripheral nervous system, where it acts preferentially on cholinergic nerve endings. Botulinum toxin blocks the release of acetylcholine at myoneural junction, causing paralysis of the affected muscles. The free toxin can be neutralized by specific antitoxin antibody. Once the toxin binds to the cell surface receptors or enters the susceptible cells, it can no longer be neutralized by the specific antibody. *(Joklik et al, p 650)*

96. (F) The staphylococcal enterotoxins, the staphylococcal pyrogenic exotoxins, and the toxic syndrome toxin share an unusual property in addition to their conventional toxic activity. These toxins serve as immunomodulators of the host defense system because of their ability to stimulate T cell to proliferate at low concentrations. They are referred to as "superantigens." *(Joklik et al, p 422)*

97. (E) *Bordetella pertussis* is the causative agent for whooping cough, which is a toxin-mediated disease. Pertussis toxin affects host cells by adenosine diphosphate-ribosylating the alpha subunits of susceptible G proteins. This action uncouples the proteins from their receptors, blocks signal transduction and causes guanosine triphosphate-dependent receptor-mediated inhibition of cellular adenylate cyclase. Since the inhibitory control is removed, basilar cyclic adenosine monophosphate (cAMP) is increased, and the cell's response to stimulatory ligands is exaggerated with increased cAMP production. For example, the production of insulin in response to glucose is increased. *(Joklik et al, p 474)*

98. **(B)** Rocky Mountain spotted fever is spread from its reservoir in nature (eg, rodents, dogs) to humans by the bite of infected ticks, primarily the wood tick (*Dermacentor andersoni*) in the western United States and the dog tick (*Dermacentor variabilis*) in the eastern areas. Tsutsugamushi disease is spread by mites, epidemic typhus is spread by human body lice, and endemic (murine) typhus and bubonic plague are transmitted by rat fleas. There is no vector in Q fever, which is acquired by inhalation of infectious particles. *(Joklik et al, pp 705–713)*

99. **(C)** Viral infection is initiated with the attachment of the viral hemagglutinin to a specific host cell membrane glycoprotein (mucopeptide) receptor. The viral particles then fuse with the membrane, and the nucleocapsid enters the cell to begin the replicative cycle. The virus enters the eclipse phase, during which no viral material can be detected in the cell by conventional procedures. During this time viral proteins and nucleic acids are being produced. The next phase is assembly, when mature virus is manufactured. Release follows, and the cycle is repeated in a new cell. *(Joklik et al, pp 824–837)*

100. **(E)** The increased metabolic activity associated with the phagocytosis of microbes by neutrophils results in the formation of such oxygen metabolites as the superoxide radical O_2^-, H_2O_2, which may be lethal for many microorganisms. H_2O_2 in the presence of cofactors, such as myeloperoxidase, and the halides chlorine, iodine, or bromine result also in microbial death. Nonoxidative mechanisms, such as the action of lactoferrin, lysozyme, and other hydrolytic phagocytic enzymes, may be directly lethal for various microorganisms. Catalase is an enzyme that degrades H_2O_2 to O_2 and H_2O. *(Joklik et al, pp 350–351)*

REFERENCES

Brooks GF, Butel JS and Ornston LN, Jawetz E, Melnick JL, Adelberg EA. *Medical Microbiology*, 19th ed. Norwalk, CT: Appleton & Lange; 1991.

Golub ES, Green DR. *Immunology*, 2nd ed. Sunderland, MA: Sinauer Associates, Inc.; 1991.

Joklik WK, Willett HP, Amos BD, Wilfert CM. *Zinsser Microbiology*, 20th ed. Norwalk, CT: Appleton & Lange; 1992.

Levinson WE, Jawetz E. *Medical Microbiology and Immunology*, 3rd ed. Norwalk, CT: Appleton & Lange; 1994.

Roitt I, Brostoff J, Male DK. *Immunology*, 2nd ed. London and New York: Gower; 1989.

Ryan KJ. *Sherris Medical Microbiology*, 3rd ed. Norwalk, CT: Appleton & Lange; 1994.

Practice Test Subspecialty List

GENERAL MICROBIOLOGY

2, 4, 7, 19, 37, 46, 48, 50, 66, 79, 83

MICROBIAL GENETICS

25, 51, 53, 85, 89

IMMUNOLOGY

1, 5, 6, 11, 15, 16, 29, 31, 36, 38, 39, 42, 52, 58, 64, 81, 87, 88, 90, 91, 92, 93, 100

ANTIBIOTICS

11, 20, 27, 43, 45, 49, 74, 75, 86, 94

MEDICAL BACTERIOLOGY

14, 18, 24, 28, 30, 33, 47, 54, 55, 60, 61, 65, 67, 69, 70, 73, 84, 95, 96, 97, 98

MEDICAL MYCOLOGY

10, 11, 27, 40

MEDICAL PARASITOLOGY

26, 76

MEDICAL VIROLOGY

3, 8, 29, 32, 34, 35, 41, 44, 45, 59, 63, 68, 71, 72, 77, 78, 79, 80, 82, 99

NAME _____
    Last   First   Middle

ADDRESS _____
            Street

_____
    City   State   Zip

DIRECTIONS   Mark your social security number from top to bottom
              in the appropriate boxes on the right.
              Use No. 2 lead pencil only.
              Mark one and only one answer for each item.
              Make each mark black enough to obliterate the letter
              within the parentheses.
              Erase clearly any answer you wish to change.

1. (A) (B) (C) (D) (E)   22. (A) (B) (C) (D) (E)   43. (A) (B) (C) (D) (E)   64. (A) (B) (C) (D) (E)

2. (A) (B) (C) (D) (E)   23. (A) (B) (C) (D) (E)   44. (A) (B) (C) (D) (E)   65. (A) (B) (C) (D) (E)

3. (A) (B) (C) (D) (E)   24. (A) (B) (C) (D) (E)   45. (A) (B) (C) (D) (E)   66. (A) (B) (C) (D) (E)

4. (A) (B) (C) (D) (E)   25. (A) (B) (C) (D) (E)   46. (A) (B) (C) (D) (E)   67. (A) (B) (C) (D) (E)

5. (A) (B) (C) (D) (E)   26. (A) (B) (C) (D) (E)   47. (A) (B) (C) (D) (E)   68. (A) (B) (C) (D) (E)

6. (A) (B) (C) (D) (E)   27. (A) (B) (C) (D) (E)   48. (A) (B) (C) (D) (E)   69. (A) (B) (C) (D) (E)

7. (A) (B) (C) (D) (E)   28. (A) (B) (C) (D) (E)   49. (A) (B) (C) (D) (E)   70. (A) (B) (C) (D) (E)

8. (A) (B) (C) (D) (E)   29. (A) (B) (C) (D) (E)   50. (A) (B) (C) (D) (E)   71. (A) (B) (C) (D) (E)

9. (A) (B) (C) (D) (E)   30. (A) (B) (C) (D) (E)   51. (A) (B) (C) (D) (E)   72. (A) (B) (C) (D) (E)

10. (A) (B) (C) (D) (E)   31. (A) (B) (C) (D) (E)   52. (A) (B) (C) (D) (E)   73. (A) (B) (C) (D) (E)

11. (A) (B) (C) (D) (E)   32. (A) (B) (C) (D) (E)   53. (A) (B) (C) (D) (E)   74. (A) (B) (C) (D) (E)

12. (A) (B) (C) (D) (E)   33. (A) (B) (C) (D) (E)   54. (A) (B) (C) (D) (E)   75. (A) (B) (C) (D) (E)

13. (A) (B) (C) (D) (E)   34. (A) (B) (C) (D) (E)   55. (A) (B) (C) (D) (E)   76. (A) (B) (C) (D) (E)

14. (A) (B) (C) (D) (E)   35. (A) (B) (C) (D) (E)   56. (A) (B) (C) (D) (E)   77. (A) (B) (C) (D) (E)

15. (A) (B) (C) (D) (E)   36. (A) (B) (C) (D) (E)   57. (A) (B) (C) (D) (E)   78. (A) (B) (C) (D) (E)

16. (A) (B) (C) (D) (E)   37. (A) (B) (C) (D) (E)   58. (A) (B) (C) (D) (E)   79. (A) (B) (C) (D) (E)

17. (A) (B) (C) (D) (E)   38. (A) (B) (C) (D) (E)   59. (A) (B) (C) (D) (E)   80. (A) (B) (C) (D) (E)

18. (A) (B) (C) (D) (E)   39. (A) (B) (C) (D) (E)   60. (A) (B) (C) (D) (E)   81. (A) (B) (C) (D) (E)

19. (A) (B) (C) (D) (E)   40. (A) (B) (C) (D) (E)   61. (A) (B) (C) (D) (E)   82. (A) (B) (C) (D) (E)

20. (A) (B) (C) (D) (E)   41. (A) (B) (C) (D) (E)   62. (A) (B) (C) (D) (E)   83. (A) (B) (C) (D) (E)

21. (A) (B) (C) (D) (E)   42. (A) (B) (C) (D) (E)   63. (A) (B) (C) (D) (E)   84. (A) (B) (C) (D) (E)

85. (A) (B) (C) (D) (E)   89. (A) (B) (C) (D) (E)   93. (A) (B) (C) (D) (E)   97. (A) (B) (C) (D) (E)

86. (A) (B) (C) (D) (E)   90. (A) (B) (C) (D) (E)   94. (A) (B) (C) (D) (E)   98. (A) (B) (C) (D) (E)

87. (A) (B) (C) (D) (E)   91. (A) (B) (C) (D) (E)   95. (A) (B) (C) (D) (E)   99. (A) (B) (C) (D) (E)

88. (A) (B) (C) (D) (E)   92. (A) (B) (C) (D) (E)   96. (A) (B) (C) (D) (E)   100. (A) (B) (C) (D) (E)